PHARMACOLOGY DEMYSTIFIED

Demystified Series

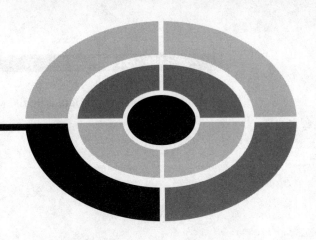

PHARMACOLOGY DEMYSTIFIED

**MARY KAMIENSKI,
PhD, RN, FAEN, FNP, CEN**

JIM KEOGH

McGRAW-HILL
New York   Chicago   San Francisco   Lisbon   London
Madrid   Mexico City   Milan   New Delhi   San Juan
Seoul   Singapore   Sydney   Toronto

The McGraw·Hill Companies

Cataloging-in-Publication Data is on file with the Library of Congress

1 2 3 4 5 6 7 8 9 0   DOC/DOC   0 1 0 9 8 7 6 5

ISBN 0-07-146208-2

The sponsoring editor for this book was Judy Bass and the production supervisor was Pamela A. Pelton. It was set in Times Roman by American Color. The art director for the cover was Margaret Webster-Shapiro; the cover designer was Handel Low.

Printed and bound by RR Donnelley.

 This book is printed on recycled, acid-free paper containing a minimum of 50% recycled, de-inked fiber.

McGraw-Hill books are available at special quantity discounts to use as premiums and sales promotions, or for use in corporate training programs. For more information, please write to the Director of Special Sales, McGraw-Hill Professional, Two Penn Plaza, New York, NY 10121-2298. Or contact your local bookstore.

CONTENTS

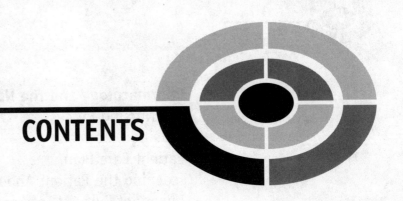

CONTENTS

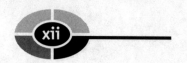

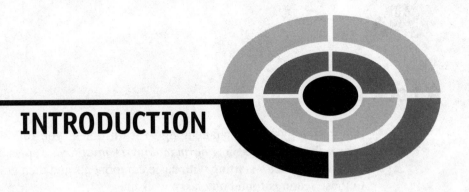

INTRODUCTION

One of the most important roles of the nurse is to administer medications. Understanding how a drug interacts with the human body will help a nurse administer drugs safely to patients.

Pharmacology Demystified shows you:

- How drugs work
- How to calculate the proper dose
- How to administer drugs
- How to evaluate the drug's effectiveness
- How to avoid common errors when administering drugs
- And much more.

You might be a little apprehensive learning pharmacology, especially if you have little, if any, experience with drugs. Pharmacology can be mystifying. However, it becomes demystified as you read *Pharmacology Demystified* because your knowledge of basic science is used as the foundation for learning pharmacology.

As you'll see in Chapter 1, each element of pharmacology is introduced by combining just the pharmacology element with facts you already know from your study of basic science.

Pharmacology is different than other basic science that you've learned—but not so different that you won't be able to quickly build upon your present knowledge base. All you need is a working knowledge of basic science—and *Pharmacology Demystified*—to become knowledgeable in pharmacology.

By the end of this book, you'll have an understanding of drugs that are used to cure common disorders. You'll know how they work, their side effects, adverse effects, and when they are not to be administered to patients. Furthermore, you'll learn how long it takes the drug to take effect and how long the therapeutic effect lasts.

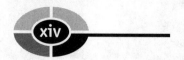
A Look Inside

Pharmacology can be challenging to learn unless you follow the step-by-step approach that is used in *Pharmacology Demystified*. Topics are presented in a systematic order—starting with basic components and then gradually moving on to those features found on classy web sites.

Each chapter follows a time-tested formula that first explains the topic in an easy-to-read style and then shows how it is used in a working web page that you can copy and load yourself. You can then compare your web page with the image of the web page shown in the chapter to be sure that you've coded the web page correctly. There is little room for you to go wrong.

CHAPTER 1: AN INSIDE LOOK AT PHARMACOLOGY

The mere mention of drugs brings all sorts of images to mind. However, these impressions are based on our experience as patients. Healthcare providers have a different view because they see drugs as an arsenal to combat disease. A drug is more than a pill. It is a compound of chemical elements that interacts with the body's chemistry causing a chain reaction of events. Healthcare providers need a thorough understanding of a drug's action in order to effectively prescribe and administer the drug to the patient. Therefore you begin in Chapter 1 learning the basic concepts of pharmacology.

CHAPTER 2: DRUG ACTION AND DRUG INTERACTIONS

Drugs are not magical. They follow proven scientific principles to interact with cells in your body to bring about a pharmaceutical response—cure your ills. In this chapter you'll learn about the scientific principles that seem to miraculously make you better when you feel rotten all over. You will learn how drugs stimulate your body's own defense mechanism to stamp out pathogens that give you the sniffles or cause serious diseases.

CHAPTER 3: PHARMACOLOGY AND THE NURSING PROCESS

Remember from your last hospital stay being awakened from a deep sleep by a nurse saying, "time to take your medicine." The nurse didn't enjoy disturbing you. It was part of standard nursing procedures used to administer medication. You'll learn about those procedures in this chapter so you too can wake up your patients to give them medication.

CHAPTER 4: SUBSTANCE ABUSE

Drugs can wipe out microorganisms that attack our body. However, some drugs can be abused resulting in an individual becoming dependent on the medication. Substance abuse is the most publicized aspect of pharmacology—and the one least understood by patients and healthcare professionals. This chapter explores drugs that are commonly abused and discusses how to detect substance abuse.

CHAPTER 5: PRINCIPLES OF MEDICATION ADMINISTRATION

Administering medication can be downright dangerous unless you follow time-tested procedures that assure that the patient receives the right drug in the right dose at the right time using the right route. In this chapter, you'll learn how this is done and how to avoid common errors that could harm your patient.

CHAPTER 6: ROUTE OF ADMINISTRATION

The way a drug is administered to a patient is called a route. Your job is to administer medication using the best route to achieve the desired therapeutic effect. This depends on a number of factors that include the type of medication and the patient's condition. In this chapter, you'll learn how to administer drugs.

CHAPTER 7: DOSE CALCULATIONS

Although a prescriber specifies a dose of a medication for a patient, a different dose may be on hand requiring you to calculate the actual dose. With intravenous medication, the prescriber usually orders a dose to be infused over a specific period of time. You must calculate the drip rate to properly set the IV. This chapter shows you how to calculate doses of medication.

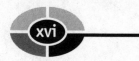
CHAPTER 8: HERBAL THERAPY

Herbal therapy is used to treat the common cold, infections, diseases of the GI tract, and about anything else that ails you. Herbs are naturally grown and don't have the quality standards found in prescription and over-the-counter medications. You'll learn about the therapeutic effect of herbal therapies in this chapter and the adverse reactions patients can experience when herbal therapy is combined with conventional therapy.

CHAPTER 9: VITAMINS AND MINERALS

Vitamins and minerals build a strong, healthy body, so you've been told when you were growing up. It is true. A balanced diet provides the vitamins and minerals you need to stay healthy. However, many patients don't have a balanced diet and therefore experience vitamin and mineral deficiencies. In this chapter, you'll learn about vitamins and minerals and how to provide vitamin therapy and mineral therapy for your patients.

CHAPTER 10: FLUID AND ELECTROLYTE THERAPY

Some diseases and treatment of disease can cause an imbalance in the body's fluids and electrolytes needed for muscle contraction and other functions. Administering electrolyte therapy to the patient restores balance. You'll learn how this is done.

CHAPTER 11: NUTRITIONAL SUPPORT THERAPIES

Nutrients are given to patients who are at risk for malnutrition caused by disease and by treatment given to cure the disease. Nutrients are also given to strengthen the patient following a trauma such as surgery. In this chapter, you'll learn about nutritional support therapies, how to prepare them, how to administer them, and how to avoid any complications that might arise.

CHAPTER 12: INFLAMMATION

Fortunately, most times the pain goes away and the inflammation subsides relatively quickly and doesn't interfere with daily activities. In this chapter,

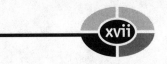
you'll learn about the process of inflammation and the medications that are prescribed to reduce the redness, swelling, warmth, and pain that is associated with inflammation.

CHAPTER 13: ANTIMICROBIALS— FIGHTING INFECTION

The immune system produces antibodies that seek out, attack, and kill microbials. However, this natural defense isn't sufficient for some patients leaving them with a runny nose, headache, and fever. They need to call in the cavalry. The cavalry is medication that kills the invading microbial. You'll learn about antimicrobial medication in this chapter.

CHAPTER 14: RESPIRATORY DISEASES

The common cold can be annoying. However, some respiratory diseases—such as emphysema—are debilitating and can slowly choke the life out of a person. In this chapter, we'll explore common respiratory diseases and learn about the medications that are used to manage the symptoms of the disease.

CHAPTER 15: NERVOUS SYSTEM DRUGS

The nervous system is our Internet over which sensory impulses travel the neural pathways to the brain where they are interpreted and analyzed for an appropriate response. Sometimes disease or other disorders cause the impulse to go astray or be misinterpreted. Drugs can be prescribed that restore the function of the nervous system. You'll learn about those drugs in this chapter.

CHAPTER 16: NARCOTIC AGONISTS

Make the pain go away. That's what most of us want when we hurt. However, pain is subjective and can be difficult for healthcare providers to manage with the appropriate medication. This chapter explores pain and how healthcare providers assess and manage pain. You'll also learn about narcotic and nonnarcotic analgesics and how they are used to treat pain.

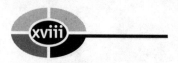
CHAPTER 17: IMMUNOLOGIC AGENTS

When the immune system is compromised through diseases including HIV, the body loses its ability to fight off microorganisms and destroys its own abnormal cells, leaving the patient to experience more episodes of infection that can ultimately lead to death. In this chapter, you'll learn about the therapies used to assist the immune system combat preventable diseases and you'll also learn about medications that inhibit the growth of HIV.

CHAPTER 18: GASTROINTESTINAL SYSTEM

Problems with the gastrointestinal system can be vomiting, ingesting toxins, diarrhea, constipation, peptic ulcers, and gastroesophageal reflux disease. Each is treatable with the proper medication. In this chapter, you'll learn about common gastrointestinal disorders and the medications that are frequently prescribed to treat these conditions.

CHAPTER 19: CARDIAC CIRCULATORY MEDICATIONS

When blood vessels become clogged and the heart is unable to pump blood sufficiently, the body loses its ability to distribute oxygen, nutrients, and hormones and remove waste products placing the patient in grave danger. Fortunately, there are medications that can be taken to treat and prevent cardiovascular disorders. In this chapter, you'll learn about drugs that affect the heart and keep the cardiovascular system humming.

CHAPTER 20: SKIN DISORDERS

Acne, dry skin, a rash, and injuries such as cuts, scrapes, puncture wounds, and burns are some disorders that affect your skin. Some of these are more annoying than endangering to your existence. This chapter discusses using medications to relieve most of the disorders.

CHAPTER 21: ENDOCRINE MEDICATIONS

Hormones are messengers that influence how tissues, organs, and other parts of your body function. An overproduction or underproduction of hormones can cause the body to function improperly. Hormones are brought back into balance by using endocrine medications, which are discussed in this chapter.

CHAPTER 22: DISORDERS OF THE EYE AND EAR

Common eye and ear disorders rarely result in loss of sight and hearing once the disorder is diagnosed and treated with the proper medication. This chapter takes a look at common disorders that affect the eyes and the ears and discusses drugs that are used to treat those disorders.

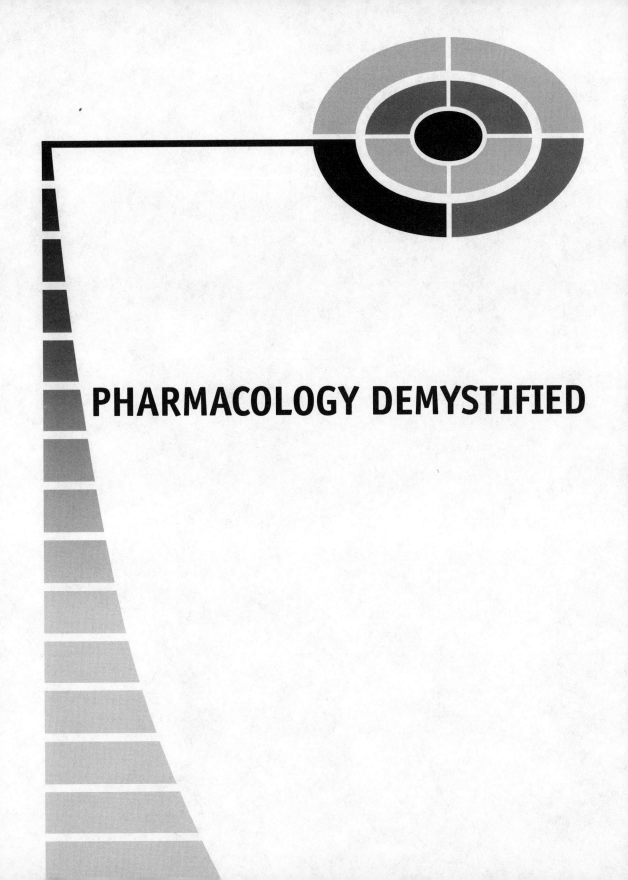

PHARMACOLOGY DEMYSTIFIED

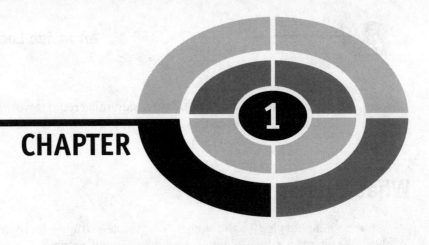

CHAPTER

1

An Inside Look at Pharmacology

Just the mention of drugs causes all sorts of images to run through our mind: the magic pill that made you feel better when you were under the weather; the stinging injection that left your arm sore for days; the handful of capsules that cost a month's pay; and even the vision of furtive street-corner exchanges.

These impressions are from our experiences as patients or consumers. Healthcare providers, however, view drugs differently because drugs are an integral component of the arsenal used to combat the diseases and physiological changes that disrupt activities of daily living.

A drug is more than a pill. It is a compound of chemical elements that interacts with the body's chemistry causing a chain reaction of events. Drugs are given to achieve a therapeutic effect. However, most drugs also have side effects. Some side affects are desirable and some are not. Healthcare providers must have a thorough understanding of a drug's action in order to effectively prescribe and administer the drug and evaluate the patient's response to the medication.

Throughout this book you'll learn about drugs: how they work; their therapeutic effects; their adverse effects; their interactions with other drugs; how they

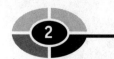

are prescribed; and how they are administered. However, before learning these details, let's begin in this chapter with the basic concepts of pharmacology.

What Is Pharmacology?

Pharmacology is the study of chemicals—drugs—on living tissues and how those chemicals help diagnose, treat, cure, and prevent disease or correct the pathophysiology of living tissues. The term pharmacology is derived from two Greek words: *pharmakon*, the Greek word for drugs, and *logos*, the Greek word for science.

Pharmacology has its roots in folklore and tradition that dates back to ancient times when knowledge of the medicinal effects of plants were passed down through generations. By 1240 AD, pharmacology moved from the realm of home remedies to a science where drug standards were established and a measuring system was developed—called the apothecary system—that was used to measure quantities of drugs. Because drugs can vary in strength and purity, pharmacological standards have been developed that govern the manufacturing and control of drugs. The United States Pharmacopeia National Formulary is the only official book of drug standards in the United States. If a drug is included in this book it has met the standards of quality, purity, and strength. These drugs can use the letters U.S.P. following the official name of the drug. Accurate dosage and the reliability of the effect the drug will have on a patient is dependent upon the purity and strength of the drug. Purity is the dilution or mixture of a drug with other materials to give it a form that can be administered. Drugs may vary in the strength of their action. The strength of drugs from plants can depend on where the plant is grown, the age at which the plant is harvested, and how the harvest is preserved. Drug packaging standards determine what information needs to be displayed on packages of drugs. You'll learn more about these later in this book.

In addition to these standards, there are a number of important laws that have been enacted to control the sale and distribution of drugs.

1938 FOOD, DRUG AND COSMETIC ACT

Before 1938 there was no control over pharmaceuticals. This changed when a drug company distributed a sulfa drug to treat pediatric patients. The drugs turned out to be a chemical similar to antifreeze. It was highly toxic and killed more than 100 people, including children.

At the urging of the public, the United States Congress passed the 1938 Food, Drug and Cosmetic Act. This act required:

- Drugs must be proven save for use before they can be sold.
- Inspections of drug manufacturing facilities.
- Safe tolerance levels be identified to prevent the patient from being poisoned.
- Cosmetics and therapeutic devices be controlled.

1952 DURHAM-HUMPHREY AMENDMENT TO THE FOOD, DRUG AND COSMETIC ACT

Until 1952, anyone could distribute drugs. With the passage of the Durham-Humphrey amendment to the Food, Drug and Cosmetic Act of 1938, a group of drugs was defined that could only be purchased if the patient had a prescription from a licensed practitioner.

1962 KEFAUVER-HARRIS AMENDMENT TO THE FOOD, DRUG AND COSMETIC ACT

The Food, Drug and Cosmetic Act of 1938 was amended once more in 1962 with the passage of the Kefauver-Harris Amendment. This amendment tightened controls on drug safety by requiring drug manufacturers to use standard labeling of drug containers. The label lists adverse reactions and contraindications or reasons why the drug should not be used.

1970 COMPREHENSIVE DRUG ABUSE PREVENT AND CONTROL ACT

By 1970, there was widespread abuse of prescription drugs. In an effort to contain this problem, Congress passed the Comprehensive Drug Abuse Prevent and Control Act. This act categorized controlled substances according to a schedule based on potential for abuse.

- Schedule I is reserved for the most dangerous substances that have no recognized medicinal use.
- Schedule II drugs have high abuse potential with accepted medicinal use.
- Schedule III drugs have high abuse potential with accepted medicinal uses.
- Schedule IV and V drugs have lower abuse potential with accepted medicinal uses.

The Source of Drugs

Ask a child where milk comes from and you might be surprised by his answer that it comes from the grocery store. The same might be true if you ask an adult where drugs come from and he answers from the drug store. Both are correct answers, but neither identifies the true source.

Drugs can be purchased from a drug store, but the origins are from one of four sources.

PLANTS

A number of plants have medicinal qualities and have been used for centuries as natural remedies for injuries and illnesses. Pharmaceutical firms harvest these plants and transform them into drugs that have a specific purity and strength sufficient to treat diseases.

An example of a drug that comes from a plant is digitalis. Digitalis is made from leaves of the foxglove plant and is used to treat congestive heart failure and cardiac arrhythmias. Digitalis also strengthens the force of the contractions of the heart.

ANIMALS

Byproducts of animals, including humans, are a source for drugs because they contain hormones that can be reclaimed and given to patients who need increased hormonal levels to maintain homeostasis.

For example, Premarin is a drug that contains estrogen that is recovered from mare urine. This is used as hormonal therapy to manage menopausal symptoms. Insulin is another hormonal drug that is used to regulate blood sugar levels in patients with diabetes mellitus. Insulin can be recovered from humans using DNA technology.

MINERALS

Our body requires trace elements of minerals in order to maintain homeostasis. Minerals are inorganic crystal substances that are found naturally on earth. Patients lacking an adequate level of these materials may take specific mineral-based drugs to raise the level of minerals.

For example, an iron supplement is a common mineral-based drug that is given to patients who suffer iron deficiency, a condition which can lead to fatigue. Iron is a natural metal that is an integral part of body proteins such as hemoglobin that carries oxygen throughout the body. Minerals are obtained from animal and plant sources.

SYNTHETIC/CHEMICAL DERIVATIVES

Great strides in molecular biology and biochemistry enable scientists to create manmade drugs referred to as synthetic drugs. A synthetic drug is produced using chemical synthesis, which rearranges chemical derivatives to form a new compound.

Sulfonamides are a common group of synthesized drugs that are used to treat many infections including bronchitis, pneumonia, and meningitis. Sulfonamides are designed to prevent the growth of bacteria.

HERBALS

Herbals are non-woody plants. Some have medicinal qualities classified as a dietary supplement—not a drug. Unlike drugs that are governed by the Food and Drug Administration, dietary supplements are not tested or regulated and can be sold over-the-counter without a prescription. This lack of monitoring means there are no standards for purity and strength for herbals. Two packages of the same herbal distributed by the same company might have different purity and strength that makes the effect of the herb unreliable. There is no control over the manufacturing process and that can lead to contamination. The law prohibits distributors of herbals from claiming that an herbal can cure a disease. They can only state the effect of the herbal on the body. For example, the manufacturer can say that an herbal increases blood flow to the heart, but cannot say that the herb prevents heart disease.

Herbals can lead to unwanted side effects and undesirable interactions with prescription drugs. For example, ginkgo inhibits platelet aggregation (grouping to form clots) if taken with coumadin, an anticoagulant. The result can be increased bleeding and stroke. Garlic interacts with protease inhibitors used to treat HIV and decreases the effectiveness of the prescribed medication. The interaction of herbals with other drugs can be unpredictable and even dangerous. Healthcare providers should encourage patients to reveal any herbal preparations they are taking.

Drugs Names

One of the most confusing aspects of pharmacology is naming drugs. A drug is given three names. Each is used in a different area of the drug industry. These names are the drug's chemical name, generic name, and brand name.

CHEMICAL NAME

The chemical name identifies chemical elements and compounds that are found in the drug. The chemical name is important to chemists, pharmacists, and researchers who work with drugs at the chemical level.

A chemical name looks strange to anyone who isn't a chemist and is difficult for most of us to pronounce. That's why names other than the chemical name are given to a drug. Here is the chemical name for a commonly used drug: N-acetyl-p-aminophenol.

GENERIC NAME

The generic name of a drug is the universally accepted name and considered the official proprietary name for the drug. The generic name appears on all drug labels and is the official name listed in official sources such as the Physicians Desk Reference (PDR). The pharmaceutical company that patents a drug has exclusive rights to sell it until the patent expires. When the patent expires, other drug manufacturers may distribute the drug under the drug's generic name or create a brand name. The generic version of a drug may be cheaper than the original drug and the cost is usually reimbursed by insurance companies. An example of a generic name for a commonly used drug is acetaminophen. The generic name is easier to read and pronounce than the drug's chemical name, N-acetyl-p-aminophenol.

BRAND/TRADE NAME

Drug companies often select and copyright a trade or brand name for their drug. This restricts the use of this name to that particular company. Many brand names may exist for the same chemical compound.

Brand name drugs may be more costly than generic drugs and are partially reimbursed or not covered at all by insurance companies.

A brand name for acetaminophen is Tylenol (patented by Johnson & Johnson Pharmaceuticals).

An example of the correct documentation of the generic and brand name of a drug is: furosemide (Lasix). This drug is a diuretic used for many patients with hypertension (high blood pressure) or cardiac (heart) disease.

Prescription versus Over-the-Counter Drugs

The 1952 Durham-Humphrey Amendment to the Food, Drug and Cosmetic Act requires that certain classifications of drugs be accessible only by prescription from a licensed practitioner. These are commonly referred to as prescription drugs or legend drugs because the drug label must display the legend "Caution: Federal law prohibits dispensing without prescription" on the label of the drug.

Drugs that fall under this classification are:

- Those given by injection.
- Hypnotic drugs (drugs that depress the nervous system).
- Narcotics (drugs that relieve pain, dull the senses and induce sleep).
- Habit-forming drugs.
- Drugs that are unsafe unless administered under the supervision of a licensed practitioner.
- New drugs that are still being investigated and not considered safe for indiscriminate use by the public.

Non-prescription drugs are called over-the-counter (OTC) drugs and are available to the public without prescription. Some over-the-counter drugs were at one time available by prescription, but later were considered safe for use by the public or reformulated for over-the-counter use. Some drugs can be sold in lower doses over-the-counter (OTC) while higher doses of the same drug require a prescription as per FDA requirements.

Drug Effects

Drugs have multiple effects on the body. Some effects are desirable and some are not. The therapeutic effect is the intended physiological effect or the reason the drug is being given. A therapeutic effect can be the drug's action against a disease such as an antibiotic destroying bacteria. Another physiological effect can be the side effects that occur in the body such as nausea and vomiting or a skin rash. A side effect is a physiologic effect that is not the intended action such as the drowsiness that occurs when a patient takes an antihistamine. Some side effects are beneficial while others are adverse effects that can be harmful to a patient.

Healthcare providers must identify all known side effects of a drug and weigh any adverse effects with the therapeutic effect before administering a drug. Patients must also be informed about expected side effects and provided instructions about how to manage adverse side effects if at all possible.

For example, female patients are instructed to drink buttermilk and eat yogurt when taking a broad-spectrum antibiotic. This counters a possible vaginal yeast infection, which is a common adverse effect of broad-spectrum antibiotics. Additionally, a female patient should be instructed to use other forms of birth control when taking this medication because antibiotics lower the effectiveness of birth control pills.

Many times patients will discontinue the use of a medication because the side effects are so unpleasant. Antihypertensive medications (blood pressure medicine) can cause side effects such as drowsiness or the inability to achieve an erection in a male. Patients may decide that this effect is undesirable and discontinue the use of the prescribed drug. Patients should be encouraged to discuss any and all side effects with the provider. Many times, there are alternative medications that can be prescribed. Abruptly discontinuing the use of a drug may not be in the best interest of a patient. Some drugs may be gradually decreased in dose and frequency. Sometimes patients discontinue taking a drug because they feel better, however, the condition being treated is still present. Some examples of these types of medication are antibiotics and antidepressants.

Drug Safety

Drugs must undergo rigorous testing before being approved by the Food and Drug Administration for use in humans. The initial testing is done with animals to determine the toxicity of the drug. Acute toxicity is the dose that is lethal or kills 50% of the laboratory animals tested. The testing is also done to determine what symptoms are experienced by the animals and the time the symptoms appear.

Subchronic toxicity studies, conducted in at least two animal species, usually consist of daily administration of the drug for up to 90 days. Physical examinations and laboratory tests are performed throughout the study and at the end of the study to see what organs may have been adversely affected by the drug.

Chronic toxicity studies, also conducted in at least two species, usually last the lifetime of the animal but the length of the study may depend on the intended duration of drug administration to humans. Three dose levels are used, varying from a nontoxic low-level dose to a dose that is higher than the expected therapeutic dose and is toxic when given over a long period of time. Physical examinations and laboratory tests are performed to determine which organs are affected and whether the drug has the potential to cause cancer (carcinogenic).

Animal studies enable scientists to develop a therapeutic index for the drug. A therapeutic index is the ratio between the median lethal dose and the median effective dose. It tells a practitioner the safe dose to give for the therapeutic effect to be achieved.

Some drugs have a narrow margin of safety and require that the blood plasma levels be frequently monitored to assure that the drug stays within the therapeutic range. Drugs that have a wide margin of safety don't require that the plasma levels be monitored. Digitalis (digoxin) is an example of a drug that has a narrow margin of safety and requires frequent monitoring of plasma levels.

Scientists also learn how the drug is absorbed, distributed, metabolized, and excreted once it is administered to the animals. This helps scientists predict how the drug will react when administered to humans.

Tests are also conducted in laboratory test tubes that can determine the metabolism of the drug in humans, which may be different from animals. These are called *in vitro* studies. Once animal studies are successfully completed, the drug is ready for human trials during which human subjects are given the drug. There are three phases of human trial.

PHASE I: INITIAL PHARMACOLOGICAL EVALUATION

In Phase I, drug trials, the drug is given to a small number of healthy volunteers to determine safe dosage levels. The purpose is to document the dose level at which signs of toxicity first appear in humans, determine a safe tolerated dose, and determine the pharmacokinetics of the drug. Pharmacokinetics will be discussed in Chapter 2. Volunteers who give consent to participate are monitored closely during this phase. Permission must be obtained from the FDA to conduct Phase I clinical trials.

PHASE II: LIMITED CONTROLLED EVALUATION

The purpose of Phase II evaluation is to monitor drug effectiveness and any side effects. Individuals with the targeted disease participate in this phase of drug trials. For example, antihypertensive (blood pressure lowering) drugs will be administered to patients who have hypertension (high blood pressure) to determine the drug's effectiveness or optimal dose response range and for side effects. The number of participants is larger than Phase I trials but usually does not exceed 100 persons and every effort is made to use only people who have no other disorders or diseases.

PHASE III: EXTENDED CLINICAL EVALUATION

Phase III drug trials include many physicians and large groups of participants. When enough information has been collected to justify continued use of the drug, a New Drug Application (NDA) is submitted to the FDA. Usually, more than 4 years has passed between the drug's selection and the filing of the NDA.

Phase IV studies are also called post-marketing follow-up. They are voluntarily conducted by pharmaceutical companies. These studies continue after the FDA has approved the drug and often include populations such as pregnant women, children, and the elderly. Manufacturers can find low-level side effects or can find that a drug is toxic and must be removed from market. The FDA continues to monitor new drugs even after they are marketed.

Drugs also undergo tests to determine the possible effects on a fetus. As a result of these tests, drugs are classified using the following Pregnancy Categories.

Category A

Adequate and well-controlled studies indicate no risk to the fetus in the first trimester of pregnancy or later.

Category B

Animal reproduction studies indicate no risk to the fetus, however there are no well-controlled studies in pregnant women.

Category C

Animal reproduction studies have reported adverse effects on the fetus, however there are no well-controlled studies in humans but potential benefits may indicate use of the drug in pregnant women despite potential risks.

Category D

Positive human fetal risk has been reported from investigational or marketing experience, or human studies. Considering potential benefit versus risk may, in selected cases, warrant the use of these drugs in pregnant women.

Category X

Fetal abnormalities reported and positive evidence of fetal risk in humans is available from animal and/or human studies. The risks involved clearly outweigh the potential benefits. These drugs should not be used in pregnant women.

Locating Drug Information

Before administering a drug to a patient (see Chapter 4), healthcare providers need to know the following information about the drug:

- Generic and trade name: The generic name is the official name of the drug while the trade name is the drug's brand name.
- Clinical uses and indications for use: Describes the purpose of the drug and when the drug is to be given to a patient.
- Mechanism of action: Describes how the drug works.
- Adverse and side effects and toxicity: Identifies the effects the drug has other than the therapeutic effect.
- Signs and symptoms to monitor: Identifies the patient's physiological response that must be evaluated after the drug is administered.
- What to teach the patient: Specifies instructions that must be given to the patient before and after the drug is administered.

This information is available in product inserts, various drug handbooks for nurses, and in computerized pharmacology databases and in the following:

- *American Hospital Formulary Service (AHFS) Drug Information:* Published by the American Society of Hospital Pharmacists, Inc. and contains an overview of every drug.
- *United States Pharmacopeia Dispensing Information:* Published by the U.S. Pharmacopeial Convention and highlights clinical information, which is the same as the drug inserts found in packages of drugs.

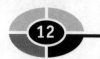

- *Physician's Desk Reference (PDR):* Published by Medical Economics with the financial support of the pharmaceutical industry and contains the same information as found in the drug inserts.
- *Physician's GenRx* published by Mosby and includes comprehensive drug information product identification charts and product ratings by the Food and Drug Administration. It also contains cost comparisons between drugs.
- *Handbook of Nonprescription Drugs:* Published by the American Pharmaceutical Association and contains comprehensive information on over-the-counter drugs including the primary minor illnesses the drug is used to treat.
- *Medline Plus (http://www.nlm.nih.gov/medlineplus/druginformation.html):* An online database produced by the U. S. National Library of Medicine and the National Institutes of Health and contains information about prescription and over-the-counter drugs and devices as well as warnings and drug recall information.

Drug Orders

A drug order, also called a medical prescription, is an instruction from a provider to give a patient medication. Providers such as a physician, dentist, podiatrist, advanced practice nurse (in most states), and other authorized licensed healthcare providers can write a drug order. Physician assistants can also write a drug order but require the co-signature of a physician.

All drug orders are written on a prescription pad or on an order sheet if written in a healthcare institution. Sometimes orders are written into a computerized drug order system. A verbal drug order is sometimes given but must be followed up with a written drug order within 24 hours.

Drug orders are written using the abbreviations shown in Table 1-1 and must contain:

- Date and time the order (prescription) was issued.
- Name of drug and whether or not a generic form of the drug can be substituted for a brand-name drug.
- Drug dose.
- Route of administration.
- Frequency and duration of administration.
- Special instructions such as withholding or adjusting dosage based on nursing assessment, laboratory results, or drug effectiveness.

- Signature of the prescriber.
- Signature of the healthcare providers who took the order and transcribed it.

Table 1-1. Commonly used abbreviations for drug orders.

Direction	L (in circle)	Left
	R (in a circle)	Right
Dose	aa	Of each
	$\bar{c}$	With
	DS	Double strength
	elix.	Elixir
	fl or fld.	Fluid
	gtt	Drop
	NS or N/S	Normal saline
	q.s.	A sufficient amount/ as much as needed/ quantity sufficient
	$\bar{s}$	Without
	$\bar{ss}$ or ss	One half
	SR	Sustained release
	XL	Long acting
	XR	Extended release
Form	amp	ampule
	aq	water
	c	Cup
	cap or caps	Capsule
	EC	Enteric coated
	mix	Mixture
	sol or soln	Solution
	supp	Suppository

Table 1-1. *(continued)*

	susp	Suspension
	syp or syr	Syrup
	tab	Tablet
	Tr or tinct	Tincture
	ung. or oint	Ointment
Method	gt or GT	Gastrostomy tube
	I.D.	Intradermal
	I.M.	Intramuscular
	I.V.	Intravenous
	IVPB	Intravenous piggyback
	IVSS	Intravenous soluset
	KVO	Keep vein open (a vey slow infusion rate)
	NGT	Nasogastric tube
	n.p.o	Nothing by mouth
	Per	Through or by
	Per os or p.o.	By or through mouth
	p.r.	By rectum
	s.c or S.C. or s.q.*	Subcutaneous
	sl or SL	Sublingual
	S&S	Swish and swallow
	vag	Vaginally
Part	A.D. or AD*	Right ear
	A.S. or AS*	Left ear
	A.U. or AU*	Both ears
	OD*	Right eye
	os*	Mouth
	OS*	Left eye

Table 1-1. *(continued)*

	OU*	Both eyes
	Rect*	Rectum
Time	ā	Before
	ad.lib	As desired
	b.i.d. or bid	Twice a day
	d.c. or D/C	Discontinue
	h or hr	Hour
	h.s.	At bed time
	min	Minute
	o.d. or OD	Once a day
	p̄	After
	p.c.	After meals
	p.r.n.	When necessary
	q.	Every, each
	q.a.m.	Every morning
	q.d. or qd*	Every day or once a day
	q.h. or qh	Every hour
	q2h, q4h	Every two hours, every four hours
	qhs or q.h.s.*	Every night at bedtime
	q.i.d. or qid	Four times a day
	q.o.d. or qod*	Every other day
	s.o.s	Once if necessary
	stat or STAT	Immediately or at once
	t.i.d. or tid	Three times a day
	t.i.w.*	Three times a week

*The Joint Commission for Accreditation of Hospitals Organization (JCAHO) has recommended that these abbreviations not be used to decrease the chance of errors. However, some hospitals and providers continue to use them when writing medications orders.

TYPES OF DRUG ORDERS

There are four types of drug orders. These are:

Routine orders: This is an ongoing order given for a specific number of doses or number of days.

Example: 1/31/05 7:30 P.M. Lasix (furosemide) 40 mg., PO, qd (signature)

This is an order to give 40 milligrams of Lasix by mouth once a day. Once a day medications are generally given around 9 A.M. or 10 A.M. based on the healthcare institution or patient choice if at home. Lasix is a diuretic.

One-time order: This is a single dose given at a particular time.

Example: Demerol 50 mg with Vistaril 25 mg IM at 10 A.M. or 2 h before call to the OR.

This is an order to give Demerol (meperidine) 50 milligrams with Vistaril (hydroxyzine) 25 milligrams intramuscularly at 10 A.M. or one hour before call to the operating room.

PRN: This is an order to give a medication if specific criteria exist, such as a headache, fever, or pain and at the patient's request.

Example: Advil 600 mg po q 6 h prm for mild to moderate knee pain.

This is an order to give Advil (ibuprofen) 600 milligrams by mouth every six hours as needed for mild to moderate knee pain.

STAT: This is a single dose order to give at once or immediately

Example: Give Benadryl 50 mg. po Stat.

This is an order to give Benadryl (dyphenhydramine) 50 milligrams by mouth immediately.

There are also protocols for administering medications. This is a set of criteria that indicates under what conditions a drug may be given. There are two types of protocols: *standing orders* or *flow diagrams* (algorithms). Standing orders are an officially accepted sets of orders to be applied by nurses, physician assistants, and paramedics in the care of patients with certain conditions or under certain circumstances. For example, if a patient is not breathing and has no heartbeat, an algorithm has been developed to administer different medications such as epinephrine and other cardiac stimulants to resuscitate the individual. Other standing orders include orders for Tylenol (acetaminophen) 600 milligrams q 4 h by mouth or per rectum for a temperature > 101.4°F.

The "Five Rights" of Drug Administration

There are five traditional right actions that should be followed when giving medication. These are to determine the right patient, right drug, right dose, right time, and right route. Five additional rights include the right assessment, documentation, education, evaluation, and the right to refuse.

RIGHT PATIENT

The right patient means that the healthcare provider gives the drug to the right patient. Each time a drug is administered, the healthcare provider must verify who the patient is by the patient's identification bracelet. This is the preferred method as opposed to identifying a patient by asking his or her name. Some patients will answer "yes" to any name and two patients can have similar-sounding names or the same name. Some patients are not mentally alert and do not remember their name. Again, check the patient's identification every time medication is administered.

RIGHT DRUG

Healthcare providers must be sure that the drug is the correct medication for the patient. This too leads to errors. Healthcare providers ask: Was this the drug prescribed on the medication order? Is the medication order legible and complete? Why is the patient receiving this medication? Is the medication consistent with the patient's condition? Does the patient have any food or drug allergies?

Providers check the expiration date and return the medication to the pharmacy if it has expired. If the medication is used past the expiration date, the effect on the patient can be unpredictable.

Healthcare providers check the medication label three times before administering the drug. First, when they take the medication from the shelf or drawer. Next, the label should be checked before pouring the drug, and third it is checked after pouring the drug before throwing away the drug packaging.

RIGHT DOSE

The dose on the medication order must be within recommended guidelines. The healthcare provider should have a general idea of the dose before performing any drug calculations. If the calculated dose varies too much from this estimated dose, check with a pharmacist or another appropriate healthcare provider. Some drug calculations should always be checked by two individuals if the calculation is complicated or the drug has the potential to be harmful if the dose is too large or too small. Medications that are wrapped and labeled or pre-filled for the exact dose are preferred and can reduce errors.

Healthcare providers should also make sure they use the proper system of measurement when calculating a dose (see Chapter 4 Principles of Medication Administration).

RIGHT TIME

Is it the correct time to administer the drug? The time is specified in the drug order and may be given a half hour before or after the stated time depending on the policy of the hospital or healthcare facility. How often a drug is given is dependent on the half life of the drug. A drug's half life is the amount of time for ½ of the drug to be eliminated from the body. A drug with a short half life must be administered more frequently than a drug with a long half-life in order to maintain a therapeutic level of the drug in plasma.

The use of military time can avoid A.M. and P.M. errors.

Check if the patient is scheduled for diagnostic or other procedures that might interfere with administration of medications. Check if the patient should receive the medication even if they are scheduled to be NPO (nothing by mouth).

Healthcare providers should also make sure that medication is given in coordination with meals. Some drugs must be given with meals while other drugs are given a specific period before or after a meal.

Where possible, the medication schedule is adjusted to conform to the patient's lifestyle, which may differ from the normal schedule. For example, Digoxin might be scheduled for 10 A.M. to conform to hospital policy, but the patient can take Digoxin any time in the morning. This becomes important once the patient is discharged and takes medication at home.

RIGHT ROUTE

The healthcare provider determines the proper routine to administer the drug so the patient's body properly absorbs it. Here are the common routes:

- Oral (by mouth): liquid, elixir, suspension, pill, tablet, and capsule
- Sublingual (under tongue): pill, tablet, and capsule
- Buccal (between gum and cheek): pill, tablet, and capsule
- Topical (applied to skin): cream, ointment, and patch
- Inhalation (aerosol sprays): liquid
- Instillation (nose, eye, ear): liquid, cream, and ointment
- Insertion (rectal, vaginal): suppository
- Intradermal (beneath skin): injection

- Subcutaneous (beneath skin): injection
- Intramuscular (in muscle): injection
- Intravenous (in vein): injection
- Nasogastric and gastronomy tubes: liquid
- Transdermal: patches

Make sure that the patient can swallow if the route of the medication is by mouth and stay with the patient until the medication is swallowed. Enteric coated or time-release drugs should not crushed or mixed. Caution should be used when administering intravenous medications because the body quickly absorbs these drugs. Therefore, healthcare providers need to know expected side effects, effects that occur when the drug is first given, effects the drug has during its therapeutic peak, and duration of the drug's action. Caution should be used when administering any medication via this route.

Self-administration of medication (SAM) is the normal practice for patients in the home and workplace. This method is also used in some acute and long-term care institutional settings. In these settings the nurse gives the patient a packet of medications with instructions that are kept at the bedside. The patient takes the medication according to the instructions and advises the nurse when he or she has done so. This practice help patients learn how to manage the medications and prepares them for discharge and use of these medications in the home. This method is often used with oncology (cancer) patients and maternity patients.

Patient controlled analgesia (PCA) is a common method of administering intravenous pain medication for many patients. This will be discussed further in a subsequent chapter.

RIGHT TO REFUSE MEDICATION

A mentally competent patient has the right to refuse medication. Refusal is documented on the patient record. Patients should be advised of the consequences of the refusal to take the medication such as a worsening of the condition. As a general rule, every effort is made to encourage the patient to take the medication. However, no one should physically force a patient to take medication.

RIGHT TO EDUCATION

The patient has the right to be told about the medication that is about to be administered. The patient is told:

- The name of the medication
- Why the medication is given
- What the medication looks like
- How much of the medication to take
- When to take the medication
- When not to take the medication
- What are the side effects, adverse effects, and toxic effects

This information is discussed in the best way the patient can understand. Healthcare providers should avoid speaking in medical terminology and, instead, use common words and expressions that are familiar to the patient—and always in the language that the patient speaks.

The patient provides feedback that he or she understands everything about the medication. It is common for the healthcare provider to ask the patient to tell in his or her own words what was told to them about the medication.

The patient is also shown how to keep track of multiple medications. Typically, the patient is encouraged to keep a list of medications. The list should have the name of the medication, dose, time the medication is to be taken and the name and phone number of the prescriber who ordered the medication.

Summary

Pharmacology is the study of drug effects on living tissue and how drugs cure, prevent, or manage diseases. Drugs are derived from plants, animals, minerals, and are synthesized in the laboratory. Each drug has three names. These are the chemical name, the generic name that is considered the official name for the drug, and the brand name, which is used by the manufacturer to market the drug.

There are two general classifications of drugs: prescription and over-the-counter drugs. Prescription drugs are also known as legend drugs and must be prescribed by an authorized healthcare provider. Over-the-counter drugs can be purchased with or without a prescription.

Drugs have three effects: these are the therapeutic effect to fight or prevent a disease; a side effect that isn't harmful; and an adverse effect that is harmful to a varying degree. Some drugs can also cause an allergic response in some patients. Healthcare providers must know about these effects before administering the medication to the patient. Furthermore, the patient must be informed of these effects.

Before a drug is manufactured and released for public use, it must undergo a series of tests that begin with animal studies and follows through to clinical studies on humans. Animal studies determine the therapeutic index for the drug. Clinical studies determine the therapeutic effect, adverse effect, and side effects the drug has on humans.

A drug is prescribed to a patient by writing a drug order or medical prescription. A drug order specifies, among other things, the name of the drug, the dose, route of administration, and frequency. Only an authorized healthcare provider can order drugs. There are four types of drug orders. These are routine orders, one-time orders, PRN orders, and STAT orders. There are also standing orders or protocols.

There are five right actions to take when giving medications. These are to give the right patient the right drug, in the right dose, at the right time, by the right route. Patients also have the right to refuse medication and the right to education about the medication.

With this overview of pharmacology under your belt, let's take a closer look at how drugs work by exploring the principles of drug action and drug interactions in the next chapter.

Quiz

1. A brand name of a drug is
   (a) the non-trademarked name given by the original drug manufacturer.
   (b) the trademarked name given by the drug manufacturer.
   (c) the official nonproprietary name for the drug.
   (d) the universally accepted name.

2. Schedule I controlled substances
   (a) cannot be prescribed.
   (b) can be prescribed only by a physician.
   (c) can be purchased over-the-counter.
   (d) are approved for medical use.

3. The 1938 Food, Drug and Cosmetic Act
   (a) established categories of drugs.
   (b) standardized labeling for drugs.
   (c) established who could prescribe drugs.
   (d) requires drug manufacturers to prove that their drugs are safe.

4. Herbals are tested and regulated by the Food and Drug Administration.
   (a) True
   (b) False

5. All drug side effects are harmful.
   (a) True
   (b) False

6. Drugs come from
   (a) animals.
   (b) humans.
   (c) plants.
   (d) all of the above.

7. P.O. in a drug order means by rectum.
   (a) True
   (b) False

8. A drug order that requires the drug to be given immediately is called a
   (a) one-time order.
   (b) PRN order.
   (c) STAT order.
   (d) standing order.

9. A patient does not have the right to refuse medication.
   (a) True
   (b) False

10. The number of times a drug is given to a patient can be determined by the half-life of the drug.
    (a) True
    (b) False

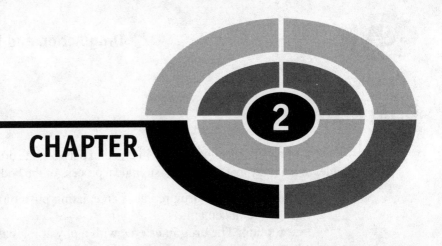

CHAPTER 2

Drug Action and Drug Interactions

"Just give me the magic pill to make me normal again." You probably said something like that the last time you felt under the weather and your home remedies didn't make you feel better. You might have even reached the point when you'd welcome an injection of a miracle drug if it would get you back on your feet quickly.

Drugs aren't miracles and have nothing to do with magic although you might think differently when your nose is running, eyes watering, and you feel rotten all over. A drug is a chemical compound specifically designed to combat disease.

In this chapter, you'll be introduced to the scientific principles that describe how drugs interact with cells in your body to bring about a pharmaceutical response that either directly attacks the pathogen that is causing your sniffles or stimulates your body's own defense mechanism to stamp them out.

Drug Actions

Drug action is the physiochemical interaction between the drug molecule and molecules in the body that alters a physiological process of the body in one of three ways.

- Replacement: The drug replaces an existing physiological process such as estrogen replacement.
- Interruption: The drug interferes with a physiological process. This occurs when an antihypertensive (high blood pressure) drug interferes with the process that constricts blood vessels and may cause blood pressure to rise. The blood vessels remain dilated and pressures remain normal or drop.
- Potentiation: The drug stimulates a physiological process as in the case of furosemide (Lasix) which is a diuretic and stimulates the kidneys to excrete urine.

A drug action begins when the drug enters the body and is absorbed into the bloodstream where the drug is transported to receptor sites throughout the body (see Pharmacokinetics, in this chapter). Once the drug hooks onto a receptor site, the drug's pharmacological response initiates. The pharmacological response is the therapeutic effect that makes the patient well.

Drugs have multiple actions. These are the desired effect and effects other than the desirable effect. The desirable effect is what makes the patient well or prevents the disease or disorder. An effect other than the desirable effect is known as a side effect. Some side effects are desirable and others are undesirable (see Side Effects, in this chapter).

The strength of a drug action is determined by how much of the drug is given, (the dose) and how often the drug is given (the frequency). For example, a patient who has a sore throat can be given a large dose of an antibiotic—a loading dose—on the first day of treatment and a normal or maintenance dose for the next five days.

Drug activity is divided into three phases. These are:

- Pharmaceutic Phase: This phase occurs after the drug is given and involves disintegration and dissolution of the dosage form.
- Pharmacokinetic Phase: This is the way the drug is absorbed, distributed, and eliminated.
- Pharmacodynamic Phase: This is the effect the drug has on the body.

PHARMACEUTIC

The pharmaceutic phase is the form of the drug such as a tablet, capsule, liquid, elixirs, or syrups. The drug in solid form must disintegrate before dissolution, which is the process by which a drug goes into solution before it becomes available for absorption. Drugs contain an active ingredient and inactive ingredients. The active ingredient is the substance that causes the pharmaceutical response. The inactive ingredient, called excipient, is the substance that has no pharmaceutical response but helps in the delivery of the drug. These are fillers and inert substances that give the drug its shape and size. The coating around tiny particles of a capsule that causes a timed-release action of the drug is an inactive ingredient.

Nearly 80% of all drugs are administered orally (P.O.) and are carried to the small intestine by the gastrointestinal tract where the drug is absorbed into the bloodstream. The time necessary for the drug to disintegrate and dissolve so it can be absorbed is called the rate limiting time.

A drug has a higher rate limiting time (Table 2-1) if it is absorbed in acidic fluids rather than alkaline fluids. Children and the elderly have a lower pH in their GI tract and therefore drugs are absorbed more slowly than in a healthy adult.

Some drugs are more effective if absorbed in the small intestine rather than the stomach. However, the stomach is more acidic than the small intestine. Therefore, pharmaceutical manufacturers place an enteric coating around the drug that resists disintegration in the stomach. The coating disintegrates in the alkaline environment of the small intestine. Enteric coating is also used to delay the onset of the pharmaceutical response and to prevent food in the stomach from interfering with the dissolution and absorption of the drug.

Tip: Never crush a capsule that contains enteric release beads or is coated for timed-release.

The form of a drug influences the drug's pharmacokinetics and pharmacodynamics.

Table 2-1.   Rate limiting time rating for drug forms.

Preparation	Absorption Rate (fastest to slowest)
Lipid soluble non-ionized liquids, elixirs, syrups	1
Water soluble ionized liquids, elixirs, syrups	2
Suspension solutions	3
Powders	4
Capsules	5
Tablets	6
Coated tablets	7
Enteric-coated tablets	8

PHARMACOKINETICS

Pharmacokinetics is the study of the drug concentration during absorption, distribution, and elimination of a drug in the patient. About 80% of all drugs are administered orally and flow through the gastrointestinal tract (GI) into the small intestine where the membrane of the intestine absorbs drug particles passing them into the bloodstream, where plasma circulates the particles, throughout the body. Drug molecules move to the intended site of action in the plasma but sometimes this journey can be limited because they have to get into the interior of a cell or body compartment through cell membranes. These membranes could be in the skin, the intestinal tract, or the intended site of action. Drug particles then attach themselves to receptor sites resulting in its therapeutic effect.

There are three ways in which drug particles are absorbed. These are:

Passive Diffusion

Passive diffusion is the flow of drug particles from a high concentration to a low concentration—similar to how water flows downstream. There is a higher concentration of water upstream than there is downstream. There is no energy expended in passive diffusion because drug particles are moving along the natural flow.

Active Diffusion

Active diffusion is how drug particles swim upstream against the natural flow when there is a higher concentration of plasma than there is of drug particles. Drug particles don't have enough energy to go against the natural flow without help. Help comes from an enzyme or protein carrier that transports drug particles upstream across the membrane and into the plasma. The enzyme or protein carrier expends energy to move drug particles.

Pinocytosis

Pinocytosis is the process of engulfing the drug particle and pulling it across the membrane. This is similar to how you eat an ice pop by engulfing a piece of it in with your mouth and swallowing it.

ABSORPTION RATE

Absorption begins where the drug is administered. This can be by mouth, injection, through the skin, and many other sites. How quickly the drug becomes therapeutic will depend on how fast the drug is absorbed. How long the drug will be effective and how much drug is needed depends on the route of administration, the dose of the drug, and the dosage form (tablet, capsule, or liquid).

The absorption rate of a drug is influenced by a number of factors that might increase or decrease the rate, This is similar to how more gasoline is used to drive at faster speeds. Absorption is affected by many factors that include pain, stress, hunger, fasting, food, and pH. Hot, solid, fatty foods can slow absorption such as eating a Big Mac before taking medication. Even exercise—which is usually good for the body—affects absorption of a drug. During exercise, circulation to the stomach is diverted to other areas of the body and drug absorption is decreased.

Circulation

Blood flow to the site of administration of the drug will help increase the rate of absorption. An area that has a lot of blood vessels and good circulation will help absorb the drug quickly and circulate it to the intended site. When a patient is in shock and has a low blood pressure due to decreased circulation (blood flow) drugs may not be absorbed very quickly.

Route of Administration

The rate at which drug particles are absorbed is determined by the amount of blood vessels there are in the area where the drug is administered. Drug particles are nearly instantaneously absorbed if the drug is injected intravenously (IV). A slower absorption rate occurs if the drug is administered intramuscularly (IM). The IM rate is dependent on the amount of blood vessels there are at the site of the injection. For example, a drug is absorbed faster in the deltoid (arm) muscle than in the gluteal (butt) muscle because there are more blood vessels in the deltoid muscle. Drugs injected in subcutaneous (SC) tissue are absorbed slower than those injected via IM injections because there are fewer blood vessels in subcutaneous tissues than in muscles.

Solubility

Drug particles dissolve in either lipid (fat) or water. Lipid-soluble drugs are absorbed more quickly than water-soluble drugs because membranes in the GI tract are composed of lipids making those membranes a perfect highway for lipid soluble drugs to move from the GI tract and into the bloodstream. However, membranes of the GI tract do not directly absorb large water-soluble molecules and a carrier must be used to transport the water-soluble drugs across the GI membrane and into the bloodstream. This additional step causes water-soluble drugs to be absorbed more slowly than fat-soluble drugs.

pH Level

The pH level of a drug determines how easily drug particles will be absorbed in the GI tract. Those drugs that are a weak acid—such as aspirin— can pass rapidly across the GI tract membrane while weak base drugs—such as an antacid—are absorbed more slowly than a weak acidic drug. Strong acids and bases destroy cells and are not absorbed.

The concentration of the drug will also affect the rate of absorption. If a high concentration of the drug is given, it will tend to be absorbed more rapidly. Sometimes larger (loading or priming) doses of a drug may be given that will be more than the body can excrete. When this is done, the drug becomes therapeutic much faster. After the first large dose, small maintenance doses will help keep the therapeutic effect.

The form (solid, liquid) the drug is given can affect the absorption rate. Drugs can be processed when they are manufactured to add other ingredients that will help or hinder absorption.

BIOAVAILABILITY

Not all drug particles reach the circulatory system. Some particles are misdirected or destroyed during the absorption process. For example, hydrochloric acid in the stomach destroys some drug particles before it can pass through the membrane and into the bloodstream.

The percentage of a dose that reaches the blood stream is called the *bioavailability* of a drug. Typically, between 20% and 40% of drugs that are administered orally reach the blood stream. This is called the first pass effect and is the beginning of the metabolism of a drug that is given orally. After a drug is absorbed in the GI tract it is carried to the liver and metabolism occurs. Sometimes very little of the drug remains available for a therapeutic effect after the first pass. Only drugs administered intravenously have a 100% bioavailability because they are directly injected into the vein.

Pharmaceutical manufacturers must consider bioavailability when determining the dose for a drug. For example, the dose for a drug administered PO (orally) might be 4 times higher than if the same drug is administered intravenously.

There are a number of factors that alter bioavailability. These are:

- Form: tablet, capsule, slow-release, liquid, transdermal patch, suppository, and inhalation.
- Route: PO (mouth), topical, parenteral, and rectal.
- GI: The ability of the mucosa (lining) in the GI tract impacts the ability to absorb drug particles and the ability to move food through the digestive tract.
- Food: Drug particles for some drugs are better absorbed if they are taken with certain foods, while other foods slow down or block absorption.
- Drugs: Some drugs increase or decrease another drug's absorption when both drugs are taken together.
- Liver metabolism: Liver dysfunction can prevent or delay the metabolism of a drug.
- Concentration: A higher portion of active ingredient in a dose increases the amount of drug particles that are absorbed.
- Cell membrane: Single layer cell membrane, such as those found in the intestine, increase absorption, while some drugs are absorbed more slowly in multiple-layers, such as skin.
- Surface area: A larger surface area, such as in the small intestine, absorbs drugs faster than a smaller area such as in the stomach.

DRUG CONCENTRATION

A drug contains an active ingredient, which produces the therapeutic effect, and other materials that give the drug form and protection. The percent of active ingredient in a dose is referred to as the drug concentration.

There are generally two levels of concentrations. These are *primary loading*—a large concentration that is used to achieve a fast therapeutic effect such as the first dose of an antibiotic, and *maintenance dose*—a typical concentration of the drug that is used to provide an ongoing therapeutic effect such as subsequent doses of an antibiotic.

DISTRIBUTION

Once absorbed, drug particles are transported in blood plasma. These are referred to as "free" drugs because they are not bound to any receptor sites. Only free drugs can cause a pharmacological response. Drugs bind to proteins in plasma, usually albumin or globulins. These drug–protein complexes decrease the concentration of free drug in the circulation. This protein–drug molecule is too large to pass through the membrane of a blood vessel and is not available for therapeutic use. This process can be reversed when free drug is excreted from the body. The drug molecule is released from the protein and it becomes free drug and can be absorbed for use. Drugs affect areas of the body with good blood supply first, such as the heart, liver, kidney, and brain and then flow to areas with less blood supply, such as muscles and fat.

Drugs accumulate in an area of the body and form a reservoir by binding to tissues. This is referred to as pooling. There are two types of pooling. These are protein binding—when a drug binds to plasma proteins, and tissue binding—fat soluble drugs are stored in adipose (fat) tissue. Inderal (propranolol) is a heart medication that is highly bound to and only about 7% of free drug is available for use at a time. Thiopental (pentothal) is an anesthetic agent that is stored in fat tissue. In addition, some drugs, such as the antibiotic Tetracycline like to be stored in bones which can interfere with growth of fetal skeletal tissues and can discolor teeth if given to children under eight years of age.

Distribution of drugs is affected by three factors.

Level of Plasma Protein

A low level of plasma protein and albumin might not provide enough binding sites for drug particles. This results in a buildup of drugs which can reach a toxic level. This happens when there is liver or kidney disease or if the patient is mal-nourished resulting in low albumin levels (hypoalbuminemia). The elderly are prone to hypoalbuminemia. Healthcare professionals should monitor a patient's plasma protein and albumin levels and the protein-binding percentage of all drugs before administering drugs to the patient.

Bloodflow

There must be adequate bloodflow to target areas of the body; otherwise, insufficient drug particles will reach affected parts of the body. Drugs can also be stored in fat, bones, muscle, and the eyes. Drugs that accumulate in fat are called lipid soluble and remain for about three hours because there is low blood flow in fat tissue.

The body also has a blood–brain barrier that enables only lipid soluble drugs—such as general anesthetics and barbiturates—into the brain and cerebral spinal fluid (CSF). The only way for nonlipid soluble drugs to enter the brain is if they are instilled intrathecally, that is, injected directly into the CSF, bypassing the blood-brain barrier.

Competing Drugs

Two drugs administered simultaneously might compete for the same binding sites making some drug particles unable to find a binding site. The result is an accumulation of free drug that could reach toxic levels. Two drugs that are highly protein bound—such as Coumadin (warfarin) and Inderal (propranolol)—will compete for the protein sites. This can cause serious problems and can result in toxic levels of one or both of the drugs when increased amounts of free drug become available.

Abscesses, exudates, body glands, and tumors hinder the distribution of drugs in the body. In addition, antibodies do not distribute well at abscess and exudates sites. The placenta metabolizes some drugs making then inactive and thereby protecting the fetus from drugs given to the mother. However, steroids, narcotics, anesthetics, and some antibiotics can penetrate the placental barrier and cause adverse effects to the fetus.

ELIMINATION

Drugs accumulate in a reservoir and are gradually absorbed and eventually eliminated by the body. This metabolism—called biotransformation—occurs in the liver where enzymes inactivate a drug by changing it into more water-soluble compounds that can be excreted from the body. Elimination occurs mainly through the kidneys, although some drugs are also eliminated in bile, feces, lungs, sweat, and breast milk.

Patients suffering from liver diseases are prone to drug toxicity because the diseased liver no longer metabolizes the drug sufficiently to allow elimination through the kidneys. The result is a buildup of the drug, which can eventually lead to a toxic effect on the body.

The amount of time for half of the drug concentration to be eliminated from the body is called the drug's half-life and is a crucial measurement used to determine how often to administer a drug. Some drugs have a short half-life (less than 8 hours) while other drugs have a longer half-life (24 hours).

For example, Digoxin has a half-life of 36 hours. This means it takes 5 to 7 days before there is a steady state of Digoxin in the serum. This is referred to as the steady state serum concentration and is the time it takes for the drug to have a therapeutic effect.

Children and the elderly might be unable to absorb and/or eliminate drugs. This can result in toxicity should additional doses be given before the previous does is eliminated from the body. Free drugs, water-soluble drugs, and unchanged drugs are filtered by the kidneys and eliminated through urine. Protein-bound drugs do not filter through the kidneys until the drug is released from the protein.

The quantity of drugs that can be excreted by the kidneys is influenced by the pH of the urine, which normally is between 4.5 and 8.0. Acidic urine (4.5) eliminates weak base drugs; alkaline urine (8.0) eliminates weak acid drugs. The pH of urine can be altered to increase the elimination of certain drugs. For example, urine can be made more alkaline by giving the patient sodium bicarbonate or made more acidic by giving the patient high doses of vitamin C or ammonium chloride.

Kidney disease decreases the glomerular filtration rate (GFR) and thereby reduces the quantity of drugs that can be eliminated by the kidneys. This can result in drug toxicity. A similar effect can be caused by a decrease in bloodflow to the kidneys.

Kidney function is tested by the creatinine clearance test. A decrease in GFR causes an increase in creatinine in serum and a decrease in creatinine in urine. The results of the creatinine clearance test vary with age and whenever there is decreased muscle mass.

In some situations, it is important to reduce the excretion of a drug to prolong the drug's therapeutic effect, such as with penicillin. Giving the patient another drug, such as Probenecid, blocks excretion of penicillin.

Drugs can be excreted artificially through the use of dialysis, which is a common treatment in certain drug overdoses. Drugs that are excreted by the kidneys can be eliminated using hemodialysis. These drugs include stimulants, depressants, and some non-narcotic analgesics.

Drugs that are metabolized by the liver are secreted into bile and then passed through the intestines and eliminated in feces. During this process, the bloodstream might reabsorb fat-soluble drugs and return them to the liver where they are metabolized and eliminated by the kidneys. This is called the enterohepatic cycle.

The lungs eliminate drugs that are intact and not metabolites such as gases and anesthetic drugs. The rate at which these drugs are eliminated corresponds to the respiratory rate. Some drugs, such as ethyl alcohol and paraldehyde, are excreted at multiple sites. A small amount is excreted by the lungs and the rest by the liver and the kidneys. Volatile drugs such as anesthetics and drugs that are metabolized to CO_2 and H_2O, are excreted through the lungs.

Sweat and salivary glands are not a major route of drug elimination because elimination depends on the diffusion of lipid-soluble drugs through the epithelial cells of the glands. However, side effects of drugs, such as rashes and skin reactions, can be seen at these sites. Some intravenously administered drugs are excreted into saliva and cause the patient to taste the drug. Eventually, drugs that are excreted into saliva are swallowed, reabsorbed, and eliminated in urine.

Many drugs or their metabolites are excreted in mammary glands. These include narcotics such as morphine and codeine. Diuretics and barbiturates, which are weak acids, are less concentrated in breast milk. However, even small amounts of drugs can accumulate causing an undesirable effect on an infant receiving breast milk.

The First Pass Effect

The most common way drugs are administered is orally, by swallowing a pill. The drug is then absorbed into the GI tract and enters the portal circulation system where drug particles are transported through the portal vein into the liver where the drug is metabolized. This is referred to as the first pass effect.

Not all drugs are metabolized in the liver. Some drugs bypass the first pass effect by sublingual administration (under the tongue) or buccal administration (between the gums and the cheek) where they are absorbed directly into the bloodstream from the mouth. These drugs do not enter the stomach where the hydrochloric acid might destroy drug particles. Other drugs go directly to the liver through the portal vein and also bypass the stomach. The drug is then metabolized in the liver and much of the drug may be eliminated and not available for a therapeutic effect. Sometimes this effect is so great that none of the drug is available for use if given by mouth. The drug must then be given in very high doses or parenterally (intramuscularly or intravenously) to bypass the liver.

Pharmacodynamics

Pharmacodynamics is a drug's effect on the physiology of the cell and the mechanism that causes the pharmaceutical response. There are two types of effects that a drug delivers. These are the primary effect and the secondary effect. The primary effect is the reason for which the drug is administered. The secondary effect is a side effect that may or may not be desirable.

For example, diphenhydramine (Benadryl) is an antihistamine. Its primary effect is to treat symptoms of allergies. Its secondary effect is to depress the central nervous system causing drowsiness. The secondary effect is desirable if the patient needs bedrest, but undesirable if the patient is driving a car.

A period of time passes after a drug is administered until the pharmaceutical response is realized. This is referred to as the drug's time response. There are three types of time responses: onset, peak, and duration.

The onset time response is the time for the minimum concentration of drug to cause the initial pharmaceutical response. Some drugs reach the onset time in minutes while other drugs take days. The peak time response is when the drug reaches its highest blood or plasma concentration. Duration is the length of time that the drug maintains the pharmaceutical response.

The response time is plotted on a time–response curve that shows the onset time response, the peak time response, and the duration. All three parameters are used when administering the drug in order to determine the therapeutic range—when the drug will become effective, when it will be most effective, and when the drug is no longer effective. It is also used to determine when a drug is expected to reach a toxic level.

For example, the time–response curve of an analgesic is used for pain management. Once the peak response time is reached, the effectiveness of the drug to block pain diminishes. The time–response curve indicates when the pharmaceutical response is no longer present requiring that an additional dose be administered to the patient.

RECEPTOR THEORY

The pharmaceutical response is realized when a drug binds to a receptor on the cell membrane. These are referred to as reactive cellular sites. The activity of the drug is determined by the drug's ability to bind to a specific receptor. The better the fit, the more biologically active the drug. Receptors are proteins, glycoproteins, proteolipids, or enzymes. Depending on the drug, binding either initiates a physiological response by the cell or blocks a cell's physiological response.

Receptors are classified into four families.

1. Rapid-Cell Membrane-Embedded Enzymes: A drug binds to the surface of the cell causing an enzyme inside the cell to initiate a physiological response.
2. Rapid-Ligand-Gated Ion Channels: The drug spans the cell membrane causing ion channels within the membrane to open resulting in the flow of primarily sodium and calcium ions into and out of the cell.
3. Rapid-G Protein-Couple Receptor Systems: The drug binds with the receptor causing the G protein to bind with guanosine triphosphate (GTP). This in turn causes an enzyme inside the cell to initiate a physiological response or causes the opening of the ion channel.
4. Prolonged-Transcription Factors: The drug binds to the transcription factors on the DNA within the nucleus of the cell and causes the transcript factor to undergo a physiological change.

A drug that causes a physiological response is called an *agonist* and a drug that blocks a physiological response is referred to as an *antagonist*. The effect of an antagonist is determined by the inhibitory (I) action of the drug concentration on the receptor site. An inhibitory action of 50 (I_{50}) indicates that the drug effectively inhibits the receptor response in 50% of the population.

Agonists and antagonists lack specific and selective effects. They are called nonspecific and have nonspecificity properties. Each receptor can produce a variety of physiologic responses. Cholinergic receptors are located in the bladder, heart, blood vessels, lungs, and eyes. A cholinergic stimulator or blocker will affect all of these sites. These drugs are called nonspecific or are said to have nonspecificity properties. A drug that is given to stimulate the cholinergic receptors will decrease the heart rate and blood pressure, increase gastric acid secretion, constrict bronchioles, increase urinary bladder contraction, and constrict the pupils. The effects may be beneficial or harmful.

Categories of Drug Action

Drugs are categorized by the type of action it causes on the body. There are four types of responses:

- Stimulation or Depression. These are drugs that either increase or depress cellular activity.
- Replacement. These are drugs that replace an essential body compound such as insulin or estrogen.
- Inhibition. These drugs interfere with bacterial cell and limit bacterial growth or eliminate the bacteria, such as penicillin.
- Irritation. These drugs irritate cells to cause a natural response that has a therapeutic effect such as a laxative that irritates the colon wall to increase movement of the colon resulting in defecation.

Therapeutic Index and Therapeutic Range

Drugs have a pharmaceutical response as long as the dose remains within the drug's margin of safety. Some drugs have a broad margin of safety. This means that a patient can be given a wide range of dose levels without experiencing a toxic effect. Other drugs have a narrow margin of safety where a slightest change in the dose can result in an undesirable adverse side effect.

The drug's Therapeutic Index (TI) identifies the margin of safety of the drug and is a ratio between the therapeutic dose in 50% of persons/animals and the lethal dose in 50% of animals. The therapeutic dose is notated as ED_{50} and the lethal dose in animals is noted as LD_{50}. The closer that the ratio is to 1, the greater the danger of toxicity.

$$TI = LD_{50}/ED_{50}$$

Drugs that have a low TI are said to have a narrow margin of safety. These drugs require that levels in the plasma be monitored and adjustments are made to the dosage in order to prevent a toxic effect from occurring.

The plasma drug levels must be within the therapeutic range, which is also known as the therapeutic window. The therapeutic range is between the minimum effective concentration (MEC) for obtaining the desired pharmaceutical response and the minimum toxic concentration (MTC). MEC is achieved by administering a loading dose, which is a large initial dose given to achieve a rapid plasma MEC.

PEAK AND TROUGH LEVELS

The plasma concentration of a drug must be monitored for drugs that have a narrow margin of safety or low therapeutic index. The concentration is measured at two points. These are the peak drug level and the trough level.

The peak drug level is the highest plasma concentration at a specific time. Peak levels indicate the rate a drug is absorbed in the body and is affected by the route used to administer the drug. Drugs administered intravenously have a fast peak drug level while a drug taken orally has a slow peak drug level because the drugs needs time to be absorbed and distributed. Blood samples are drawn at peak times based on the route used to administer the drug. This is usually ½ to 1 hr after drug administration.

The trough level is the lowest plasma concentration of the drug and measures the rate at which the drug is eliminated. Blood should be drawn immediately before the next dose is given regardless of the route used to administer the drug.

Side Effects

A drug can have a side effect in addition to its pharmaceutical response. A side effect is a physiologic effect other than the desired effect. Sometimes side effects are predictable and other times they are not and may be unrelated to the dosage. Some side effects are desirable and others are undesirable.

A severe undesirable side effect is referred to as an adverse reaction that occurs unintentionally when a normal dose of the drug is given to a patient. For example, an adverse reaction might be anaphylaxis (cardiovascular collapse)

Some adverse reactions are predictable by age and weight of the patient. Young children and the elderly are highly responsive to medications because of an immature or decline in hepatic and renal function. Body mass also influences the distribution and concentration of a drug. The dosage must be adjusted in proportion to body weight or body surface area.

Drug effects can also be related to other factors. These include:

Gender. Women typically are smaller than men and have a different proportion of fat and water which affects absorption and distribution of the drug.

Environment. Cold, heat, sensory deprivation or overload, and oxygen deprivation in high altitude create environmental factors that might interact with a drug.

Time of administration. A drug might be influenced by the presence or absence of food in the patient's gastrointestinal tract or by the patient's cortiocosteroid secretion rhythm. In addition, circadian cycle, urinary excretion pattern, fluid intake, and drug metabolizing enzyme rhythms all might influence a drug's effect.

Pathologic state. A drug can react differently if the patient is experiencing pain, anxiety, circulatory distress, or hepatic and/or renal dysfunction.

Idiosyncracy. This is an abnormal response that is unpredictable and unexplainable that could result from the patient overresponding or underresponding to the drug or the drug having an effect that is different from what is expected.

Tolerance. The patient has a decreased physiologic response after repeated administration of the drug. This is common with tobacco, opium alkaloids, nitrites, and ethyl alcohol. The dosage must be increased to achieve the pharmaceutical response.

Drug dependence. This can be either a physical or psychological dependency. With a physical dependency, the patient experiences an intense physical disturbance when the drug is withdrawn. With psychological dependency, the patient develops an emotional reliance on the drug.

Drug interaction. The administration of one drug increases or decreases the pharmaceutical response of a previously administered drug.

Synergism. A more desirable pharmaceutical response is achieved through the interaction of two drugs that are administered.

Potentiation. Concurrent administration of two drugs increases the pharmaceutical response of one of those drugs.

Toxic effect. This occurs when the administered drug exceeds the therapeutic range through an overdose or by the drug accumulating in the patient.

Tachyphylaxis. The patient builds a tolerance to the drug due to the frequency in which the drug is administered. This occurs with narcotics, barbiturates, laxatives, and psychotropic agents. The patient may eventually need more of the drug to reach the desired effect.

Placebo effect. The patient receives a psychological benefit from receiving a compound that has no pharmaceutical response. A third of patients taking a placebo experience the placebo effect.

Pharmacogenetic effect. A drug varies from a predicted response because of the influence of a patient's genetic factors. Genetic factors can alter the metabolism of the drug and results in an enhanced or diminished pharmaceutical response.

Allergic reactions. If the patient was previously sensitized to the drug, a drug might trigger the patient's immunologic mechanism that results in allergic symptoms. Antibodies are produced the first time the drug is introduced to the patient creating a sensitivity to the drug. The next time the drug is given to the patient, the drug reacts with the antibodies and results in the production of histamine. Histamine causes allergic symptoms to occur. The patient should not take any drug that causes the patient to have an allergic reaction.

There are four types of allergic reactions. These are:

- Anaphylactic. This is an immediate allergic reaction that can be fatal.
- Cytotoxic reaction. This is an autoimmune response that results in hemolytic anemia, thrombocytopenia, or lupus erythematosus (blood disorders). In some cases, it takes months for the reaction to dissipate.
- Immune complex reaction. This is referred to as serum sickness and results in angioedema, arthralgia (sore joints), fever, swollen lymph nodes, and splenomegaly (large spleen). The immune complex reaction can appear up to three weeks after the drug is administered.
- Cell mediated. This is an inflammatory skin reaction that is also known as delayed hypersensitivity.

Summary

A drug has a physiochemical action with the physiological process of the body resulting in a pharmaceutical response. Drugs replace a missing element such as a hormone, interrupts a physiological process or stimulates a physiological process to occur. In addition to a therapeutic effect, drugs may have side effects that can be desirable or undesirable.

The strength of a drug action is determined by the dose administered to a patient and how frequently the dose is administered. The first dose is called a loading dose or priming dose and consists of a large concentration of the drug. Subsequent doses are called maintenance doses and consist of a normal concentration of the drug.

Drug activity is divided into the pharmaceutic phase, pharmacokinetic phase; and the pharmacodynamic phase. The pharmaceutic phase is the disintegration and dissolution of a drug taken orally. The pharmacokinetic phase is the mechanism used to absorb, distribute, and eliminate a drug. The pharmacodynamics is a drug's effect on the physiology of the cell and the mechanism that causes the pharmaceutical response.

Drugs bind to receptors on the cell membrane called reactive cellular sites. Receptors are proteins, glycoproteins, proteolipids, or enzymes. Depending on the drug, binding either initiates a physiological response by the cell or blocks a cell's physiological response. A drug that causes a physiological response is called an agonist. A drug that blocks a physiological response is called an antagonist.

The safety of a drug is identified by the drug's therapeutic index. A low therapeutic index means a drug has a narrow margin of safety requiring that that the drug's peak level and trough levels be closely monitored. A high therapeutic index means a drug has a broad margin of safety and does not require frequent monitoring of the patient and the serum drug level.

Now that you have a good understanding of the theory of how drugs work, in the next chapter we'll turn our attention to the practical aspect of pharmacology and see how pharmacology is used in the nursing process.

Quiz

1. The pharmacokinetic phase is
   (a) the form of the drug.
   (b) the way the drug is absorbed, distributed, and eliminated.
   (c) the effect the drug has on the body.
   (d) none of the above.

2. The ingredient in a drug that causes a physiological response is called
   (a) D-fill.
   (b) excipient.
   (c) D-active.
   (d) particle.

3. The method in which a drug is absorbed by flowing from a high concentration to a low concentration is called:
   (a) active diffusion.
   (b) pinocytosis.
   (c) passive diffusion.
   (d) absorption rate.

4. All drugs are absorbed immediately when they are administered.
   (a) True
   (b) False

5. Lipid soluble drugs are absorbed more quickly than water-soluble drugs.
   (a) True
   (b) False

6. Bioavailability is
   (a) the quantity of drug in a vial.
   (b) the quantity of drug injected into the body.
   (c) the number of drug particles in a dose.
   (d) the percentage of a dose that reaches the bloodstream.

7. Primary loading is the first measured quantity of drug that is eliminated from the body.
   (a) True
   (b) False

8. A drug that causes a nonspecific physiological response is called a(n)
   (a) agonist.
   (b) metabolite.
   (c) protein.
   (d) molecule.

9. Insulin is a type of inhibition drug.
   (a) True
   (b) False

10. Therapeutic index identifies the margin of safety of the drug
    (a) True
    (b) False

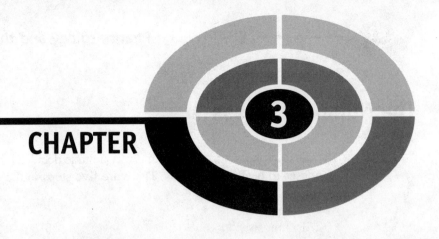

Pharmacology and the Nursing Process

Anyone who has spent a few nights in a hospital bed remembers being awakened from a sound sleep by a nurse saying, "Time to take your medication." Try as you might to ignore the request you can't win. The voice simply becomes more insistent until you have no choice but to open your eyes.

Patients are also awakened sometimes so the nurse can check vital signs. This is to determine if the medication is having an effect or if the patient is experiencing an undesirable side effect. In cases where the patient is being treated with a narrow spectrum antibiotic, blood may be drawn to determine if the antibiotic is working on the infection.

Administering medication, evaluating the patient's response, and determining if the drug is working as planned are pharmacology activities that are part of the nursing process. You were introduced to pharmacology in previous chapters. This chapter takes a look at the nursing process as it relates to giving medications.

The Nursing Process

The nursing process is a systematic way a nurse decides how to treat the patient's responses to health and illness. There are five steps in the nursing process:

1. Assessment
2. Diagnosis
3. Planning
4. Intervention/Implementation
5. Evaluation

Assessment is data collection. During the assessment step, the nurse is gathering subjective and objective data from the patient that will later be used to arrive at a nursing diagnosis. Subjective data is information that is reported by the patient such as, "I'm feeling warm." Objective data is information that can be measured or observed, such as the patient's temperature or the color of the patient's skin.

Diagnosis is the patient's problem, which is determined by analyzing data collected during the patient's assessment. The data could lead the nurse to determine that the patient has more than one problem. This diagnosis is referred to as a nursing diagnosis. A nursing diagnosis is different from a medical diagnosis. For example, a nurse might diagnose an alteration in mobility in a patient who has had a stroke. A physician or advanced nurse practitioner determines the medical diagnosis, which is cerebral vascular accident (CVA). The nurse might also determine this patient has a potential for alteration in nutrition because he or she is having difficulty swallowing because of the stroke.

The *plan* is how the nurse proposes to treat the nursing diagnosis. The plan takes the form of a care plan that itemizes the patient's nursing diagnosis. Each nursing diagnosis will have an expected outcome or goal. The care plan contains at least one nursing intervention for each nursing diagnosis, the expected outcome for each intervention, and how the nurse will evaluate the outcome. For example, the final outcome goal for an alteration in mobility might be to have the patient get out of bed and ambulate without assistance. However, the interventions will begin with getting the patient out of bed and to the chair or assisting the patient to walk short distances each day.

The *intervention* is executing the plan. For example, the nurse will assist the patient to the chair the first time and might delegate the task to a nursing assistant thereafter if the patient does not have any problems.

The *evaluation* step of the nursing process determines if the intervention worked. For example, the nurse evaluates the patient's response to getting out of bed and also determines if the patient continues to get out of bed on a daily basis. If the patient continues to have no problems getting out of bed, the nurse may change the interventions to include walking short distances in addition to getting out of bed and increase those distances each day. When the patient is able to get out of bed and walk without assistance, the final goal will have been achieved.

The nursing process is circular. If the nurse determines during the evaluation step that the intervention didn't work or the expected outcome has been achieved, the nurse begins the nursing process again, starting with the assessment step and then revises the care plan as the patient's problem changes. The nursing process is repeated until the patient's problem(s) is resolved.

ASSESSMENT RELATED TO DRUGS

During the assessment phase, the nurse systematically collects, verifies, and analyzes patient-related data. A portion of the assessment process directly relates to administering medication to the patient.

Before medication is given to a patient, the nurse must make the follow assessments.

Is the drug order valid?

A drug order must be written by a physician, dentist, physician assistant, or advanced practice nurse and contain:

- The date and time the order is written
- The name of the drug
- The dosage
- The route of administration
- The frequency of administration
- The duration (how long the patient is to receive the drug)
- The signature of the prescriber

Identify the brand and generic name for the drug

Drugs are known under several names. These are

- The chemical name used by pharmacists and researchers
- The generic name, which is the official (proprietary) non-proprietary name that is universally accepted

- The brand name, which is the name chosen by the drug manufacturer
- The official name that appears in the *USP-NF*

When is the drug used?

The nurse is required to know why the drug is given to the patient and what symptoms a patient exhibits to indicate that the drug should be administered. The nurse cannot rely solely on the prescriber because the patient's condition might have changed since the patient was assessed. Furthermore, there is always a potential that the order is in error. There are a variety of reasons an order can be in error. These include, but are not limited to, writing an order or a prescription for the wrong patient, for a drug to which the patient is allergic, for a drug that will interact badly with another drug the patient is taking, a dose that is too small or too large for the patient based on weight, or simply the wrong drug. Medication errors can be reduced or eliminated if everyone involved in the process uses critical thinking skills and checks and double checks the orders, the patient, and the medication.

How does the drug work?

It is critical that the nurse understands how the drug is absorbed, distributed, metabolized, and eliminated before administering the drug to the patient. One of these mechanisms might be malfunctioning. For example, the patient might have lower than expected urinary output and is unable to excrete the drug in normal volume resulting in a potential toxic buildup in the body.

The nurse must also know the drug's onset of action, peak action, and duration of action. As you'll recall from the previous chapter, onset is the time period when the drug reaches the minimally effective concentration in the plasma. The peak action is when the drug reaches the maximum concentration in the plasma. The duration is the length of time the therapeutic action will last.

What interacts with the drug?

The effectiveness of a drug can be influenced by interactions with food, herbal remedies, and other drugs that alter or modify the drug's action. Such interactions might increase the drug's effectiveness, decrease it, or neutralize it. The nurse must be aware of known interactions in order to avoid them.

What are the side effects and toxicity of the drug?

A side effect is a physiological response in the patient's body that is not re-lated to the drug's primary action. Some side effects are beneficial while side effects—such as nausea and vomiting—are undesirable. By knowing a drug's possible side effects, the nurse can prepare to manage them before the patient is given the drug.

The nurse must also know the toxicity of a drug. A drug's toxicity is the drug concentration in plasma and accumulation in tissues that exceeds the drug's therapeutic range.

What signs and symptoms must be monitored?

The nurse must note the signs and symptoms that indicate the patient is having an adverse reaction to a drug or that the drug has reached toxic levels. These indications may not be present for minutes, hours, and even days after the drug is administered.

What must a patient know about the drug?

Many drugs are self-administered by patients after they leave the healthcare facility. Therefore it is important that the nurse identify information about the drug that the patient needs to know to properly administer the drug.

Is the drug available? Has the drug expired? How much does the drug cost?

The drug that is ordered may not be available in the healthcare facility. The nurse must make sure the drug is available and make sure that the drug on hand hasn't expired if it is available. For example, some healthcare facilities might have a very low requirement for a particular drug and the stock of the drug might be old and have passed the expiration date.

The cost of the drug is important to know for a number of reasons. Some drugs are not covered by the patient's health insurance because they are expensive. The insurance company may cover the cost of a similar medication that costs less. In addition, many patients do not have insurance to cover medications and they can-not afford to have an expensive prescription filled. Nurses should ask patient's about their insurance coverage and if they can afford to buy the medication if they don't have coverage. Many patients might stop taking an important medication because they don't have enough money.

Patient information

Before administering a drug, the nurse must review information about the patient to assure that the patient will not have an adverse reaction to the drug. The nurse must determine:

- Does the patient have any allergies to the drug or to food that might be given along with the drug?
- Has the patient's condition changed since the drug was ordered?
- What is the patient's age?
- What is the appropriate dose of the drug based upon the patient's weight?
- What is the patient's gender?
- Is the patient pregnant?
- What is the patient's primary language?
- Are there any religious or cultural influences that would cause the patient to resist taking the medication?
- Does the patient know and understand the purpose of the medication?
- Does the patient's history include taking vitamins, birth control pills, and herbal remedies?
- Does the patient use illegal drugs or alcohol?
- Does the patient have a tolerance for the drug that is being administered?
- Are there any genetic factors that might cause an adverse reaction by taking the medication?
- Are there any emotional factors that can affect the patient's ability to take the drug?
- Are there any contraindications for the medication that are indicated by taking vital signs and reviewing current laboratory and diagnostic tests?
- Is the patient's mental status sufficient so that the patient understands why medication is being administered? Is there someone available to monitor the patient?
- Can the patient afford the medication?
- Will family members or friends be with the patient to monitor for side effects and toxicity?
- Is the patient scheduled for tests, procedures, or other activities at the same time he or she is scheduled to receive medication?
- Is the patient scheduled to receive medication during visiting hours?
- Is the patient required to have a procedure performed, such as insertion of an IV or feeding tube before medication is administered?

Getting this information may sound overwhelming to the new nurse. However, a lot of this information has already been obtained when the patient is admitted or arrived at the office or clinic for care.

Nursing Diagnosis

The nurse develops a nursing diagnosis after analyzing information gained from assessing the patient. A nursing diagnosis is a statement that describes the patient's actual or potential response to a health problem that the nurse is licensed and competent to treat. The North American Nursing Diagnosis Association (NANDA) developed a guide used by many nurses to arrive at a nursing diagnosis.

A physician or advanced practitioner uses the medical diagnosis to prescribe a treatment for combating the disease. This might involve medication and/or a change in the patient's lifestyle. A nurse uses the nursing diagnosis to develop a comprehensive quality care plan to restore the patient to a state where the patient can return to activities of normal living.

For example, a physician might diagnose a patient as having diabetes and prescribes glucose monitoring and insulin injections to control the disease. The nursing diagnosis might be a knowledge deficit about the disease and the medications to treat it. The nurse teaches the patient how to monitor glucose and give injections as well as how to identify adverse side effects of the medication and of the disease. Furthermore, the nurse determines if the patient has the financial, social, and mental capacity to self-medicate. The nurse then develops a plan to enlist the healthcare team to assist the patient if the patient lacks the capacity.

The nursing diagnosis consists of a problem statement that identifies the potential or actual health problem that the nurse is licensed and accountable to treat. A nursing diagnosis may also include the cause of the problem—such as alteration in mobility related to right sided paralysis—which are factors related to or associated with the patient's problem and symptoms that manifested the problem.

A common nursing diagnosis related to drug therapy might be:

- Knowledge deficit of disease and medication related to inability to understand English

This occurs when the patient doesn't understand the language used by healthcare professionals such as when healthcare is provided in English and English is the patient's second language.

- Risk for injury related to side effects of drug

The patient may be given medication such as narcotic analgesics for pain that impairs the patient's activities of normal daily life such as driving a car.

- Alteration in thought processes related to drug action

Some drugs such as barbiturates, sedatives, and mood-altering medication interrupt the patient's normal thought process, which could confuse the patient (and the patient's family and friends) if they are unaware of such a side effect of the drug.

- Constipation related to drug action or side effect

Morphine sulfate and other opioids cause a reduction in intestinal movement resulting in constipation that might make the patient uncomfortable. Knowing this, the nurse might instruct the patient about foods and fluids that might increase intestinal motility such as bran and increased water intake.

- Fluid volume deficit related to drug action

Diuretic medication such as furosemide (Lasix) causes the patient to lose more than the normal volume of fluid in an effort to counteract a disease that results in the retention of fluids. The nurse alerts the patient to the likely increase in urination and also monitors the patient's fluid intake and output to assure that the patient maintains an adequate fluid level.

- Breathing pattern ineffective related to drug side effects

Opioids, such as morphine sulfate, can reduce the patient's breathing to a level where the patient's respiration is no longer effective. It might mean not moving enough air or blowing off too much CO_2. The nurse should monitor the patient's respiratory rate on a regular basis.

Patient Care Plan

Once a nursing diagnosis is reached, a care plan is developed that describes how the healthcare team will address the patient's problems. It contains

- Nursing diagnosis
- Expected outcomes—Goal statement
- Interventions based on a scientific and medical rationale needed to achieve the goal
- How to measure each outcome

GOAL STATEMENT

At the heart of the care plan is a goal statement that specifies an expected out-come of the health care team's intervention with the patient. Think of a goal statement as what you want to happen to the patient. For example, a typical goal is that a patient will report a reduction in pain from 8 to 4 on a scale of 0 to 10 in three hours.

A goal statement is a *nursing order* that must be patient centered and specify a desired behavior to occur at a specified time. The behavior must be observable and measurable and the goal statement must specify criteria for measuring the behavior.

Ideally, both the nurse and the patient develop and accept the goal. If the patient's decision-making ability is impaired, then the patient's family or another support person becomes the patient's advocate in the planning process. It is critical that the patient adopts the goal statement; otherwise, the goal might not be achieved. For example, if the patient doesn't believe in taking pain medica-tion, then a goal of reducing pain by taking analgesics will not be met. The nurse will then have to explore alternatives to pain medication such as a massage or imagery. The care plan should be shared with the patient's family, the healthcare team and others who are caring for the patient so that everyone is working toward the same goals.

DEADLINES AND MEASUREMENT

It is important that the care plan establish realistic deadlines for reaching the goal, otherwise the patient and those caring for the patient will become frustrated when the goal is not met. For example, it isn't realistic to say that the patient will no longer cough after taking dextromethorphan (Robitussin DM) simply because the medication isn't an instant cure for coughing. A more realistic goal is for the frequency of the patient's coughing to decrease after each dose. The deadline might be that the patient will take dextromethorphan for 48 hours and report a decrease in frequency of coughing and experience uninterrupted rest. This goal is both observable and measurable since the nurse can observe if the patient is cough-ing and measure the frequency of the cough to determine if the goal is reached.

INTERVENTIONS

The care plan must also specify the intervention for each goal statement. An intervention is a clear statement that specifies the action that must be taken to achieve the goal statement. An intervention must complement the goal statement, use available resources, follow protocols established by the healthcare facility, and always keep the patient's safety in mind.

There are three types of intervention.

Nurse-initiated intervention

A nurse-initiated intervention is a nursing order performed independently by the nurse based on a scientific rationale that benefits the patient in a predicted way, such as removing a blanket to lower the patient's temperature.

Physician or advanced practice intervention

This type of intervention is a dependent function issued by a physician or an advanced practitioner that is carried out by a nurse, such as administering prescribed medication to the patient.

Collaborative intervention

A collaborative intervention is an activity performed among multiple healthcare professionals, such as physical therapy for the patient.

EVALUATION

Each outcome on the care plan must be evaluated to determine if the goal is achieved. Once all goals on the care plan are reached, the care plan no longer exists. The patient no longer exhibits symptoms of the nursing diagnosis. However, if one or more goals are not realized, reassessment or data collection should occur. This would include reassessing the patient and other factors, such as schedules, availability of resources, and developing new goals, interventions, and evaluations.

Teaching the Patient About Drugs

A critical nursing responsibility is to educate the patient and the patient's family about the medication that is administered to the patient or that is self-administered by the patient. Teaching should be conducted in a comfortable environment in a language that both the patient and the patient's family understand. Use appropriate charts, graphs, audio, and videotapes as necessary. Always provide enough time for questions and answers. Avoid rushing. If the information cannot be presented in one session, plan several sessions. It is always a good idea to give the patient and family members material that they can take home and review at their leisure. It is very important that written information be at a reading level that can be understood by the patient and family.

Demonstrate how the patient or family members are to administer medication. For example, show the proper injection techniques if the patient requires insulin injections or the correct use of bronchodilator inhalers for asthma. Don't assume that they can administer the medication after seeing you do it. Make sure to have the patient and family members show you how they plan to give the medication. This is especially critical when medication is given using a syringe, topical drugs, and inhalers. The patient and the caregiver must have visual acuity, manual dexterity, and the mental capacity to prepare and administer medication.

Prompt the patient and family members to give you feedback from your lesson and demonstration by asking:

- What things help you take your medicine?
- What things prevent you from taking your medication?
- What would you do if you forget to take your medication?
- What would you feel if you are taking too much of the medication?
- What could you feel that are side effects of taking the medication?
- Is there anything you can do to reduce side effects of the medication?

It is very important that the patient and family members be informed about the signs and symptoms of an allergic response to the medication such as urticaria (hives), swollen lips, hoarse voice, difficulty breathing, and shortness of breath—an indication of life threatening anaphylaxis.

In addition to the signs and symptoms of an allergic response, you must also discuss side effects and toxic effects of the medication and any dietary considerations the patient must follow while on the medication.

Some patients require several medications. Therefore, the nurse needs to develop a medication plan to help the patient manage the medication schedule. Common techniques include:

- A multicompartment dispenser to hold a daily or weekly supply of medication
- A timer to remind the patient when to take medication
- Color-coded envelopes where each color represents an hour or a day
- A written record when medication should be administered and when it was administered

Impact of Cultural Influences in Drug Administration

The cultural background of the patient and of the patient's family can impact the administration of medication. Cultural influences are learned values, beliefs, customs, and behavior. These influences include the patient's belief about health such as:

- What healthcare can do for the patient
- The patient's susceptibility to disease
- The benefits of taking steps to prevent disease
- What makes a patient seek healthcare
- What makes a patient follow healthcare guidelines

For example, a patient who is a coal miner may believe that all coal miners will eventually have lung cancer. In that case, the patient feels there is no benefit to stop smoking. Another patient may avoid taking pain medication for fear that they might become addicted.

Some cultures have their own beliefs about how to prevent and cure disease. For example, although garlic does lower blood pressure, taking garlic as an herbal cure might be dangerous if the patient is also taking antihypertensive medication because the patient's blood pressure could be lowered too much. Herbal remedies are preferred by some cultures over traditional Western medicine and some patients continue herbal treatment even when a mild illness progresses to a critical level.

Healthcare providers can have different beliefs than their patients. A patient may refuse any treatment because of the sole belief in the healing power of prayer. Healthcare providers must be nonjudgmental and tolerate alternative beliefs in healthcare even if those beliefs are harmful to the patient. When confronted with cultural differences that can result in an adverse effect to the patient, healthcare providers can educate the patient about the benefits of medications and treatment and the risk that the patient is exposed to by not following recommended treatment. This information is sometimes best given while the healthcare provider is assessing the patient. The nurse should be careful to remain nonjudgmental about the patient's decisions.

Cultural beliefs can also influence who makes healthcare decisions for the family. In most cultures, women are typically responsible for managing the family's health. However, in some cultures, although the female is responsible for providing and obtaining care, the oldest male is seen as the head of the family and the authority figure for making overall decisions such as when to access healthcare.

The way the patient communicates with healthcare providers is greatly influenced by individual culture. Here are factors to consider when communicating with a patient:

- Eye contact might not be appropriate.
- Ask the patient how he or she should be addressed. Always address the patient formally until the patient gives permission to be addressed informally.
- Know how the patient perceives time (e.g., day/night, sunrise/sunset). Otherwise, the patient may be unable to comply with the appropriate medication schedule.
- Maintain the patient's personal space. Always ask permission to invade the personal space to perform a procedure. In some cultures, patients don't want anyone standing or sitting too close and they feel uncomfortable if someone touches them.
- Consider food beliefs and rituals as related to illnesses. Some patient's believe that the more you eat, the healthier you will become. Other people restrict certain foods for religious reasons.
- Evaluate the family's attitude toward the elderly. The elderly are revered in some cultures and the family goes to great lengths to care for them. In other cultures, the family leaves the elderly to die peacefully without interference.

ETHNIC CONSIDERATIONS

Besides cultural differences, there are also ethnic and racial differences in the physiological response to drugs. As you'll recall from Chapter 2, pharmacogenetics is the study of the influence genetics have on a drug response. For example children with Reyes Syndrome, which is a liver disease, cannot metabolize aspirin because of a genetic defect.

Likewise, a genetic factor in African-Americans makes them less responsive to beta-blocking agents used in cardiac and antihypertensive medications. Asians have a genetic factor that causes undesirable side effects when given the typical dose of benzodiazepines (diazepam [Valium]) alprazolam [Xanax], tricyclic antidepressants, atropine, and propranol [Inderal]. Therefore, a lower dose must be given.

Mother and the Fetus

Many drugs cross the placenta, but only some of them can have an adverse effect on the fetus because of the immature fetal metabolism and slower excretion rates. Waste products are excreted into the amniotic fluid and then absorbed by the mother or swallowed by the fetus.

Alcohol, barbiturates, and narcotics—such as diphenhydramine (Benadryl), amobarbital (Amytal), diazepam (Valium), codeine, heroin, methadone, morphine, propoxyphene (Darvon)—that are used during pregnancy can lead to harmful effects on the newborn. Use of these drugs during pregnancy can create an addiction in the newborn. The baby will go into withdrawal from the drug when they are born. This can result in hyperactivity, crying, irritability, seizures and even sudden death.

When taken by the mother during the first trimester, some drugs have a teratogenic effect on the fetus resulting in fetal defects. This includes mutagenic (genetic mutation) or carcinogenic (causing cancer) effects. These drugs include Thalidomide, which causes abnormal limb development, and cocaine, which causes miscarriages, fetal hypoxia (lack of oxygen), low-birth-weight infants, tremors, strokes, increase in stillbirth rates, congenital heart disease, skull defects, and other malformations.

Adverse side effects of the drug on the fetus can be avoided by carefully checking the Pregnancy Category of the medication before the medication is administered to a pregnant woman. Regardless of the Pregnancy Category of the drug, always carefully observe the pregnant patient after administering medication to assure that the patient doesn't show any observable adverse response.

Pediatrics

Special care must be given when administering medication to pediatric patients because their organs are immature and they might have difficulty absorbing, distributing, and excreting the medication. This is especially true with neonatal patients. Neonatal patients can receive some medication through breast milk. However, because the mother has already metabolized and excreted the medication, less than the original dose is passed into breast milk.

Other medications cannot be given to a mother who is breastfeeding because of the toxic effect the medication has on the baby (unless breastfeeding is interrupted for 24 hours to 72 hours).

These medications include amphetamines, bromocriptine, cocaine, cyclophosphamide, cyclosporine, doxorubicin, ergotamine, gold salts, lithium, methotrexate, nicotine, and phenindione.

Organs in the neonate might be unable to handle the normal dose of some medications. For example, the stomach lacks acid, gastric emptying time is prolonged, the liver and kidneys are immature, and there is a decrease in protein binding.

ADMINISTERING MEDICATION TO PEDIATRIC PATIENTS

There isn't a standard dose for pediatric patients. The dose is calculated using the patient's weight or the patient's body surface area. Some over-the-counter medications specifies a dose based on the child's age, but these are really based on the average weight of a child within that age range. The dose can become problematic if the child's weight is lower or higher than that of the age group. If a child with a very low weight receives an age-related dose it might result in an undesirable adverse affect from the medication. When a child who is heavier than average receives a dose related to age, the drug may not have a therapeutic effect.

Before administering medication to a pediatric patient consult with the parents to assess if the patient has allergies to food, medications, and the environment, a family history of allergies, an experience with medications and illnesses, or is taking any other medication or herbal remedies.

Elderly

More than 30% of all prescriptions and more than 50 percent of all over-the-counter medications in the United States are consumed by patients who are over 60 years of age. It is this group of patients who are three times more likely to be admitted to a healthcare facility for an adverse reaction to medication.

Fifty-one percent die from these reactions; 70 to 80 percent of the adverse reactions are dose related.

There are several important reasons for such a high occurrence of adverse response to medication. These include:

- Polypharmacy (multiple medications are prescribed without discontinuing current medication, causing an interaction between drugs);
- Medication can impair the mental and physical capacity leading to accidental injury;
- Age can increase the sensitivity to drugs and drug-induced disease;
- Absorption of medication is altered due to an increase in gastric pH;
- Distribution of the medication is affected because of a decrease in lean body mass, increased fat stores, a decrease in total body water, decreased serum albumin, and a decrease in blood flow and cardiac output;
- Metabolism changes as enzymatic activity decreases with age, and liver function;
- Excretion is impaired due to decreased kidney function.

ASSESSING THE ELDERLY

Begin assessing an elderly patient by obtaining a complete history of medications used by the patient. This includes all prescription drugs, over-the-counter drugs, home remedies, vitamins, and herbal treatments. Make sure that you determine the medications that have been prescribed and medications that the patient actually takes. Include those that are taken at the patient's discretion. Some patients don't take all of the medications that are prescribed to them because of the cost of the medication or some unpleasant or undesirable side effects. Also note how often the medications are taken.

List all practitioners who prescribed medications for the patient, including the patient's primary physician, orthopedist, and cardiologist. Create a list of all pharmacies providing medication to the patient. Review the expiration dates for all medications. Ask the patient how they self-medicate, if they maintain a medication schedule, and if they ever forget to take their medication. If they do, ask what medications they've skipped and what they do when they forget or skip a dose.

Determine if the patient has any barriers to taking medication safely such as allergies, physical handicaps, memory loss, cultural beliefs, and financial constraints. Also, learn if the patient has support from family, friends, and neighbors. Most importantly, be aware of the cost of medication prescribed to the patient. The elderly typically live on a fixed income and may be unable to purchase expensive medications—even if the benefit outweighs the cost. Always keep medication for the elderly simple and to a minimum.

Summary

There are five steps in the nursing process. These are assessment, diagnosis, planning, intervention, and evaluation. The assessment step collects data about the patient that is analyzed to arrive at a nursing diagnosis. A care plan is then developed that describes what must be done to address the symptoms of the nursing diagnosis. The care plan is then enacted during the intervention step and the results are then evaluated. The care plan terminates if the goals of the plan are achieved or revised if the goals are not achieved. Before any medication is given to a patient, the nurse must assess a number of factors that include the drug order, drug actions, interactions, and contraindications.

Educating the patient about medication is an important responsibility for the nurse. The nurse must explain why the medication is given and how the patient can self-medicate. The nurse must also make sure that the patient and the family know the signs and symptoms of adverse side effects from the medication as well as any toxic effects and dietary considerations to follow while taking the medication.

Cultural factors typically influence the patient's belief about health and can impact medication prescribed to treat a patient's illness. The nurse must put aside his or her own opinion about those beliefs and work within those limitations when caring for the patient.

Genetic, ethnic, and racial differences play a role in the physiological response to drugs. Some groups of patients are less responsive to certain medications because of genetic factors; other groups of patients can experience a toxic effect because of hereditary traits.

Drugs can have different effects on the very young and the elderly because of physiological changes in their bodies. The very young have immature organs that are not yet able to metabolize, absorb, distribute, and excrete certain drugs.

Likewise, the elderly have mature organs that might have lost the capability to properly process medication. Furthermore, the elderly may require multiple medications simultaneously that can result in drug interactions that produce adverse side effects.

Quiz

1. A medical diagnosis
   (a) is the same as a nursing diagnosis.
   (b) identifies the disease that inflicts the patient.
   (c) is a problem statement that identifies the potential or actual health problem.
   (d) None of the above.

2. An expected outcome is
   (a) the patient's condition after a care plan is executed.
   (b) the goal of a care plan.
   (c) adverse reaction to a medication.
   (d) a side effect to a medication.

3. After the patient is shown how to self-medicate, the nurse should
   (a) show a film to the patient on self-medication.
   (b) make sure the patient's family is shown how to medicate the patient.
   (c) make sure the patient has the prescription for the medication.
   (d) ask the patient to demonstrate how he or she will self-medicate.

4. A healthcare provider should administer medication to a patient even if the patient's cultural beliefs disagree with receiving medication.
   (a) True
   (b) False

5. A infant receives a full dose of the drug given to its mother when the infant breastfeeds.
   (a) True
   (b) False

6. A dose for a pediatric patient is determined by
   (a) the patient's weight.
   (b) the patient's height.
   (c) the patient's age.
   (d) the patient's sex.

7. Adverse reaction to medication is a leading cause of death in elderly patients.
   (a) True
   (b) False

8. Which of the following is a type of intervention?
   (a) Nurse-initiated
   (b) Physician or advanced practitioner initiated
   (c) Collaborative
   (d) All of the above

9. Knowledge deficit related to language difficulties is a common nursing diagnoses related to drug therapy.
   (a) True
   (b) False

10. NANDA is a guide to nursing diagnosis.
    (a) True
    (b) False

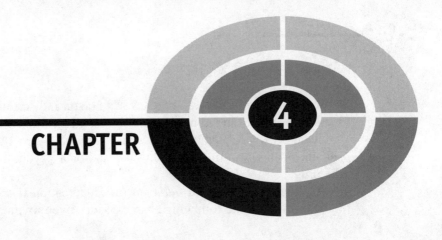

4

Substance Abuse

Substance abuse is probably one of the most publicized aspects of pharmacology—and the least understood by patients. Patients who are in pain frequently avoid taking medication because they are fearful of becoming addicted to the drug. Rarely do patients become addicted. However, should a dependency develop, the medication is gradually reduced until the dependency subsides. Patients—and healthcare professionals—can become dependent on medication. This chapter explores drugs that are commonly abused and discusses how to detect substance abuse.

Drug Misuse and Abuse

Substance abuse affects all socioeconomic groups and has become a major medical, social, economic, and interpersonal challenge for society. According to the Centers for Disease Control, one in 68 people in the United States is a substance abuser and 19.5 million people over the age of 12 use illegal drugs resulting in 19,000 deaths per year.

A medication is *misused* whenever a person indiscriminately uses the medication (such as when an individual uses medication that was prescribed for someone else). A medication becomes *abused* when the person continually self-medicates resulting in a physical and/or a psychological dependence on the drug.

A person is considered *addicted* to a medication if the person experiences three or more of the following characteristics over six months.

TOLERANCE

Tolerance occurs when an increasingly larger dose of the medication is required to achieve the same physiological reaction. It is important to realize that tolerance is not addiction. In some treatments, patients commonly develop a tolerance for a drug, but don't become addicted to it. The prescriber increases the dose to achieve the same therapeutic effect. The medication is discontinued once the treatment is completed.

WITHDRAWAL

Withdrawal is a physiological and/or psychological reaction a person experiences when a medication is no longer administered. Prescribers properly manage treatment by gradually decreasing the dose and/or frequency of administration of the drug to avoid withdrawal symptoms in a patient.

INCREASED DOSAGES

A person who is addicted tends to regularly increase the dosage of the medication expecting to increase the physiological reaction of the drug such as reaching a higher state of euphoria for a longer period of time.

UNCONTROLLABLE USE

A person addicted to drugs is unable to control the urge to self-medicate. The desire for the drug must be met as quickly as possible.

TAKING THE DRUG IS A SCHEDULED EVENT

The person spends a lot of time to acquire the drug, self-medicate, and recover from the effects of the drug. This is evident with a patient who is addicted to sedatives whose thoughts are focused on how to get the next dose. Time in the day must then be set aside to administer the medication and to avoid contact with other people until the visible effects of the drug have worn off.

PRIORITY OVER ACTIVITIES OF DAILY LIFE

Daily activities are scheduled around times when the patient acquires, uses, and recovers from the effects of the drug. Everything else, including family and work, takes a backseat to the addiction.

ADDICTION CONTINUES DESPITE NEGATIVE CONSEQUENCES

The person continues to self-medicate regardless of the repercussions. Individuals who are addicted to drugs will begin to be late for work and gradually begin to miss entire days until they lose the job. However, the self-medication will continue.

Behavioral Patterns of Addiction

Besides the clinical signs of addition mentioned in the previous section, there are behavioral patterns that are common in a person who abuses medication. These behavioral patterns deviate from what is considered normal behavior.

For example, a substance abuser fails to keep to a routine and will be late to work or school or not go at all. The person may have poor hygiene and appear disheveled—especially when compared with others. Family and social relationships become strained as craving for the drug or being under the influence of the medication makes it nearly impossible to interact normally. The person is also in frequent need of medical attention as a result of self-medication. The medication itself might disrupt normal bodily functions or place the person in a state that exposes him or her to harm.

For a variety of reasons, a substance abuser experiences more legal problems than the average person. The police might arrest the person for illegally obtaining or possessing the medication or for driving while under the influence of the drug. A substance abuser is exposed to unsavory characters who are involved in the illicit drug trade. These interactions can create unsafe and violent situations for all involved.

Denial is the most common behavior exhibited by drug abusers. Because the addiction may be gradual and often the abuser is in an altered mental state as a result of the effects of the drug, the individual may be unable to recognize the addiction. As the addiction worsens, the drug abuser is unwilling to admit to the problem and the denial continues.

Healthcare Professionals and Substance Abuse

Fans of the television show "ER" will recall how Dr. John Carter became dependent on pain medication that was legally prescribed to treat pain from a nearly deadly attack he experienced in the emergency room. His dependency drove him to steal drugs from the hospital to feed his addiction.

"ER" is fiction, but its depiction of a healthcare professional becoming a substance abuser is well founded as up to 15 percent of overall addiction to opioids have been attributed to healthcare professionals for more than 130 years. Many healthcare professionals who become drug abusers feel they can self-medicate without becoming addicted because they know when to stop taking the medication. Craving for the drug quickly overshadows their critical thinking.

Healthcare professionals self-administer drugs for a number of reasons.

PERFORMANCE ENHANCEMENT

Some healthcare professionals such as interns and residents are on duty for 36 hours at a stretch during which they make many critical decisions. Some feel they need a boost to maintain a high performance level especially after being on duty for so many hours without sleep.

SELF-TREATMENT

A healthcare provider knows how to recognize symptoms of a disease and knows what medications are used to treat the disease so it makes sense to self-treat when he or she becomes ill. This is especially true when the healthcare provider is depressed, anxious, or is in pain. The information used to diagnose personal illness is subjective and as the craving for the medication increases it interferes with the objective reasoning that the healthcare provider normally uses when assessing patients.

EASY ACCESSIBILITY TO DRUGS

Drugs are available to many healthcare professionals especially in a healthcare facility where they administer medication. Even under tight controls, drugs can be diverted by healthcare professionals with little chance of being caught. For example, they may give the patient half the prescribed dose and keep the other half for themselves.

RECREATIONAL USE

After a long shift, healthcare professionals need to relax. The fastest way to get to that state of mind may be to take a pill or inject a drug. However, additional doses may be needed to remain in that state. Eventually, the healthcare professional may become addicted to the drug.

Detecting Substance Abuse

The term "substance abuser" conjures images of an unkempt, malnourished person who sleeps on the streets. In reality, the person working alongside you or living in the house across the street from you could be a substance abuser because many substance abusers go to great lengths to hide their addiction.

However, no matter how well substance abusers try to conceal their addiction, eventually the addiction causes them to change and it is those changes that become signs of substance abuse. Here are those signs.

DISORGANIZATION

Many of the drugs used to alleviate pain or anxiety can lead to addiction. These drugs alter the thinking process. Consequently, individuals are unable to think clearly and logically. Simple tasks can become overwhelming and eventually an addicted individual will become scattered or disorganized. For example, taking a medication for pain creates a sense of distance from the real world. Trying to add a column of numbers or serve food to customers will become confusing and an individual may be unable to decide what to do first.

FREQUENT ABSENCES

Some drugs can create periods of wakefulness that lead to a "crash." The individual may sleep because of fatigue or to sleep off the effects of a pain- or anxiety-relieving drug that causes drowsiness. Individuals simply don't wake up to go to work or experience periods of withdrawal from reality that result in an inability to remember to go to work or school.

INABILITY TO GET ALONG WITH COLLEAGUES

As the addiction worsens, individuals have difficulty with interpersonal relationships for several reasons. One reason is the simple fact that nothing really matters anymore except getting more of the drug. In addition, the disorganization and frequent absences make a drug abuser an unpopular colleague. Co-workers begin to suspect there is a problem and put pressure on the individual to "clean up their act." This can deteriorate into very unpleasant episodes at work and at home.

CHANGES IN APPEARANCE AND PERSONAL HYGIENE

The altered mental state experienced by drug abusers also changes their perception of themselves. The addicted individual may be unaware of how they look or even forget to take a shower and change clothing regularly. The need to find more of the drug can also be time consuming and interfere with regular activities that include personal hygiene.

SLURRED SPEECH OFF HOURS

A side effect of the most abused drugs is slurred speech and staggering gait. Responses are slowed and the individual may appear to be intoxicated. Frequently a drug abuser will make a great effort to appear normal during working or school hours. However, after hours may become the time to take more of the drug and the side effects are more pronounced or obvious.

Delayed Action

Drug abuse in the healthcare field can go undetected because of the structure of the healthcare industry. Healthcare providers may be less supervised than in other industries. For example, physicians work independently and come under scrutiny only in a healthcare facility setting. Furthermore, healthcare professionals have the capability to self-diagnose and to self-treat and may not have another provider complete an objective assessment which might reveal substance abuse. Acknowledging substance abuse may put the individual at risk of suspension or revocation of the license to practice.

There can also be a "white wall of silence" among healthcare professionals when it comes to reporting a colleague for substance abuse. Although they want to help their colleague, no one wants to be responsible for a colleague losing his or her license—or expose themselves to inadvertently making false accusations.

Silence is not the right course of action. First, there is an ethical obligation to report suspected abuse to protect patients who are being treated by the healthcare provider. Healthcare facilities and regulatory boards are sensitive to the need to maintain confidentiality during the handling of the allegation and subsequent inquiry. Second, the addicted person actually becomes a patient and should be given the best and most appropriate care. That care includes treatment for the addiction. Keeping silent about suspicion of addiction is actually harmful to the substance abuser and violates the ethical responsibilities of the healthcare provider.

Substance abuse is considered a handicap. Therefore, the healthcare provider who is employed by a healthcare facility may be protected by state and federal employment discrimination laws such as the Rehabilitation Act (29USC, Section 706). This Act requires employers to continue employment of a substance abuser as long as the employee can perform their job function and is not a threat to safety or property. This means that the healthcare provider's responsibility might be temporarily reassigned until treatment is completed.

DRUG TESTING

Drug testing is the most common method used to detect if a person has taken medication recently. Many businesses, government agencies, and healthcare facilities require prospective employees to be screened for drugs. In addition, employees might be required to undergo random drug testing or drug testing under special circumstances (such as medication unaccounted for in their work area).

Testing for drug overdose or poisoning is best done with blood. The immediate levels found can determine what treatment should occur. Screening to determine if someone is using drugs inappropriately is commonly done with urine testing. Urine testing can detect drugs used days or even a week before the test is performed. As false positive and false negative results can occur, caution should be used when interpreting the results. When asked if they are taking any kind of medication, individuals should include prescription, over-the-counter, and herbal remedies. For example, traces of diphenhydramine (Benadryl)—a commonly used antihistamine medication—will be found in urine and will cause the person to test positive for methadone.

Whenever the result of a urine test is found to be positive for drugs, the person should undergo another test for that specific medication to confirm the results. The second test is used to identify a false positive that might be generated by the first test. Again, urine testing is done but the request is to screen only for the specific drug identified in the first test. Blood levels may also be obtained to determine immediate use of drugs.

Drug testing only gives evidence that the individual has used or been exposed to a drug but does not indicate any pattern of drug use or the degree of dependency. Table 4-1 shows the length of time that traces of popular drugs remain in the body. The most commonly misused and abused drugs are listed in Table 4-2.

Table 4-1.   Days substances remain in urine.

Drug	Days Detectable in Urine
Alcohol	Less than 1 day
Amphetamines	Up to 1–3 days
Barbiturates	Up to 1 day short acting 2–3 weeks long acting
Cocaine	Up to 2–4 days
Methadone	Up to 3–5 days
Marijuana	
Single use	Up to 3–5 days
Chronic use	Up to 29 days
Opioids—Short-acting	Up to 3–4 days
PCP	2–4 days

Table 4-2. The most commonly misused and abused drugs as reported by the National Surveillance Agency Drug Abuse Warning Network (DAWN).

Drug	Description
Xanthines	A class of drugs that include caffeine and are used in coffee, tea, chocolate, and colas. These drugs affect the central nervous system (CNS). Most frequently abused drug.
Nicotine	Used in tobacco products. This drug affects the central nervous system (CNS). One of the most frequently misused and abused drugs.
Ethyl alcohol	Used in distilled spirits and beverages. This drug affects the central nervous system (CNS). One of the most frequently misused and abused.
Anticholinergics	A class of drugs that includes Robinal, which is referred to as the "date rape" drug. This drug affects the central nervous system (CNS).
Steroids	A performance enhancing drug that affects the central nervous system.
Amphetamines	A class of drugs that includes dextroamphetamine, "dexies," and methamphetamine (commonly referred to as "speed" and "crystal meth"). This drug affects the central nervous system (CNS).
Pentazocine	Creates a morphine-like effect. Also known as Talwin. This drug affects the central nervous system (CNS).
L-dopa	Used to alleviate some of the symptoms of Parkinson's disease. This drug causes an alteration in feelings, thoughts, and perceptions.
Cocaine	A leading drug resulting in visits to the emergency department. This drug can cause tachycardia (fast heart rate), increased blood pressure, chills, fever, agitation, nervousness, confusion, inability to remain still, nausea, vomiting, abdominal pain, increased sweating, rapid breathing, large pupils, and advance to CNS hemorrhage, congestive failure, convulsions, delirium, and death.
Heroin	A leading drug resulting in visits to the emergency department. Heroin is a pro-drug and is converted in the liver to morphine with the same side effects.
Morphine	A leading drug resulting in visits to the emergency department. Morphine is an opioid narcotic analgesic. Side effects include sedation, decreased blood pressure, increased sweating, flushed face, constipation, dizziness, drowsiness, nausea and vomiting.

Table 4-2. *(continued)*

Drug	Description
Acetaminophen	Commonly known as Tylenol. A leading drug resulting in visits to the emergency department. This medication is commonly used in overdoses and can cause serious kidney problems and death.
Aspirin	A leading drug resulting in visits to the emergency department. Aspirin abuse can cause gastric (stomach) irritation which can lead to ulcers and subsequent gastric hemorrhage (bleeding).
Alprazolam	Known as Xanax, is an antianxiety and antipanic agent. Several of the side effects include episodes of violent and aggressive behavior, seizures, delirium, and other withdrawal reactions.
Marijuana/hashish	These are cannabis drugs that seem to act as a CNS depressant. The effects are mental relaxation and euphoria and decreased inhibitions.
Diazepam	Commonly known as Valium it is used for short-term relief of anxiety symptoms. Side effects include drowsiness, fatigue, and ataxia (muscular incoordination). Overdose can result in somnolence (sleepiness), confusion, diminished reflexes, and coma.
Ibuprofen	This is a commonly used nonsteroidal anti-inflammatory drug. Side effects and overdose can result in gastrointestinal bleeding or a metabolic acidosis.
PCP/PCP combinations	PCP is a hallucinogenic drug that can cause violent and aggressive behavior.
Lorazepam	Commonly known as Ativan. This causes an alteration in thoughts, feelings, and perceptions.
Benzodiazepines	This medication can cause an alteration in thoughts, feelings, and perceptions.
Amitriptyline	Commonly known as Elavil. This medication is a mood elevator and can cause an alteration in thoughts, feelings, and perceptions.
Clonazepam	Commonly known as Klonopin. This medication is used to inhibit seizure activity. Side effects can be mild drowsiness, ataxia, behavioral disturbances that are manifested as aggression, irritability, and agitation.
d-propoxyphene	Commonly known as Darvon. This is an opioid analgesic that can cause an alteration in sensory perception which includes euphoria, dizziness, drowsiness, hypotension, nausea, and vomiting.

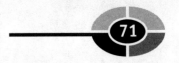

Substances that Can Be Abused

Nearly all drugs that are abused produce a desirable effect such as altering the state of the mind and filling a void in a person's life. Some professionals believe a person who has a low threshold for frustration, a fear of failure, and a feeling of inadequacy are more prone to abuse drugs. Those who abuse drugs do so because they are:

- Bored,
- Pressured by their peers,
- Seeking pleasure,
- Affluent and want to experiment,
- Seeking to escape from reality,
- Feeling inadequate,
- Feeling ashamed and depressed,
- Seeking relief from conflicts.

There are four characteristics that describe drugs that are frequently abused.

1. The drug creates an altered state of consciousness.
2. Prolonged use of the drug creates a tolerance for the drug.
3. The desirable effect is quick.
4. Withdrawal symptoms develop if the drug is stopped after prolonged use. Administering the drug is a fast way to treat withdrawal symptoms.

Dependence versus Tolerance

There is an important difference between drug dependence and drug tolerance although sometimes these terms are used interchangeably. Drug dependence occurs when the patient has a psychological and/or physical dependence on the drug that results in withdrawal symptoms that can become unbearable for the patient to endure. Relief comes only when the patient is administered a dose of the drug.

Tolerance occurs when the concentration of a drug no longer has a continuing therapeutic effect. This happens because receptor sites in the effective tissues adapt to the prescribed level of drug. The only way to regain the therapeutic effect is to increase the concentration of the drug.

Tolerance also has a metabolic effect commonly referred to as pharmacologic tolerance. Prolonged exposure to a drug increases the excretion of the drug from the body. This means there is a lower concentration of the drug in plasma that is distributed throughout the body.

Pathophysiologic Changes Occurring in Substance Abuse

Drug abusers frequently exhibit pathophysiologic changes that require treatment along with the patient's drug addition. These debilitating changes are malnutrition, dehydration, and hypovitaminosis.

In addition, these patients can experience respiratory diseases such as pneumonia, blood clots (pulmonary emboli), and abscesses.

In addition, drug abusers rarely use aseptic techniques for administering drugs intravenously which can lead to localized and systemic infections such as endocarditis (infection of the lining of the heart), HIV, and sepsis (infection of the entire circulatory system). Drug abusers also incur cellulitis (infection in the tissues), sclerosis (scaring of the veins), phlebitis (irritation of veins), and skin abscesses.

Drug abusers are always at risk of overdosing because the active ingredient in illegal drugs are frequently adulterated with dangerous substances such as amphetamines, benzodiazepines, hallucinogens, and alcohol. This makes the potency of the drug unreliable and the risk of death from an accidental overdose is high.

Cultural Aspects of Substance Abuse

The views of drug use differ among cultures around the world. Some drugs considered illegal in one culture are accepted in another culture. Alcohol, caffeine, and nicotine are addictive drugs that are widely accepted in the United States and elsewhere throughout the world.

Cannabis, on the other hand, is illegal in the Untied States and in many other countries. Hallucinogens that affect the auditory and visual senses such as peyote are used by Native Americans as part of religious rituals. Coca leaves that contain cocaine are brewed or chewed by people in the mountainous regions of the Andes to decrease hunger, increase work performance, and create a sense of well being.

Commonly Abused Substances

There are five groups of drugs that are commonly abused in the United States and in other developed countries. These are heroin, cocaine, cannabis, hallucinogens, and inhalants. Heroin is a Schedule I drug (see Chapter 1) that has no accepted medical use in the United States. Cocaine stimulates the central nervous system (see Chapter on CNS). Cannabis includes drugs such as marijuana and hashish.

Hallucinogens are drugs that alter perception and feeling. These include LSD, mescaline, psilocybin, and PCP. Inhalants are aerosols and volatile hydrocarbons such as airplane glue and paint thinner that give the drug abuser a "buzz" or feeling of euphoria.

CANNABIS DRUGS

Cannabis is an extract from the leaves, stems, fruiting tops, and resin of the hemp plant (*Cannabis saliva*). The most common form of cannabis is hashish. Hashish is the resinous material of the cannabis plant. Other forms of this drug include banji, ganga, charas, kif, and dagga.

Hashish is classified as a controlled substance although it isn't a narcotic derivative. Hashish also has sedative-hypnotic, anesthetic, or psychedelic properties and is capable of altering perception, thought, and feeling.

Hashish is administered orally using pipes or cigarettes and can be injected subcutaneously, however the most potent route is inhalation. Many drug abusers prefer smoking hashish through a water pipe to reduce the irritating effect of the acidic smoke. Some drug abusers grind hashish into a powder and mixed it with foods in order to delay the absorption of the drug by the body.

Hashish acts to depress the central nervous system and causes mental relaxation and euphoria that occurs within 15 minutes and lasts up to four hours. The drug abuser experiences a loss of inhibitions. The person's time and space perception is altered and causes a free flow of ideas to occur. These ideas, however, are disconnected. The person can experience blanks or gaps in memory similar to an epileptic episode. The user may also have palpitations, loss of concentration, lightheadedness, weakness, tremors, postural hypotension, ataxia (staggering gait) and a sense of floating. As the dose increases, the effects of the drug progresses from relief to dis-inhibition, excitement, and anesthesia. Respiratory and vasomotor depression and even collapse can occur with high doses.

Hashish is metabolized in the liver and is eliminated in bile and feces. Only a trace amount of hashish is detectable in urine. Hashish may affect the metabolism of drugs that require protein binding. These include ethyl alcohol, barbiturates, amphetamines, cocaine, opiates, and atropine.

Hashish has withdrawal symptoms. These include minor discomfort for a few days. Insomnia, anxiety, irritability and restlessness may persist for a few weeks. The person may have intermittent craving for a few months, which is best treated by exercise. No pharmacological intervention should be given.

HALLUCINOGENS

Hallucinogens are natural and chemically manufactured drugs that alter perception and feeling. These drugs alter the mind and change a person's perception of time, reality, and the environment. Hallucinogens disrupt the normal activity of serotonin, which is a neurotransmitter that sends signals throughout the brain. Hallucinogens cause abnormal activation of serotonin in the part of the brain responsible for coordinating and processing hearing and sight. The result is that people taking hallucinogens hear voices and see images that don't exist.

Researchers are unsure if hallucinogens permanently alter the brain's chemistry, however, some patient's who have taken hallucinogens experience chronic mental disorders.

The following are commonly used hallucinogens.

LSD

Lysergide, better known as LSD, is a potent hallucinogenic that results in a psychoactive effect that heightens perception, creates distortions of the body, and causes visual hallucinations. The person taking LSD can experience unpredictable mood swings from euphoria to depression and panic, which is commonly referred to as a "bad trip." LSD also causes hypertension, dilated pupils, hyperthermia, and tachycardia (rapid heart rate).

LSD takes effect within 20 minutes and lasts up to two hours altering the user's state of consciousness. This can lead to psychosis and trigger flashbacks called "latent psychosis." The experience is frequently unpleasant.

Acute panic and paranoia is a common side effect that can lead to homicidal thoughts and actions. The toxic effect of LSD causes impaired judgment and toxic delirium. This results in a stage of exhaustion and feeling of emptiness where the person is unable to coordinate thoughts. This fall into depression increases the risk of suicide. Some people who take LSD also enter into a long-term schizophrenic or psychotic reaction. LSD stimulates the uterus and could induce contractions in a pregnant woman.

Healthcare providers treat a person who is under the influence of LSD by using a "talk-down" approach where they talk the patient through the episode in a quiet, relaxed environment. If this approach fails, drug therapy is employed using a benzodiazepine such as diazepam (Valium). Drugs should only be used along with crisis intervention therapy.

Avoid using phenothiazines such as chlorpromazine (Thorazine). These can exacerbate the patient's panic reaction and cause postural hypotension (low blood pressure when standing). Also avoid large doses of tranquilizers, using restraints, and isolating the patient because these interventions are more traumatic than therapeutic.

Mescaline

Mescaline is an alkaloid that is extracted from the flowering heads (mescal buttons) of the peyote cactus. Mescaline causes subjective hallucinogenic effects similar to LSD. The extract is a soluble crystalline power that can be dissolved into tea or placed in capsules for ingestion.

This drug takes effect almost immediately and lasts about six hours before it reaches its half-life and is excreted into the urine. People taking mescaline experience anxiety, hyperreflexia, static tremors, and psychic disturbances with vivid visual hallucinations. They also feel abdominal pain, nausea, and diarrhea.

Psilocybin

Psilocybin is extracted from Mexican mushrooms. It produces a subjective hallucinogenic effect that is similar to mescaline, but of shorter duration. Psilocybin takes effect in a half hour to an hour after the drug is administered and its effect can last up to six hours.

People who take this drug experience a pleasant mood although some users become apprehensive. This results in impaired performance and poor critical judgment. Some exhibit hyperkinetic (compulsive movements) behavior and inappropriate laughter. The pupils dilate and the person experiences vertigo

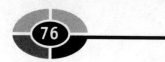

(dizziness) and ataxia (stagger). They also have paresthesias (numbness, tingling) and muscle weakness. The drug also induces drowsiness and sleep.

PCP

PCP is a controlled substance called phencyclidine that causes hallucinations. Usage can result in assaults, murders, and suicides. PCP was developed in the late 1950s as a dissociative anesthetic that leaves a patient awake but detached from surroundings and unresponsive to pain. Once the drug's hallucinogenic effect was discovered, PCP was withdrawn from use in humans, but continued to be used in veterinary medicine. PCP picked up the street name "hog" because of its use with animals.

PCP metabolizes rapidly in the liver and forms a high concentration in urine if taken in large quantities. A small dose of PCP has a half-life of between half an hour and 1 hour. Larger doses can have a half-life of 1 to 4 days.

Patients who are under the influence of PCP are flushed and sweat profusely. They have nystagmus (rapid eye movements), diplopia (double vision), and ptosis (drooping eyelids). These patients also appear sedated and under the influence of an analgesic. They also exhibit the effects of alcohol intoxication with ataxia (staggering gait) and generalized numbness of the extremities.

Patients undergo three stages of psychological effect when using PCP. The first stage is a change in body image and a feeling of de-personalization. This follows with the second stage when the patient's hearing and vision become distorted. The third stage occurs when the patient feels apathy, estrangement, and alienation.

The patient's thoughts become more disorganized. Attention span is impaired as is motor skills and overall sense of body boundaries. The drug's hallucinatory effects can occur long after the patient's acute symptoms are gone. These are unpredictable and can happen months after the drug was taken.

The patient can experience psychotic disturbances which are exhibited by paranoid behavior, self-destructive actions, random eye movement, and excitation. These are combined with physiological changes such as tachycardia, hypertension, respiratory depression, muscle rigidity, increased reflexes, seizures, and an unconscious state with open eyes.

There is no known chemical antidote to PCP. The only treatment is to keep the patient quiet, in a dark room, away from sensory stimuli, and protected from self-inflicted injury. Don't attempt to talk the patient down as the patient can perceive any interaction as a personal attack and may become very violent. The patient is commonly given diazepam (Valium) or haloperidol (Haldol) for their antianxiety and antipsychotic effects.

PCP is very toxic and nurses should be aware of the severity of the drug's effects. These include hypertensive crisis, intracerebral hemorrhage (bleeding

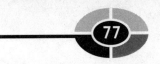

into the brain), convulsions, coma, and death. Patients who have used PCP should be closely monitored.

Inhalants

Inhalants are not drugs. They are volatile hydrocarbons and aerosols that are used to dispense a variety of chemical products that create a euphoric effect when inhaled. These products include airplane glue, paint thinner, typewriter correction fluid, lighter fluid, nitrous oxide, xylene, toluene, and include over 1000 household and commercial products. Treatment of abuse of inhalants uses a symptomatic approach rather than a pharmacological approach because there are no specific antidotes to these products. When inhaled, the intoxication can last a few minutes or several hours. If used repeatedly, the individual can lose consciousness; high concentrations can cause heart failure or death. Some of the products can replace oxygen in the body and the individual can suffocate. Each of these side effects needs to be treated separately. The permanent health effects caused by the use of these inhalants can include hearing loss, peripheral neuropathies (numbness, tingling) or spasms of arms and legs, CNS or brain damage and bone marrow damage, that results in blood problems. Kidney and liver damage can also occur.

Nursing Assessment

Patients who abuse drugs require a careful and complete assessment which includes vital signs (temperature, blood pressure, heart rate, and respiratory rate). Pupil size is inspected and the skin is examined for needle marks and abscesses. The patient's nutrition, elimination, and sleep patterns are noted, too. Determine if the patient has a past medical history of drug use, drug abuse, and related drug illnesses such as HIV, cellulitis, endocarditis, and pneumonia or other respiratory problems.

The following are commonly used nursing diagnoses for drug abuse patients:

- Knowledge deficit related to denial of problem
- Ineffective individual coping related to lack of support system
- Risk for violence to oneself or others related to drug use
- Altered health maintenance related to drug dependency
- Ineffective management of therapeutic regimen

The plan of care for a patient who is a drug abuser will depend on the reason for hospitalization. The physical response to drug use should be monitored and any infections or disease states must be treated. The plan should also include treatment for the abuse in a supportive and rehabilitative setting. This may include counseling, psychotherapy sessions, and medications to overcome the withdrawal symptoms.

Nursing implementation may focus on managing the patient's acute intoxication and withdrawal and then monitoring the effectiveness of therapy to treat the patient's substance abuse problem.

The evaluation of the effectiveness of the treatment centers on how well the patient is successfully detoxified and withdrawn from the drug and how well the patient refrains from re-abusing the substance. It is important for nurses to realize that overcoming a drug addiction is a long and sometimes lifetime task. Patients may have many relapses along the way and the process can seem frustrating and hopeless. However, the nurse should remain non-judgmental and objective when caring for substance abuse patients.

Summary

Substance abuse is one of the most widely misunderstood areas of pharmacology and has led some patients to avoid narcotics and pain-relieving drugs for fear of becoming addicted to the drug.

Substance abuse is the indiscriminant misuse of medication that results in a physical and/or psychological dependence on the drug. A person is considered addicted to a drug if over a six month period they develop dependence for the drug, they experience withdrawal symptoms when the drug is no longer administered, and they require increased doses of the drug to experience the same therapeutic effect.

An addicted person also has an uncontrollable urge to use the drug and self-medication interferes with activities of daily life and continues despite the negative consequence of using the drug.

Drug abusers exhibit common behavioral patterns such as being unable to maintain a normal routine, have poor hygiene, and strained family and social relationships. They also have more legal problems than the average person. And most importantly, they are frequently in denial that they have a problem.

Healthcare professionals are especially prone to drug abuse because drugs can enhance performance during long shifts, drugs are easily accessible, and healthcare professionals know how to self medicate. Furthermore, revealing your own abuse of drugs places the healthcare provider's license and livelihood in jeopardy.

There are tests available to determine if a person has taken drugs, however those tests are not foolproof. There is a chance that the results will be a false positive or false negative.

Commonly abused drugs fall into one of five groups. These are heroin, cocaine, cannabis, hallucinogens, and inhalants. Although many of the drugs that are in these groups are illegal in the United States, some of them are legal in other countries.

Quiz

1. Tolerance to a drug occurs when
   (a) a drug is no longer effective.
   (b) a person becomes addicted to a drug.
   (c) a higher dose is required to achieve the same therapeutic effect.
   (d) None of the above.

2. A patient undergoing withdrawal from hashish is treated by
   (a) administering a lower dose of hashish.
   (b) administering a sedative.
   (c) doing nothing.
   (d) prescribing exercise.

3. When a patient is withdrawing from LSD,
   (a) provide massive doses of tranquilizers.
   (b) restrain the patient.
   (c) talk down the patient.
   (d) isolate the patient.

4. A patient who only takes prescription drugs cannot become dependent on the drug.
   (a) True
   (b) False

5. Some drugs increase a person's performance.
   (a) True
   (b) False

6. Psilocybin is
   (a) extracted from Mexican mushrooms.
   (b) extracted from coca leaves.
   (c) extracted from coca resins.
   (d) extracted from the stalk of the coca plant.

7. Prolonged exposure to a drug increases the excretion of the drug from the body.
   (a) True
   (b) False

8. A licensed practitioner can help prevent a patient from becoming dependent on a drug by
   (a) using a prescribed management routine.
   (b) limiting treatment to one month.
   (c) providing the patient with psychological counseling.
   (d) All of the above

9. A healthcare professional is ethically expected to report another healthcare professional if there is a suspicion of drug abuse.
   (a) True
   (b) False

10. Some healthcare providers use drugs for recreational purposes.
    (a) True
    (b) False

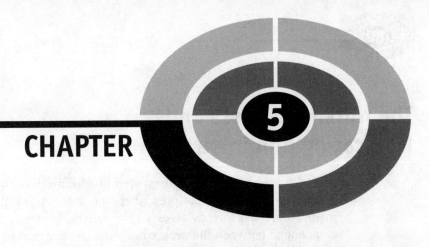

Principles of Medication Administration

Administering medication to a patient can be tricky and outright dangerous unless special precautions are followed to assure that the patient receives the right drug, given at the right time, using the right route.

In this chapter you'll learn the proper way to administer medication and how to avoid common errors that frequently result in improper medication administration that harms the patient. You'll also learn how to assess the patient to determine if the patient experiences the therapeutic effect of the medication.

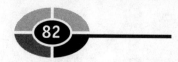
The Nursing Process and Medication Administration

Assessing the patient is the first step in administering medication. This might seem unusual because the prescriber—prior to writing the prescription for the medication—has already assessed the patient. However, the patient's condition can change between the prescriber's assessment and the time the medication is administered. Assessing the patient also provides a baseline from which you can compare the patient's reaction to the medication after administering the medication.

The assessment is divided into two areas. First is a general assessment that is necessary for every medication. Then there is an assessment that is required for specific drugs. The general assessment must determine:

- *Is the therapeutic action of the drug proper for the patient?*

This, too, appears unusual since the prescriber has already made this determination. However, the nurse is responsible to independently verify that the drug is proper for the patient. You do this by reading the patient's diagnosis in the patient's chart and looking up the medication in the drug manual where it will state the approved use of the drug.

If the drug isn't used for the patient's condition, then the nurse should contact the prescriber. Nurses may not administer drugs that are being used for purposes other than those approved by the FDA. It is important to realize that in some situations, the prescriber will be using the drug for a secondary therapeutic effect that addresses the patient's condition which is acceptable if that purpose is FDA approved.

- *Is the route proper for the patient?*

Some drugs can be administered using more than one route. Although the prescriber specifies a route in the medication order, the patient's current condition might indicate a different route is appropriate.

For example, the prescriber might order antibiotics PO. However, the patient might have a very high fever that needs immediate relief by administering antibiotics IV. In another situation, the patient might be experiencing stomach pains and vomiting, which is a clear indication that PO isn't the desired route. If the route is no longer appropriate, then the nurse should contact the prescriber and obtain an order to use an alternate route that is appropriate for the patient's condition.

• *What is the proper dose for the patient?*

The prescriber will specify the dose in the medication order. Sometimes the dose doesn't match the prepared dose that the nurse has on hand requiring the nurse to calculate the dose. For example, the prescriber might write a medication order for 800 mg of ibuprofen. The nurse might have on hand 200 mg tablets and will have to calculate that the patient must be administered 4 tablets of 200 mg of ibuprofen.

With some drugs the prescriber will order a dose based on the weight of the patient. It is the nurse's responsibility to calculate the actual dose after weighing the patient. For example, the prescriber orders Depakote 10 mg/kg. The patient weights 176 lbs. The nurse has 200 mg/5 mL on hand and calculates that the correct dose for the patient is 20 mL. (You'll learn how to perform this calculation in Chapter 7).

• *Assess for contraindications.*

The patient might have developed a condition since being assessed by the prescriber that makes it inappropriate to receive the medication. The nurse must review the drug's profile in the drug manual to determine the drug's contraindications and then determine if they apply to the patient. If so, then the nurse must contact the prescriber to advise of the patient's condition. This is particularly important since different healthcare professionals might prescribe the patient drugs.

For example, the patient might be scheduled for an angiogram in 24 hours and the prescriber has a standing medication order for Glucophage. Glucophage reacts with contrast dyes and therefore cannot be administered to the patient within 24 hours of any dye procedures such as an angiogram. However, withholding medications should only be done after the healthcare provider has been notified.

• *Assess for side effects and adverse reactions to the drug.*

Drugs can have known side effects—some of which the patient can tolerate and others that result in an adverse reaction. The nurse must review the profile of the drug in the drug manual to determine any side effects and adverse reactions that it might cause and monitor the patient for such signs and symptoms. The nurse should alert the patient to the possible side effects before administering the medication. In addition, the nurse can prepare to deal with a possible adverse reaction the patient might have to a medication.

For example, some opioids such as morphine sulfate can cause respiratory depression. Narcan (naxalone) can reverse the effects of opioids. Keeping narcan available when administering morphine sulfate in high doses or to a patient who has never had morphine might avoid an adverse reaction.

Assessment Required for Specific Drugs

Besides contraindications for a drug, the drug's profile in the drug manual also provides the nurse with the pharmacologic response of the drug (see Chapter 2)—how the drug works in the body. Knowing this, the nurse can assess the patient to determine if the patient's body will be able to metabolize and eliminate the medication.

Here are the areas that the nurse needs to consider:

- *Absorption*

The patient must be able to absorb the medication. For example, PO medication is absorbed in the GI tract (stomach and small intestine). A patient with GI disturbances such as vomiting or diarrhea will not be able to absorb the medication.

- *Distribution*

Once absorbed, the medication must be distributed throughout the body. In order for this to occur, some drugs must bind to protein, which carries drug particles through the veins and arteries. If the patient has low protein levels, some drug particles are unable to bind to the protein and the unbound drug particles are free drug which can possibly result in a toxic effect.

For example, Dilantin binds to albumin. If the patient has a low albumin level, there will be less Dilantin bound to protein. The patient will be receiving the proper therapeutic dose but because much of it is not bound to protein, the serum levels of free drug will be too high—causing toxicity.

- *Metabolism*

The liver breaks down drugs so they can be excreted from the body. If the patient's liver isn't functioning properly, then the drug particles are not metabolized and cannot be excreted from the body. This results in a buildup of the drug and can possibly cause toxicity in the patient. It is important to remember that inadequate liver function is not always caused by liver disease. Age influences liver function. For example, newborns have an immature liver while the elderly have decreased liver function.

- *Excretion*

    The kidney is the main organ that excretes medication although some medication is excreted in bile, feces, respiration, saliva, and sweat. The patient is unable to excrete drugs if these routes are not functioning properly. The nurse should be aware of the route in which the drug is excreted from the body and then determine if that route is fully functional before administering the medication to the patient.

    In addition to the pharmacologic response of the drug, the nurse must also assess other aspects of the patient and the medication. These are:

    o *Age*

    The very young and the elderly are more sensitive to drugs than the average adult because there is a decrease in gastric secretion resulting in poor absorption through the GI tract. The elderly are particularly sensitive to barbiturates and central nervous system depressants. Therefore, it is critical that the nurse assess the patient's age before administering medication and carefully monitor very young and elderly patients afterwards for adverse side effects.

    o *Body Weight*

    The prescriber might order medication given at the recommended dose. However, the recommended dose is typically for a patient whose body weight is within the average range (70 kg for an adult). The medication might have a different effect if the patient's body weight falls outside this range. For example, the recommended dose might be too strong for a very thin patient resulting in a toxic effect. Likewise, the recommended dose might be too low for an obese patient and never reach the therapeutic level. This is particularly important to assess when administering medications such as antineoplastics (anti-cancer drugs) where a low therapeutic level can have a non-therapeutic effect for the patient—resulting in an undesirable outcome. Using body weight to determine drug dose will avoid this problem.

    o *Pharmacogenetic*

    Genetic factors might have a serious influence on the response to a drug. Depending on the medication, a patient might have a genetically based adverse reaction to the drug. Therefore, in assessing the patient, the nurse must determine if parents, siblings, or other close relatives have had an adverse reaction to the medication.

○ *Time*

Medication must be given to the patient at the most opportune time during the day to assure that the therapeutic effect is attained. Some drugs are effective only if taken with meals while other medication cannot be taken with meals. Likewise, certain drugs are more effective if taken at bedtime.

○ *Food-drug interaction*

Certain types of foods can adversely effect the drug's therapeutic effect by increasing absorption, delaying absorption, and even preventing absorption of the medication. Furthermore, food may cause the patient to experience an adverse reaction as in the case with phenelzine sulfate (Nardil), which is an MAO monoamineoxidase inhibitor anti-depressant. Nardil cannot be given with foods that use bacteria or molds in their preparation or for preservation of those that contain tyramine, such as cheese, sour cream, beer, wine, figs, raisins, bananas, avocados, etc. The nurse must assess if the drug has a contraindication with food and educate the patient about this food-drug interaction.

○ *Drug-drug interaction*

The nurse should be aware that the combination of drugs administered to the patient may have a negative effect. Some drugs when administered together might increase or decrease the therapeutic effectiveness of either or both medications by competing for the same receptor sites in the body. Furthermore, a combination of some medications produce toxicity or a fatal condition such as anaphylaxis. Sometimes there is more than one provider prescribing medications. The prescribers should be notified before medications are administered if there is a possibility of a drug-drug interaction.

○ *Drug History, Tolerance, and the Cumulative Effect*

Continued use of a medication might lessen the therapeutic effect of the drug because the patient's body becomes tolerant of the medication. The nurse must assess the patient's drug history and monitor the patient for signs and symptoms that the drug is having a therapeutic effect. One such example would be the absence of seizures if the patient is taking phenytoin (Dilantin), an antiseizure medication. Another concern is the drug buildup in the patient's body. The patient may be unable to metabolize and excrete the medication as fast as new doses are administered. The result is a cumulative effect that can result in toxicity. The patient should be monitored for signs of drug build-up. For example, ataxia (muscular incoordination), nystagmus (rhythmic oscillation of eyes), and double vision are signs of toxic levels of Dilantin.

Administering Medication

Medication can be administered once the nurse assesses the patient and determines that the medication can be administered safely. The nurse follows implementation procedures for administering medication.

- *Check the prescriber's medication order*
  The initial step in administering medication is to read the medication order that is written by the prescriber to make sure that the proper medication and dose is administered to the patient. The prescriber's medication order is found in the patient's chart.

- *Check the Medication Administration Record (MAR)*
  The medication administration record is a transcription of the prescriber's medication order. Many times the MAR is a computer-generated document, but sometimes there will be handwritten entries in the MAR. Compare the MAR with the prescriber's medication order to assure that the proper medication, dose, and other aspects of the medication order have been properly transcribed.

- *The nurse should check all medications prescribed to the patient even if he or she will not be administering all of the medications while taking care of the patient.*
  The MAR lists all medication that the patient receives including those already given to the patient and medication that has been discontinued. It is critical for the nurse to review all medications and not just those that will be given on the nurse's shift because previous medications may still be active in the patient's body. Remember that some drugs have a long half-life making them still a potential conflict with other medication days after it was administered to the patient.

- *Check the patient's allergies*
  Although the patient's chart might indicate that the patient does not have any allergies to medication or food, the nurse must review whether or not the patient has allergies before administering medication. Sometimes the patient may not have recalled any allergies when the patient's history was taken, but will recall an allergy after being questioned again by the nurse.

- *Create your own medication administration worksheet*

  Although the MAR lists medications and the times they are to be administered, the patient may be scheduled for tests and procedures that conflict with the medication schedule. It is best to create a medication administration worksheet that schedules both medication and the patient's other activities so there is one schedule for the patient.

- *Check PRN (as needed) medications*

  It is common for some medications to be administered to the patient by the nurse on an as needed basis (PRN) such as analgesics (pain medication). PRN medication isn't scheduled on the MAR but is listed in a different section of the MAR. Therefore, the nurse must determine when PRN medication was administered and what PRN medication was administered before giving any medication. This avoids any potential interaction between medications.

PREPARING THE MEDICATION

Once the nurse is assured that the medication can be administered properly to the patient, the nurse can administer it by following these steps:

1. Wash hands. This is the best way to prevent infection.
2. Prepare medication that you are going to give at this time. Don't prepare all medications at once. It is possible that someone else may have to administer the other medications. Nurses should NEVER give medication that someone else has prepared.
3. Prepare medications in a quiet area so you are not interrupted.
4. Double check your math when calculating doses. Have a colleague verify your calculations if necessary.
5. Make sure that all of the patient's medications that will be administered during the shift are in the patient's medication drawer. Compare the contents of the patient's medication drawer against the MAR. The medication and dose in the drawer should match the MAR.
6. Compare the medication with that listed on the MAR. Sometimes the pharmacy substitutes a generic drug for a brand name drug. Always look up the medication in the drug manual if you do not recognize the name of the drug.
7. Check the name of the medication three times: 1) when you remove it from the drawer; 2) when you prepare the medication; and 3) before returning the medication to the drawer or disposing of the wrapper or container. If

the medication is wrapped, then bring the wrapper with you to the patient's room and check the wrapper again before administering the medication to the patient.

AT THE PATIENT'S BEDSIDE

After medication is prepared, it is taken to the patient's room where the nurse administers the medication to the patient. In doing so, the nurse must follow precautions to assure that the medication is administered safely. Here's how it is done:

1. Wash your hands.
2. Introduce yourself to the patient.
3. Ask the patient to state his/her complete name. Don't assist the patient by saying, "are you Mr. Jones." The patient should say his/her name without your help if possible.
4. Compare the patient's name and number on the patient's identification band against the patient's name and number on the MAR.
5. Ask the patient if he or she has any allergies to food or medication. The patient may be aware of food allergies such as shellfish, but unaware of allergies to medication. However, patients who are allergic to shellfish are also allergic to some medications.
6. Examine the patient's identification band to see if the patient has allergies. Allergies may be noted on the identification band.
7. Assist the patient into a comfortable position to administer the medication.
8. Ask the patient if he/she knows about the medication and why the medication is being administered. The patient's response provides insight into knowledge the patient has about his/her condition and treatment. This gives the nurse a perfect opportunity to educate the patient about his/her condition, treatment and medication.
9. Make sure that the patient sees the medication if it is a tablet or liquid. Stop immediately if the patient doesn't recognize the medication as the drug the patient received previously. Recheck the order. The dose may have changed, a different medication was substituted, or there is an error in the medication.
10. Make sure you have baseline vital signs, labs, and other patient data before administering the medication. To determine the patient's reaction to the drug, the baseline can be compared to vital signs, labs, and other patient data taken after the patient receives the medication.

11. Instruct the patient about side effects of the medication and take precautions to assure the patient's safety such as raising the side rails and instructing the patient to remain in bed until the side effects subside.

12. Stay with the patient until all the medications are swallowed. Remember that the patient has the right to refuse medication. Notify the prescriber if this occurs.

13. Properly dispose of the medication and supplies used to administer the medication. Don't leave the medication at the patient's bedside unless required by the medication order.

14. Wash hands before leaving the patient's room.

15. Document in the MAR that you administered the medication to the patient.

HANDY TIPS WHEN ADMINISTERING MEDICATION

Medication can taste bad. You can minimize this adverse effect by giving the patient ice chips prior to administering the medication. Ice chips numb the taste buds so the patient is unable to taste the medication.

Give bad-tasting medications first followed by pleasant-tasting liquids. This shortens the time the patient experiences the bad taste. The patient is left with the taste of the pleasant tasting medication in his/her mouth. Use the liquid form of the medication where possible because patients find it easier to ingest a liquid. Offer water after giving a medication if it is not contraindicated.

Administer medication to a patient who needs extra assistance taking the medication after you give medication to your other patients. In this way, you can devote the necessary time to assist this patient without being pressured to administer medication to your other patients.

AVOID MEDICATION ERRORS

Medication errors are the most common cause of patient injuries in a hospital. It is therefore critical that the nurse avoid situations that frequently result in medication errors. If an error occurs, assess the patient and notify the nurse in charge and the physician. Follow your hospital's policy for preparing an incident report. Review the steps that caused the error to occur.

Here are ways to avoid common errors:

- Avoid distractions when preparing medication.
- Avoid conversations while preparing medication.
- Only administer medications that you prepare.
- Only pour or prepare medication from containers that have full labels that are easy to read.
- Don't transfer drugs from one container to another container.
- Don't pour medications directly into your hand.
- Don't give medications that have expired.
- Don't guess about medication and doses. Always ask the prescriber.
- Don't administer drugs that are discolored, have sediment, or are cloudy unless this is a normal state for the medication.
- Don't leave medications by the bedside or with visitors.
- Keep medications in clear sight.
- Don't give medication if the patient says he/she has allergies to the drug or the drug group or if the patient says it does not look the same as the drug they normally take.
- Use both the patient's name and patient's number on the identification band to identify the patient.
- Don't administer medication with food or beverages unless the medication can be given with food and beverages.

PROPERLY DISPOSE OF MEDICATION

Hospitals have strict policies that govern how unused medications and supplies used to administer medication are handled. Here are steps typically found in hospital policies.

- Don't recap needles.
- Discard needles and syringes in an appropriate container that prevents others from receiving a needle prick.
- Dispose of medication in the sink or toilet and not in the trash.
- Return controlled substances to the pharmacy.
- Dispose of controlled substances in the presence of another licensed health-care worker who will sign as a witness to the disposal.
- Discard unused solutions from ampules before discarding the ampule.

ADMINISTERING MEDICATION AT HOME

The nurse is responsible for educating the patient on how to self-medicate at home by providing the do's and don'ts of administering the medication. The nurse must explain the following:

- Store the medication properly. Some medication, such as insulin, must be refrigerated.
- Always label the date and time when the medication was opened.
- Keep the medication in a locked cabinet away from the reach of children.
- Explain the reason the patient is taking the medication and how often the medication is given.
- Explain what to do if the patient misses a dose.
- Describe the signs and symptoms of the toxic effect of the medication if the patient takes more than the prescribed dose.
- Describe the signs and symptoms of side effects and adverse reactions that might occur when taking the medication.
- Explain negative interactions the medication might have with certain foods.
- Develop a system for self-medication for patients who have poor eyesight and decreased mental capacity. For example, the patient can use specially marked containers for each day of the week. A relative or friend can fill those containers with the appropriate medication. The patient is then taught to open the proper container each day.
- Give the patient a list of medication, dose, and frequency and the name of the prescriber so the patient can keep the list in a wallet or pocketbook.
- Suggest that the patient wear a MedicAlert bracelet or other jewelry that identifies the patient as having allergies or chronic illnesses.

Evaluating the Patient After Administering Medication

The nurse must assess the patient after the patient is given medication to determine if the medication has had the desired therapeutic effect. To do this, the nurse compares the patient's current vital signs, labs, and other pertinent patient data with baseline information. The patient should also be assessed after the medication has reached its onset and peak time. Early or late assessments could be misleading and provide false information about the effectiveness of the drug.

The nurse must suspend administering further doses of the medication if the patient shows the signs and symptoms indicating an adverse reaction to the medication. The prescriber must be immediately notified of the patient's condition.

The nurse must also note any side effect of the medication experienced by the patient and how well the patient tolerates the side effect. If the patient has a low tolerance to the side effect, then the nurse needs to notify the prescriber. The prescriber might substitute a different medication or prescribe other medication to alleviate the side effect.

The nurse must determine if the patient is receiving the therapeutic effect from the medication. This is critical when giving pain medication. Doses are often ordered for the average-weight patient. Patients who are very thin or obese may be receiving too much or too little medication. Prescribers are also concerned about patients developing tolerance to or dependency on pain medication and may underprescribe the dose or how often it may be given. If the nurse accurately assesses the patient's response to the drug, the dose or frequency may be adjusted to provide appropriate relief from pain.

Controlling Narcotics

Special precautions are necessary for storing and handling narcotics because the manufacture, sale, and use of narcotics are controlled by federal legislation. Here are the steps that must be taken to secure narcotics.

- Keep narcotics in a double-locked drawer or a closet.
- One nurse per shift must keep the keys to the narcotic drawer on his/her person.
- A sign-out sheet must be used to control the inventory of narcotics.
- Document on the MAR or similar records when a patient is given a narcotic.

Controlled substances (narcotics) are generally counted at least once per shift. The amount of the drug available is compared with the numbers that have been used for patients and signed for on the narcotics form. Each agency has a policy to govern this activity and to determine what action should be followed if the count is not accurate.

Summary

Assessing the patient is the first step when administering medication. Assure that the patient is receiving the proper medication and proper dose because the patient's condition might have changed since the prescriber assessed the patient.

The assessment is divided into two areas. First, a general assessment is required and then assess for specific medications. The general assessment determines several factors that include the right drug, dose, and route for the patient. The assessment also determines contraindications, side effects, and adverse effects, of the medication. The specific assessment examines the pharmacologic response of the medication in relation to the patient's capability to absorb, distribute, metabolize, and excrete the medication.

Once the nurse has determined that medication is proper for the patient, the nurse prepares to administer the medication by verifying the prescriber's medication order and comparing it to other medications that the patient received to determine potential interactions. The nurse also determines if the patient has allergies to the medication.

The medication is prepared in a quiet place without any interruptions. At the bedside, the nurse follows safety procedures that assure the medication is being administered to the proper patient. The nurse verifies the patient's identity and that the patient knows why the medication is being given. Baseline data (such as vital signs, and labs) is obtained by the nurse. They will be compared to similar data collected after the onset of the medication.

The nurse will monitor the patient after the medication is administered and look for signs and symptoms of adverse reactions to the medication.

Now that you have a good understanding of how to administer medication, in the next chapter we'll take a look at the different routes used to administered medication.

Quiz

1. The desired action of a medication is called
   (a) its medication reaction.
   (b) its safety action.
   (c) its therapeutic action.
   (d) none of the above.

2. What can inadvertently cause a patient to receive an insufficient dose of a medication?
   (a) genetic substitution of a brand medication
   (b) allergies
   (c) obesity
   (d) under weight

3. Why should Narcan be on hand when administering an opioid?
   (a) It reverses the narcotic effect.
   (b) It can be substituted for the narcotic.
   (c) It is mixed with a narcotic to extend the peak time of the narcotic.
   (d) It is mixed with a narcotic to shorten the narcotic's onset.

4. The body weight of a patient can never influence the dose of a medication.
   (a) True
   (b) False

5. A patient who is allergic to shellfish is likely to be allergic to some medications.
   (a) True
   (b) False

6. The purpose of collecting baseline patient data is
   (a) to adhere to legal requirements.
   (b) to legally protect the nurse.
   (c) so it can be compared to the patient's condition after the medication is administered to determine the patient's reaction to the medication.
   (d) to determine the patient's condition before administering the medication.

7. It is acceptable to administer medication to a patient that is prepared by another licensed practitioner.
   (a) True
   (b) False

8. Ice chips are given to the patient prior to administering bad-tasting medication because
   (a) the ice chips dilute the medication.
   (b) the ice chips numb the taste buds.
   (c) the ice chip moisturizes the oral cavity.
   (d) none of the above.

9. The prescriber's medication order is compared to the MAR to assure that the medication has been properly transcribed to the MAR.
   (a) True
   (b) False

10. A prescriber's medication order is always accurate and should not be questioned.
    (a) True
    (b) False

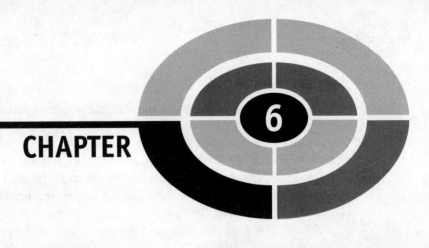

CHAPTER 6

Route of Administration

The patient has the right to receive the proper medication and have that medication administered using the best route to achieve the desired therapeutic effect. The route is based on the form in which the medication is given to the patient.

The best route depends on a number of factors that include the nature of the medication and the patient's condition. In this chapter you'll learn the routes and how to administer medication using each route.

Medication and Routes

The last time that you had a headache and took an aspirin you were using the oral route to get rid of your headache. The oral route is just one of 11 different routes that are used to administer medication.

As the name implies, the oral route means that the patient ingests the medication. Sublingual and buccal are two other routes that also involve the patient's mouth but instead of ingesting the medication, the medication is absorbed within the oral cavity from beneath the tongue (sublingual) or between the cheek and gum (buccal).

You probably rubbed hydrocortisone on an insect bite to relieve itching. Itching subsides as the skin absorbs the hydrocortisone. This is the topical route. Medication is also absorbed by the skin using the transdermal route, which is commonly known as the "patch."

Medication that you place in your eyes, ears, or in your nose is administered using the instillation route in the form of drops, ointment, and sprays. Patients with lung problems sometimes receive medication using the inhalation route. Medication is delivered using an inhaler that changes liquid medication into a spray.

Patients who have upper gastrointestinal (GI) disturbances might have a tube inserted via the nasal passage into the stomach (nasogastric tube) or a tube inserted directly into the stomach through the skin and stomach wall (gastrostomy tube) that is used to bypass the upper GI tract and provides a direct path to the stomach. Both tubes can be used to introduce medication into the patient.

The suppository route is used to administer medication through the rectum and the vagina. A route that few patients look forward to is the parenteral route because medication is given using injections or directly into the vein, the intravenous (IV) routes.

ORAL ROUTE

Oral medications are in the form of tablets, capsules, and liquids and most are absorbed in the small intestine and have a peak time of between 1 and 3 hours. Tablets can be divided using a tablet cutter into half or quarters to reduce the dosage that is given to the patient. Some tablets can also be crushed so that the medication can be mixed with food such as applesauce. Capsules must be taken whole because they are enteric-coated so that the medication isn't released until it reaches the intestines. Some capsules contain timed-release medication.

Here are the precautions that must be taken when the oral route is prescribed.

- No oral medication is given to patients who are vomiting, who lack a gag reflex, or who are in an unresponsive state.
- Do not mix oral medication with large amounts of food or liquid because it can alter the effectiveness of the medication. Food and liquid might interfere with the patient's ability to absorb the medication depending on the drug. In that case medication should be given while the patient's stomach is empty.

LIQUID MEDICATION

Liquid medication takes one of three forms: elixirs, emulsion, and suspensions. An elixir is a sweet, pleasant-smelling solution of alcohol and water used as a vehicle for medicine. Robitussin, a commonly used cough preparation, is an elixir. An emulsion is a suspension of small globules of one liquid in a second liquid with which the first will not mix, such as milk fats in milk. And a suspension is a preparation of finely divided, undissolved particles dispersed in a liquid, such as bismuth subsalicylate (Pepto-Bismol).

When administering liquid medication:

- Dilute, shake, or stir the medication only if required (follow the directions on the label).
- Read the meniscus at the lowest fluid mark to determine the dose while pouring the liquid. This is best done at eye level.
- Refrigerate open or reconstituted (mixed) liquid medication as per the medication label. Date and label the time the medication was opened or reconstituted.

SUBLINGUAL AND BUCCAL MEDICATION

These medications are quickly absorbed into the circulatory system because the tissues beneath the tongue and between the cheek and gum consist of a thin layer of epithelium cells and a vast network of capillaries. Nitroglycerin can be administered sublingually.

When administering sublingual or buccal medication:

- Do not permit the patient to ingest food or liquid if the medication is administered sublingually (under the tongue) or bucally (between the cheek and gum) until the medication is completely absorbed.
- Sublingual medication such as nitroglycerin can be administered to a non-responsive patient. Sublingual medication dissolves quickly with minimal chance of aspiration.

TRANSDERMAL ROUTE

The transdermal route is commonly referred to as "the patch" because the medication is contained in a patch that is absorbed through the skin. There are an increasing number of drugs that are administered using this route. These include cardiovascular medication such as nitroglycerin, neoplastic drugs (cancer), and hormones (estrogen and birth control medications). In addition, analgesics (Fentanyl), medication used to treat allergic reactions, and smoking cessation drugs such as Nicotrol are also administered through the transdermal route.

Transdermal patches provide a consistent blood level and less absorption problems in the gastrointestinal tract that are commonly experienced by patients who take oral medications.

When administering transdermal medication:

- Check the prescriber's order.
- Don't cut the patch in half.
- Remove the patch before applying another patch.
- Apply the patch onto the specified area of the body. Nitroglycerin is placed on the chest or upper arm. The nicotine patch is applied to the trunk or upper arm. Fentanyl is positioned on the chest, flank, or upper arm.
- Alternate the sites of the patch on the patient's body.
- Wear gloves when administering the patch because the nurse can easily absorb the medication, which can cause an undesirable reaction.
- Place the patch on a clean, dry, hairless area where the skin is intact.
- Some transdermal medication is available in a tube with an accompanying pad of paper patches. The paper has measurement lines on it and the medication is squeezed onto the paper in the amount ordered. For example, nitroglycerin $\frac{1}{2}$ inch. Label the patch with the date, time and your initials.

TOPICAL ROUTE

The topical route refers to applying medication to the skin for a local effect. There are three ways to administer topical medication. These are with a glove, with a tongue blade, or with a cotton-tipped applicator. Never apply topical medication with an ungloved hand because medication may be absorbed into your body as well as into the patient's body.

When administering a topical medication:

- Check the prescriber's order.
- Use clean or sterile technique if applying the medication to skin that is broken or burned.
- Stroke the medication firmly onto the skin.
- Be sure the patient is comfortable when applying medication to painful areas of the skin.

- Don't use a light, feathery touch when administrating medication to an area that is pruritic (itchy) because this makes the itch worse.

INSTILLATION ROUTE

Instillations are liquid medications that are administered to the eyes and ears as drops, ointment, or sprays. You'll need to take special precautions when administering an instillation to prevent spreading the disease.

Here's what you need to do to administer installations in the eye:

- Check the prescriber's order.
- Wash hands and then apply clean gloves. You don't need sterile gloves.
- Position the patient so that the patient is looking toward the ceiling.
- Gently pull down the skin below the infected eye to expose the conjunctival sac.
- If eye drops,
  - Administer the prescribed number of drops into the center of the conjunctival sac.
  - Don't touch the eyelids or the eye lashes with the dropper.
  - Release the skin and gently press the lacrimal duct (inner corner of the eye) with sterile cotton balls or tissues for 1–2 minutes. This prevents the systemic absorption of the medication through the lacrimal canal.
- If eye ointment,
  - Squeeze about a half-inch of ointment onto the conjunctival sac.
  - Tell the patient that he or she might experience blurred vision temporarily.
- Instruct the patient to keep his or her eyes closed for 1–2 minutes.
- Avoid placing medication on the cornea since this can cause discomfort and possibly damage the cornea.

Here's what you need to do to administer eardrops:

- Check the prescriber's order.
- Wash hands and then apply clean gloves.
- Make sure the medication is at room temperature.
- Position the patient so his or her head is tilted slightly toward the unaffected side.
- Straighten the external ear canal by pulling the auricle up and back for a patient who is 3 years of age and older and down and back for a patient under three years of age. (Hint: Children are shorter than adults, so you pull down.)

- Instill the prescribed number of drops into the ear.
- Don't touch the ear with the dropper; the dropper will become contaminated.
- The patient should remain with his or her head tilted for 2–3 minutes.

When administering nose drops and sprays:

- Check the prescriber's order.
- Ask the patient to blow his or her nose.
- For nose drops.
  - Position the patient's head back if the infection is in the frontal sinus.
  - Position the patient's head to the affected side if the infection is in the ethmoid sinus.
  - Administer the prescribed number of drops.
  - tIlt the patient's head backwards for five minutes after administering drops.
- For nose sprays,
  - Tell the patient to close the unaffected nostril.
  - Ask the patient to tilt his or her head to the side of the closed nostril.
  - Spray the medication.
  - Ask the patient to hold his or her breath or open the closed nostril and breathe through it per the medication instructions.

INHALATION ROUTE

The inhalation route is used to have the patient inhale the medication using an inhaler. This is a common route used to administer bronchodilators to patients with breathing problems such as asthma, pneumonia, and chronic obstructive pulmonary disease.

The medication enters the lower respiratory tract where it is rapidly absorbed in the bronchioles providing the patient with relief from bronchospasms, wheezing, asthma, or allergic reactions.

Inhalation is used to deliver antibiotics, steroids and mucolytic agents (drugs that thin secretions making it easier to clear the bronchi). The patient can experience side effects such as tremors, nausea, tachycardia, palpitations, nervousness, and dysrhythmias (see Chapter 14).

There are two commonly used inhalers. These are the hand-held nebulizer and the hand-held metered-dose device. The hand-held nebulizer changes liquid medication into a fine spray. The hand-held metered dose device is a small, metal container about 5 to 6 inches high, with a push button spray device on the top to release the medication.

Inhalers are not a very efficient way of delivering medications to the lungs because only 9% of the medication reaches the lungs. The efficiency increases by using a spacer, which delivers 21% of the medication to the lungs. The spacer is a funnel-like device that attaches to the mouthpiece of the metered dose inhaler (MDI). The medication is released into the spacer and then the patient inhales slowly and deeply to get the drug into the airway.

When administering medication using an inhaler:

- Check the prescriber's order.
- Position the patient in a semi- or high-Flower's position (sitting up).
- Teach the patient to wait 2 minutes between puffs of an MDI if the prescriber orders more than one puff.
- The patient should rinse his or her mouth with water and expectorate (spit) following inhalation of steroids because steroid inhalants promote oral fungal infections.

NASOGASTRIC AND GASTROSTOMY TUBE ROUTE

Nasogastric and gastrostomy tubes are used for patients who are unable to swallow or ingest anything orally. The nasogastric tube is passed through the nose and into the stomach opening with direct access to the stomach through which medication can be administered to the patient. The nasogastric tube is also used as a temporary feeding tube and to remove stomach contents. The gastrostomy tube is inserted through the skin and directly into the stomach and is used primarily as a permanent feeding tube that can also be used to administer medication.

When administering medication through the nasogastric tube and the gastrostomy tube:

- Check the prescriber's order.
- Be sure that the tube is in the proper position by one of two methods:
  1. Attach syringe to free end of NG tube; inject 1 or more 20 mL bursts of air into the tube. Aspirate gastric contents and check pH with test paper. If it is 0–4 the tube is in the stomach.
  2. Inject 10 mL of air through NG tube and listen with the stethoscope over the stomach for a rush of air. This is not done with a gastronomy tube.
- Remove the plunger from a syringe and pour medication into the syringe.
- Close the clamp on the nasogastric or gastrostomy tube.
- Attach the syringe to the nasogastric or gastrostomy tube.
- Open the clamp, pour the medication into the syringe and hold the tube up, allowing the medication to flow down the tube.

- Flush the tube with 30 to 50 mL of water.
- Close the clamp and remove the syringe.

SUPPOSITORIES ROUTE

Suppositories are used to administer medication via the rectum or the vagina, depending on the nature of the patient's condition or the type of medication. Rectal suppositories are the preferred route to administer medication when the patient's upper GI tract is not functioning properly or when the medication has an offensive taste or foul odor. It is also used when digestive enzymes change the chemical integrity of the medication.

The rectum promotes absorption of the medication because it contains many capillaries and can produce a high blood concentration of the medication.

When administering a suppository rectally:

- Check the prescriber's order.
- Provide the patient privacy.
- Position the patient in the Sims position (left side lying).
- Wash hands and then apply clean gloves.
- Lubricate the suppository, if necessary.
- Ask the patient to breathe through his or her mouth. This relaxes the anal sphincter.
- Insert the suppository.
- ask the patient to remain in the Sims position for 20 minutes.

When administering a suppository vaginally:

- Check the prescriber's order.
- Wash hands and then apply clean gloves.
- Place the patient in the lithotomy (on back with legs flexed at the knees) position.
- Insert the suppository using an applicator.
- Clean the vaginal area after the suppository is inserted.

PARENTERAL ROUTE

The parenteral route is where medication is injected into the patient using a syringe. There are four commonly used parenteral routes: intradermal (ID), subcutaneous (SC), intramuscular (IM), and intravenous (IV).

The choice of which of the parenteral routes to use is determined by the prescriber based on the nature of the medication, the desired onset of the therapeutic effect, and the patient's needs. For example, the test for TB is performed by injecting the purified protein derivative intradermally, which is under the skin. Insulin is injected subcutaneously, although regular insulin can also be administered intravenous. Medications administered intravenously have a faster onset of therapeutic effect than other parenteral routes. Vaccinations, some antibiotics, and other medications are injected intramuscularly.

INTRADERMAL

Intradermal injections are given in hairless areas of the body that are lightly pigmented and thinly keratinized so that the nurse can observe any reaction to the medication. These are:

- Inner aspect of forearm or scapular area of back.
- Upper chest.
- Medial thigh sites.

Medication injected intradermally has a localized effect because it does not enter the bloodstream. It usually causes a wheal (blister) to appear at the injection site. Injections are given using a 26–27 gauge needle and a 1 mL syringe calibrated in 0.01 mL increments. The typical injection is between 0.01 to 0.1 mL.

Here's how to administer medication intradermally:

- Check the prescriber's medication order.
- Wash hands and then put on clean gloves.
- Properly identify the patient.
- Cleanse the area of the site in a circular motion using alcohol or betadine, depending on the medication and agency policy.
- Hold the skin taut.
- Position the bevel up and insert the needle at a 10- to 15-degree angle. You should be able to see the outline of the needle through the skin.
- Inject slowly to form a wheal.
- Slowly remove the needle.
- Don't massage the area.
- Mark the site with a pen.
- Tell the patient not to wash the mark until a healthcare provider assesses the site for a reaction between 24 to 72 hours after the injection.

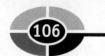
- Assess the patient in 24 to 72 hours. If the patient is allergic to the medication, then the diameter of the wheal should increase. If the patient is tested for TB, assess the hardness of the wheal and not the redness of the area.

SUBCUTANEOUS

The subcutaneous injection is suited for medications that need to be absorbed slowly to produce a sustained effect, such as insulin and heparin. Subcutaneous medications are absorbed through capillaries and the onset of the medication is slower than intramuscular and intravenous routes.

Choose an injection site that has an adequate fatpad. To prevent lypodystrophy, sites must be rotated if injections are given frequently. Lypodystrophy is a loss of the fat area under the skin causing ineffective absorption of insulin.

These sites are: abdomen, upper hips, upper back, lateral upper arms, and lateral thighs.

Subcutaneous injections are given using a 25–27-gauge needle that is $1/2$ or $5/8$ inches in length and with a 1 to 3 mL syringe calibrated 0.5 to 1.5 mL. However, syringes used for insulin are measured in units and not mL.

Here's how to administer medication subcutaneously:

- Check the prescriber's medication order.
- Wash hands and then put on clean gloves.
- Properly identify the patient.
- Cleanse the area of the site in a circular motion using alcohol, betadine, or soap and water as per agency policy.
- Pinch the skin.
- Insert the needle at 45–90-degree angle. 45 degree is preferred when the patient has a small amount of subcutaneous tissue.
- Release the skin.
- Inject the medication slowly.
- Quickly remove the needle.
- Gently massage the area unless heparin is injected.
- Apply a band aid as necessary.

INTRAMUSCULAR

Intramuscular injections are used so that the medication is rapidly absorbed into the patient's body. The absorption rate depends on the patient's circulatory state.

Usually no more than 5 mL of medication is injected for an adult and 3 mL for a child. If the prescriber orders a higher dose, divide the dose into two syringes.

Choose an injection site based on the size of the muscle with a minimum number of nerves and blood vessels in the area. These sites are:

- Ventrogluteal (hip)
- Dorsogluteal (buttocks)
- Deltoid (upper arm)
- Vastus lateralis (front of thigh)

See Table 6-1 for more details.

Intramuscular injections use a 20 to 23-gauge needle that is 1 to 1.5 inches in length and a 1 to 3 mL syringe that is calibrated with 0.5 mL to 1.5 mL.

Here's how to administer medication intramuscularly:

- Check the prescriber's medication order.
- Wash hands and then put on clean gloves.
- Properly identify the patient.
- Cleanse the area of the site in a circular motion, using using alcohol or betadine as per the agency guidelines.
- Flatten the skin at the injection site using your thumb and index finger.
- Insert the needle at a 90-degree angle into the muscle between your thumb and index finger.
- Release the skin.
- Slowly inject the medication.
- Quickly remove the needle.
- Gently massage the area (unless this is contraindicated by the medication).

Z-Track Injection Technique

The Z-Track inject technique is used to prevent medication from leaking back in the subcutaneous tissue after the medication has been injected into the patient. This technique is used whenever the medication—such as dextran (iron)—might cause a visible and permanent skin discoloration. The gluteal muscle is the preferred site for a Z-Track injection.

Here's how to administer medication using the Z-Track technique:

- Check the prescriber's medication order.
- Wash hands and then put on clean gloves.

Table 6-1.   Injection sites.

Injection Site	Description
Ventrogluteal	• Relatively free of major nerves and vascular branches. • Well-defined bony anatomic landmarks. • For IM or Z-Track injections. • Locate the site by placing the heel of your hand on the greater trochanter of the femur with the thumb pointed toward the umbilicus. The index finger marks the anterosuperior iliac spine. The middle finger traces the iliac crest curvature. The space between the index and middle fingers is the injection site.
Dorsogluteal	• Good site for IM and Z-track injections. • Danger to major nerves and vascular structures near site. • Easy to give subcutaneously by mistake when trying to give an IM because the fat is often very thick.
Deltoid	• Preferred site for vaccines. • Easily accessible. • Muscle mass is small compared to other sites. • Use a $5/8$ inch to 1.5 inch long needle • Locate the acromion process of the scapula and the deltoid. Measure 2 to 3 fingers below the acromion process on the lateral midline of the arm to identify the proper site. Inject at a 90-degree angle.
Vastus lateralis	• Preferred site for infants younger than 7 months. • It has a relatively large muscle mass. • Free from major nerves and vascular branches. • Site is a hand's breadth below the greater trochanter and above the knee. • Inject at a 45-degree angle toward the knee.

- Properly identify the patient.
- Cleanse the area of the site in a circular motion using alcohol or betadine as per the agency guidelines.
- Pull the skin to one side and hold it.
- Insert the needle at a 90-degree angle.
- Inject the medication as you hold the skin to one side.
- Withdraw the needle.
- Release the skin.

Tips for Minimizing Pain

Receiving medication via injection is a painful process for the patient. However, you can minimize the discomfort by following these tips:

- Encourage the patient to relax. The more they tense their muscle, the more the injection hurts.
- Replace the needle with a new needle after you withdraw medication from a vial or if the medication is irritating.
- Position the patient on his or her side—with knees flexed if you are using the ventrogluteal site. Position the patient flat on the abdomen with toes turned inward if you are using the dorsogluteal site. Use the same technique if the patient prefers to stand.
- Don't inject into sensitive or hardened tissues.
- Compress tissues at the injection site.
- You can prevent the antiseptic (e.g., alcohol wipe) from clinging to the needle during the injection by waiting for the antiseptic to dry before injecting the medication.
- Dart the needle to reduce puncture pain.
- Inject the medication slowly.
- Withdraw the needle quickly and straight.
- Use the Z-Track technique.
- Ask the patient to cough on the count of three. Inject the medication when the patient coughs.

INTRAVENOUS

Intravenous injections are used to provide rapid onset for a medication because the medication is directly injected into the circulatory system (IV push [IVP]). IVs can be placed in the cephalic or cubital vein of the arm or the dorsal vein of the hand. However, cubital veins should be avoided except in emergency situation because cubital veins are used for withdrawing blood specimens for laboratory testing. Start an IV at the hand and then work toward the cubital vein.

IV injections use a 21- to 23-gauge needle that are 1 to 1.5 inches in length. Use the larger bore for viscous (thicker) drugs. IV lines are inserted with a butterfly needle or with an angiocatheter that ranges from 14 gauge for whole blood or fractions of blood to 23 gauge for rapid infusion. Medication may be administered directly into the vein with a syringe, into an intermittent catheter inserted into the patient's vein, or injected into intravenous fluids such as 5% Dextrose in Water (D_5W) and delivered as an intravenous drip called a piggy back.

Here's how to administer medication IV:

- Check the prescriber's medication order.
- Wash hands and then put on clean gloves.
- Properly identify the patient.
- Cleanse the area of the site in a circular motion using alcohol or betadine as per the agency guidelines.
- Apply a tourniquet above the site.
- Insert the butterfly or catheter into the vein until blood returns through the butterfly or catheter.
- Remove the tourniquet.
- Stabilize the needle or catheter.
- Dress the site according to your healthcare agency's policy.
- Monitor the flow rate of the IV fluid, distal pulses, skin color (redness [infection]), skin temperature, insertion site for infiltration (swelling), and side effects of the medication since the action of the medication occurs rapidly.
- Follow policy agency policy regarding adding medications to the fluid in the bottle or bag, piggy back technique, and intravenous push.

Summary

Medication is given to a patient using one of several routes depending on the nature of the medication and the patient's condition. The prescriber selects the route, which is written in the medication order.

The oral route is used for tablets, capsules, liquids, suspensions, and elixirs. Don't use this route if the patient cannot swallow or is not conscious or alert.

The sublingual and buccal routes are used for rapid absorption of medication because blood vessels are close to the surface of the tongue and gums. The transdermal route is used for medication that can be absorbed through the skin by the use of a patch. The topical route is used to apply medication locally. The instillation route is used to administer medication through drops and sprays. Medication is directed to the lungs by using the inhalation route where the patient uses an inhaler.

If the patient has disruption of the upper GI tract, then the prescriber will order a nasogastric or gastrostomy tube. The nasogastric tube is inserted through the nose and into the stomach. The gastrostomy tube is inserted through the skin and directly into the stomach. Both of these tubes can be used to deliver medication to the patient.

The suppository route is used to absorb medication directly into the rectum or vagina. The parenteral route is used to inject medication directly into the dermal or subcutaneous tissue, muscle, or into the veins.

Quiz

1. A patient who is administered medication sublingually
   (a) has upper GI problems.
   (b) should ingest food or liquid to help absorption of the medication.
   (c) shouldn't eat or drink until the medication is absorbed.
   (d) None of the above.

2. If the dose of a transdermal patch is more than the prescriber's medication order
   (a) cut the patch to an appropriate length.
   (b) contact the prescriber.
   (c) do nothing.
   (d) give the patient the patch anyway.

3. When giving ear drops to a two-year-old,
   (a) pull the earlobe downward and back.
   (b) pull the earlobe upward and back.
   (c) pull the earlobe upward and forward.
   (d) pull the earlobe downward and forward.

4. A rectal suppository can be used if the patient cannot absorb medication in the upper GI tract.
   (a) True
   (b) False

5. The inner aspect of the forearm is the good site for an intradermal injection.
   (a) True
   (b) False

6. The Z-Track injection is used
   (a) to prevent medication from leaking back onto the tissue.
   (b) to prevent dislodging the needle.
   (c) to ease the pain of the injection.
   (d) None of the above.

7. Withdrawing a needle slowly decreases the pain of an injection.
   (a) True
   (b) False

8. A piggyback is inserted
   (a) into the IV tube.
   (b) into the patient's arm.
   (c) into the patient's leg.
   (d) None of the above.

9. The nurse should massage the site after giving a heparin injection.
   (a) True
   (b) False

10. Pinch the skin when giving an insulin injection.
    (a) True
    (b) False

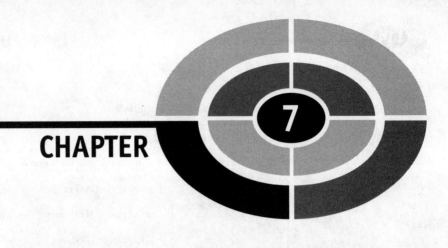

CHAPTER 7

Dose Calculations

Calculating the proper dose of medication is a critical aspect of administering medicine to a patient. Although the prescriber specifies a dose in the medication order, the dose prescribed may not be the same as the dose that is on hand, requiring the nurse to calculate a comparable dose based on available medication.

With intravenous (IV) medications, the prescriber might order a dose to be infused into the patient over a specific amount of time. The nurse must use this information to calculate the drip rate, which is used to set the IV so medication is administered at the proper rate.

Some medication orders prescribe a dose according to the patient's weight. The nurse is responsible for weighing the patient and then applying a formula provided by the prescriber to calculate the actual dose.

This chapter teaches you how to perform on hand calculations, IV calculations, and weight calculation in order to determine the proper amount of medication to administer.

The Metric System and Medication

Medication is prescribed in measurements of the metric system. Some students become anxious at just the mention of calculations. If you feel anxious and panicky, relax. We'll show you the easy way to perform these calculations.

Table 7-1. Units and their equivalents.

Unit	Purpose	Equivalents
Gram	Weight	1 kilogram (kg) = 1000 grams (g)
		1 gram (g) = 1000 milligrams (mg)
		1 milligram = 1000 micrograms (mcg)
		1 kilometer = 1000 liters
Liter	Volume	1 liter (L) = 1000 milliliters (mL) = 1000 cubic centimeters (cc)
		1 milliliter (mL) = 1 cubic centimeter (cc)

Medication calculation requires you to know how to multiply and divide. You'll also need to know six metric measurements and five household measurements (ounces, teaspoon, tablespoon, cup and drop).

Let's begin with the metric system. The metric system uses grams to measure weight and liters to measure volume as shown in Table 7-1. Prefixes are used to indicate the number of grams and liters. Table 7-2 shows the commonly used prefixes that you'll see when calculating medication.

Each prefix indicates the value. The prefix is placed before the unit of measure such as 1 kilogram or 1 milliliter. Look at Kilo in Table 7-2. The factor is 1000, which is larger than a gram or liter. Therefore, you multiple the gram or liter by 1000. That is, a kilogram is 1000 grams and a kiloliter is 1000 liters. The important point to remember is that the prefix of the measure implies the size of the measurement.

Table 7-2. Prefixes used in medication.

Unit	Purpose	Equivalents
Kilo	1000	One thousand times
Centi	0.01	One hundredth part of
Milli	0.001	One thousandth part of
Micro	0.000001	One millionth part of

HOUSEHOLD MEASUREMENTS

Household measurements are used for liquid medications that are given to patients in the home setting. An example is two teaspoons of cough medication. Nurses encounter household measurements when providing home healthcare services and when determining a patient's fluid intake and output in the hospital setting. Nurses also use pounds when calculating a dose that is based on a patient's weight. Patients should use measuring spoons for medication administration at home and avoid using tableware.

Patients are usually more comfortable self-administering medication if the dose is in household measurements. However, medication is recorded using metric measurements. Therefore, a nurse must be able to convert household measurements to metric measurements.

Let's say that the patient drinks an 8-ounce glass of orange juice. The nurse must convert that to milliliters (mL) or cubic centimeters (cc) in order to record the intake volume in the patient's fluid input and output chart. (Remember 1 mL = 1 cc.)

Table 7-3 contains commonly used conversion factors for household measurement and metric measurement.

Table 7-3.   Commonly used conversion factors for household measurement and metric measurement.

Household System	Metric System
Weight	
2.2 pounds (lb)	1 kilogram (kg)
Volume	
1 ounce	30 mL = 30 cc
16 ounces	500 mL = 500 cc
32 ounces	1000 mL = 1000 cc
1 liter	1000 mL = 1000 cc
Household Measurement	
60 drops (gtt)	1 teaspoon (tsp)
1 teaspoon (tsp)	5 mL = 5 cc
1 tablespoon (tbs)	15 mL = 15 cc
2 tablespoons (tbs)	1 ounce = 30 mL = 30 cc

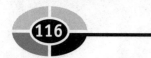

Converting Metric Units

Let's take a look at how to convert units of the metric system. You'll need to learn how to convert from one metric unit to another (e.g., grams to milligrams) in order to arrive at like units when calculating a dose. For example, if the dose is in milligrams and the prescriber's medication order specifies grams, you'll need to convert grams to milligrams before calculating the dose.

Converting from one metric unit to another metric unit isn't difficult if you remember these three rules.

1. Determine if the desired measurement is larger or smaller than the given measurement. Remember that gram, liter, and meter are larger units and milligram, milliliter, and millimeter are smaller units.
2. If you are converting from a smaller unit to a larger unit, then you multiply by moving the decimal three places to the left.
3. If you are converting from a larger unit to a smaller unit, then you divide by moving the decimal three places to the right.

Suppose the medication order is 300 mg and you need to convert this to grams. A milligram is smaller than a gram. You are converting from a smaller unit (a milligram) to a larger unit (a gram). Therefore, you divide by moving the decimal three places to the left, as shown here.

$$300 \text{ mg} \div 1000 = 0.3 \text{ g}$$

If the prescriber ordered 0.9 grams and the dose that you need is in milligrams, you are converting from a larger unit (a gram) to a smaller unit (a milligram). Therefore, you multiply by moving the decimal three places to the right, as shown here.

$$0.9 \text{ g} \times 1000 = 900 \text{ mg}$$

One of the most common conversions that you'll perform is converting milliliters into cubic centimeters. This is also the easiest conversion because one milliliter (mL) is equal to 1 cubic centimeter (cc).

Always place a zero to the left of the decimal when the quantity is not a whole number. This avoids errors when reading the number.

Incorrect: .9
Correct: 0.9

CONVERTING HOUSEHOLD UNITS AND METRIC

You'll find yourself having to convert between household and metric units when you calculate a patient's input and output volume and when you provide home healthcare to a patient. There, you'll use a teaspoon, tablespoon, or cups measured in ounces to administer medication.

When converting from milliliters or cubic centimeters to ounces, divide by 30, as shown here: [Remember 30 cc (30 mL) = 1 oz.]

$$240 \text{ mL} \div 30 = 8 \text{ oz}$$
$$60 \text{ cc} \div 30 = 2 \text{ oz}$$

When converting from ounces to milliliters or cubic centimeters, multiple by 30, as shown here:

$$2 \text{ oz} \times 30 = 60 \text{ mL}$$
$$4 \text{ oz} \times 30 = 120 \text{ mL}$$

When converting from pounds to kilograms, divide by 2.2, as shown here: Remember 2.2 lbs = 1 kilogram

$$22 \text{ lbs} \div 2.2 = 10 \text{ kilograms}$$

When converting from kilograms to pounds, multiple by 2.2, as shown here:

$$63 \text{ kg} \times 2.2 = 138.6 \text{ pounds}$$

Formulas for Calculating the Desired Dose

In the ideal world, the prescriber will write a medication prescription that has a dose that is available in the hospital. For example, the medication prescription is for a 15-mg tablet of Inderal and the hospital has on hand a 15-mg tablet of Inderal.

In the real world, the dose specified in the medical prescription may not be available. The hospital might have 10-mg tablets of Inderal and not the 15-mg tablets prescribed. Instead of asking the prescriber to change the medication order, the nurse calculates the proper medication to give the patient based on the medication order and the dose that is on hand.

In this example, the nurse calculates that the patient should receive 1.5 tablets of Inderal. This means that the nurse must divide one tablet into halves.

There are two methods nurses can use to calculate the desired dose. These are the formula method or the ratio-proportion method. Either method will produce same result. When applying either method, make sure that all the terms are in the same units before calculating the desired dose. For example, the medication order might be in grams and the dose on hand might be in milligrams. The nurse will need to convert the grams to milligrams before calculating the desired dose to give. Always convert to the unit of the "have" dose.

The formula method uses the following formula to determine the correct dose.

$$\frac{D}{H} \times V = A$$ Quantity (Desired dose divided by dose you have multiplied by vehicle of drug you have equals the amount calculated to be given to the patient)

D = desired dose
H = dose you have
V = vehicle you have (tablets or liquids)
A = amount calculated to be given to the patient

Ratio and proportion method

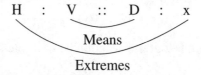

H is the drug on hand (available)
V is the vehicle or drug form (tablet, capsule, liquid)
D is the desired dose (as prescribed)
x is the unknown amount to give, and
:: stands for "as" or "equal to."

Multiply the means and the extremes. Solve for x; x is the divisor.

Example: Give 500 mg of ampicillin sodium by mouth when the dose on hand is in capsules containing 250 mg.

500 mg divided by 250 mg multiplied by 1 capsule = 2 capsules

Formula method:

$$\frac{500\,mg}{250\,mg} \times \frac{capsule}{1} = 2 \text{ capsules}$$

Example: Give 375 mg of ampicillin when it is supplied as 250 mg/5mL.

375 mg divided by 250 mg multiplied by 5 mL = 7.5 mL

Example: Diltiazem (Cardizem) 60 mg PO b.i.d. On hand are 30 mg tablets.

$$\frac{60\,mg}{30\,mg} \times tablet = 2 \text{ tablets}$$

Ratio and Proportion Method:
Prescribed: Amoxicillin 100 mg PO q.i.d.
Available: Amoxil (amoxicillin) 80 mL

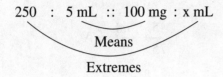

250   :   5 mL :: 100 mg : x mL

Means

Extremes

250x = 500
  x = 2mL

Answer: Amoxicillin 100 mg = 2 mL
Prescribed: Aspirin/ASA gr x, q4h, PRN for headache
Available: Aspirin 325 mg/tablet

a. Convert to one system and unit of measure. Change grains to milligrams

b.

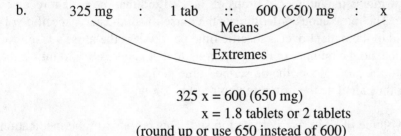

325 mg   :   1 tab   ::   600 (650) mg   :   x

Means

Extremes

325 x = 600 (650 mg)
x = 1.8 tablets or 2 tablets
(round up or use 650 instead of 600)

Be sure to label all the terms in the formula with the appropriate unit. This will help to prevent errors. For example, use mg following a value in the formula if the value is in milligrams.

Parenteral Medications

Parenteral medication is a medication that is administered to a patient by an injection or by an intravenous flow. The dose for an injection is calculated using the formula method or the ratio-proportion method that is described previously in this chapter.

For example, the prescriber might order Demerol 45mg IM prn to alleviate the patient's pain. The Demerol label states 75 mg/mL. This is the dose you have. The nurse must calculate the number of milliliters that should be administered to the patient.

Using the basic formula $\left(\dfrac{D}{H} \times V = A\right)$ here's the calculation:

$$\frac{45\,mg}{75\,mg} \times \frac{1\,mL}{1} = A$$

$$\frac{45}{75} \times \frac{1\,mL}{1} = A$$

$$\frac{45\,mL}{75} = .6\,mL$$

CALCULATING THE IV FLOW RATE FOR CONTINUOUS OR INTERMITTENT (PIGGYBACK) INFUSIONS

The IV flow rate is the number of drops of the IV fluid that the patient receives in a minute. The intravenous order directs the nurse to administer a specific volume of fluid to the patient over a specific time period. It is the nurse's responsibility to calculate the number of drops per minute that is necessary to infuse the IV fluid into the patient over the prescribed time period.

In order the calculate the drip rate you need to know:

- The volume of fluid that is to be infused. This is found in the medication order in milliliters (mL) or cubic centimeters (cc).
- The amount of time over which the infusion is to take place.
- The drip factor, which is specified on the IV tubing that is used for the infusion.

Here's how to calculate the drip rate. It is important to remember that although we use milliliters in the following examples, you can substitute cubic centimeters (cc) for milliliters (mL) if cc is specified in the order. Always express gtt/min in whole numbers. Always carry out to the tenth then round to nearest whole number. If a volumetric pump is used to deliver the IV fluid, then you'll need to use cc per hour.

Total fluid multiplied by drip factor and divided by the infusion time in minutes.

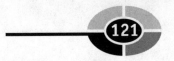

Medical prescription: 250 ml 5% D/W to infusion over 10 hours. Drip factor 60.

Total fluid = 250 mL(cc)

Drip factor = 60 gtts/min

Infusion time in minutes = 600 min

$$\frac{250\,\text{mL} \times 60\,\text{gtts}/\text{min}}{600\,\text{minutes}} = \frac{15,000\,\text{mL}}{600\,\text{min}} = 25\,\text{gtts}/\text{minute}$$

Heparin infusion

Heparin is a medication that inhibits the formation of platelets and can be administered either as a subcutaneous injection or as a continuous intravenous infusion. The proper dose of heparin is always calculated using either the formula method or the ratio-proportion method.

Example: Medical prescription: Heparin 7500 Units SC

Available Heparin 10,000 Units per mL

Using the formula method:

$$\frac{7500\,\text{units}}{10,000\,\text{units}} \times \text{mL} = .75\ \text{mL}$$

Summary

The dose specified in a medication order may not be the same dose for the medication that you have on hand. Therefore, you must calculate a new dose that is proportional to the prescribed dose.

All doses are calculated using the metric system. You must be able to convert within the metric system and convert between household measurements and metric because patients are likely to self medicate using household measurement—such as a teaspoon—rather than using metric measurements.

Converting between metric units is performed by moving the decimal to the left or right depending on whether you are moving from a smaller metric unit to a larger metric unit or vice versa. Converting between household measurements and metric is achieved by multiplying or dividing using a conversion factor. This depends on whether you are converting from household measurements to metric or vice versa.

There are two methods that are used to calculate a dose. These are the formula method and the ratio-proportion method. Both use the on hand dose of a medication to determine the desired dose based on the medication prescription.

The formula method and the ratio-proportion method are also used to calculate parenteral medications. Alternatively, parenteral medication can be administered through a vein either as a bolus or an infusion. If infusing through an intravenous line, the nurse must calculate the number of drops per minute the IV should run to deliver the amount of medication ordered.

We'll leave the topic of preparing medications and explore medications that are available in nature in the form of herbs. You'll learn about herbal therapy in the next chapter.

Quiz

1. Prescribed: Duricef 0.4G PO QID. On hand: Duricef 200 mg capsules. How many capsules do you need?
   (a) 1 capsule
   (b) 2 capsules
   (c) 5 capsules
   (d) 20 capsules

2. Prescribed: Ceclor 150 mg. On hand: Ceclor 300 mg tablets. How many tablets do you need?
   (a) 30 tablets
   (b) 5 tablets
   (c) 50 tablets
   (d) 0.5 tablets

3. Prescribed: 1000 mL of 0.9% normal saline (NS) intravenously every 8 hours. The intravenous tubing delivers 15 gtts/mL. How many gtts/min (drops per minute) will be infused?
   (a) 31 gtts/min
   (b) 44 gtts/min
   (c) 25 gtts/min
   (d) 28 gtts/min

4. Prescribed: Diabenese 600 mg. On hand: Diabenese 300 mg tablets. You need 2 tablets.
   (a) True
   (b) False

5. Ordered: 1 liter of NS q 7h. Available 1 liter of NS and IV tubing with a drip factor of 10. You would regulate the IV at 23.8 gtts/min.
   (a) True
   (b) False

6. Prescribed: Heparin 1000 units/hour intravenously. Available: Heparin 25,000 units/hour in 250 cc D5W. How many mL/hr should be administered to give the correct dose?
   (a) 0.10 mL/hr
   (b) 1.0 mL/hr
   (c) 10 mL/hr
   (d) None of the above

7. Prescribed: 1 liter of D5W q8h. Available: 1 liter of D5W and IV tubing 10 gtts/mL. You regulate the IV at 20.8 gtts/min.
   (a) True
   (b) False

8. Prescribed: 1000 mL of IV fluid q12h. Available: 1000 mL of IV fluid and microdrip tubing. How many gtts per minute will you regulate the IV?
   (a) 83 gtt/min
   (b) 83.3 gtt/min
   (c) 8.33 gtt/min
   (d) 0.833 gtt/min

9. Prescribed is Prilosec 4.4 mg/kg for a child who weights 88 lbs. Available is Prilosec 50 mg/5 mL. You would give the child 1.76 mL.
   (a) True
   (b) False

10. Prescribed is Ceclor 2 mg/kg for a child who weighs 20 lbs. Available is Ceclor 20 mg/2 mL. You would administer 1.8 mL.
    (a) True
    (b) False

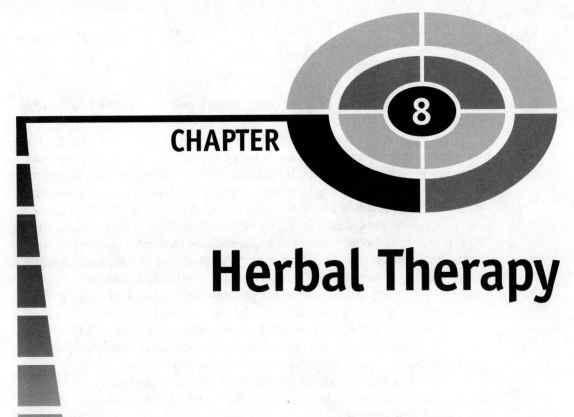

CHAPTER 8

Herbal Therapy

Ever wonder how people survived centuries ago when there wasn't a local pharmacy and the local physician was several days travel? They used plants—called herbs—as medicine to treat the common cold, infections, diseases of the GI tract, and anything else that ailed them.

Today, herbal therapy has made a comeback as an alternative to prescription medication and OTC remedies. Herbs continue to elicit a therapeutic effect on patients. However, patients are exposed to risk. There isn't a quality standard for herbal therapy and many herbs can cause adverse reactions when combined with prescription and OTC medication.

In this chapter, you'll learn about the therapeutic effect of herbal therapies and about the nursing process that should be implemented to prevent patients from developing an adverse reaction to herbal therapy when combined with conventional therapy.

Inside Herbal Therapy

In recent years, herbal therapies have gained popularity as multimillion-dollar businesses have capitalized on the therapeutic properties of natural herbs and the fact that herbs are exempt from the government regulations imposed on the pharmaceutical industry.

Herbs are plants or parts of plants that have a proven therapeutic effect. These were the "original" medicines. Even today, physicians in Germany and other countries prescribe herbs as the first choice when combating certain diseases.

However, herbs are not typically prescribed in the United States for a number of reasons. Few pharmacy schools offer courses in botanical remedies and some nursing pharmaceutical courses focus more on misuse of herbal therapies than their proper use. Probably the most leading reason that herbs are not prescribed is that health insurance in the United States does not pay for these therapies.

Herbal therapies cannot be patented, which is a likely reason why the pharmaceutical industry hasn't pushed the government and the medical community to use herbal therapies as treatment for diseases and symptoms of diseases.

The Food and Drug Administration is not required to approve herbal therapies. This creates an open and unregulated market for herbal therapies that lacks quality standards found in the pharmaceutical industry.

In 1992, Congress instructed the National Institutes of Health to develop an Office of Alternative Medicine to support research studies of alternative therapies—including herbals.

Interestingly, herbs are the raw material of old and new pharmaceutical medication. For example, the herb foxglove is the source for digitalis and the herb salicin is the source for aspirin. The breast-cancer-fighting drug Taxol comes from the pacific yew tree.

Although the therapeutic effect of herbs have been well known for thousands of years, there seems to be a lack of uniform information about them that describes their use, dosage, side effects, and contraindications. This is information that is available for all prescription and OTC pharmaceutical medications.

In addition, there aren't any qualitative monographs that provide guidelines for compounding and standards of purity for herbal medication. That is, there isn't a well-defined measurement for purity and manufacturing of herbal medication as there is for prescription and OTC pharmaceutical medications.

An effort has been launched by the United States Pharmacopeia (USP), the World Health Organization (WHO), American Herbal Phamarcopeia (AHP), and others to develop herbal therapeutic monographs that provide this information for herbal therapies.

One in five people in the United States who have taken prescription medication also have taken herbal medications. And while herbal preparations can be therapeutic, the lack of quality standards and contraindication with prescribed and OTC medication exposes patients to potential toxicity and other adverse side effects.

Forms of Herbal Therapies

Herbs are plants or parts of plants that contain medicinal qualities. Some herbs can be taken as whole. One such herb is fresh aloe, which can be used topically to treat burns and minor cuts. Other herbs must be transformed into a form that is suitable for ingestion.

Herbs are living organisms that have a very short life after they are removed from their source of nutrition (that is, picked from the ground). Enzyme activity begins to cause the herb to decay immediately after the herb is harvested. Therefore, steps must be taken to preserve the herb by drying it in sunlight or by using another heat source. Drying removes moisture and lowers the enzyme activity. This enables the herb to retain its therapeutic qualities for up to six months.

Extraction techniques are used to remove the therapeutic material from an herb. The most commonly used extraction technique is to first isolate the part of the herb that contains the therapeutic material and then soak that part in alcohol or water. This helps to produce a reliable dose.

Some extractions take the form of oils. Herbal oil is prepared by soaking the dried herb in olive oil or vegetable oil and heating the herb for an extended period of time. Oils promote the concentration of the therapeutic material and, if properly stored, extend the therapeutic life of the material for months.

Herbal therapies also come in the form of salves. Salves are semi-solid fatty preparations such as balms, creams, and ointments. They are prepared in a way similar to herbal oils except once the dried herb is soaked in oil, melted wax is mixed with the oil. It is left to cool and harden to form the therapeutic balm, cream, or ointment.

Herbal tea is another popular form of herbal therapy. Herbal tea is made by soaking fresh or dried herbs in boiling water. Once the herb blends with the water, the resulting tea can be stored in the refrigerator for later use as a drink, bath water additive, or applied topically in a compress to the skin.

Herbs are also available as tinctures. Chaparral tincture, for example, contains important ingredients that cannot be dissolved in water. Tinctures are also a convenient way to take herbs that does not require kitchen preparation. Disagreeable-tasting herbs can be swallowed more quickly and can be masked with juice. Tinctures are made by soaking fresh or dried herbs in water or alcohol causing the water-soluble and fat-soluble components of the herb to concentrate. The concentrate is the desired form. Water is used for people who do not consume alcohol. Alcohol is used to preserve the herbal concentrate for a year.

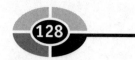

Herbal capsule is another common form of herbal therapy. The herb is dried and pulverized into a powder that is placed inside the capsule. Some herbal capsules contain oil-soaked herbals or herbal juices.

Herbal tablets are similar to herbal capsules except the dried, pulverized herb is combined with stabilizers and binders and then compressed into a tablet. A stabilizer is an ingredient that assures that the herb maintains its therapeutic effect. A binder is an ingredient that acts like glue to hold together the powdery mixture of herb and stabilizer.

Herbal therapy can also take the form of syrup. Syrups are made by drying the herb and soaking it in water or oil and then adding a sweetener to the mix. The sweetener is usually honey or sugar. The sweetened mixture is then heated until the syrup forms. Herbal syrups are used to treat colds, cough, and sore throat.

Hazards of Herbal Therapeutics

Herbal therapies have a therapeutic effect and are acceptable interventions for diseases and symptoms. However, the lack of standards in manufacturing and lack of oversight by regulatory agencies exposes patients to potential hazards.

Pharmaceuticals approved for distribution in the Untied States have undergone rigorous testing that identifies the purity and concentration of the active ingredient that delivers the therapeutic effect. This also identifies the toxic levels that can cause serious and potentially lethal toxic effects. In addition, testing also identifies the effect a pharmaceutical has when combined with other prescribed or OTC medications.

Herbal therapies lack this testing for a number of reasons. These include the expense of these tests and the lack of regulation. Anyone can sell herbal therapy without having to receive approval from a governmental agency or from the medical community.

A major concern is the effect herbal therapy has on the patient who is also taking prescribed medications. Medication interaction is always a risk. A prescriber should always ask what medication the patient is taking and review the patient's chart before prescribing another medication.

For example, a patient who takes cascara—a laxative for constipation—and senna—also a laxative—along with Digoxin—which is used to treat an irregular heart rhythm—can develop a toxicity. Likewise, taking juniper—a diuretic that causes increased urination—and dandelion—also a diuretic—along with

Lithium, which is a commonly prescribed psychiatric medication, elevates the therapeutic effect of Lithium and can result in a toxic level.

Another hazard is the route in which herbal therapy is administered. For example, comfrey is used as an ointment to relieve swelling that is associated with abrasions and sprains. However, internal use can cause liver damage. Some comfrey therapies are designed for internal use. One such use is treating a cough using comfrey as an expectorant.

The herbal dietary supplement ephedra, commonly known as ma huang, is used as an energy boost and for losing weight. Ephedrine and pseudoephedrine are components of ephedra that have a stimulant and bronchodilation effect. However, ephedra has an adverse effect of palpitations—which can result in stroke.

Herbal Therapy and the Nursing Process

Nurses need to include a discussion about the patient's use of nonconventional therapeutic agents by name, dosage, frequency, side effects and why the patient is taking this remedy in the nursing assessment. This assessment should include information about all prescription and over-the-counter medications taken by the patient and why the patient is taking these drugs. Herbal medications, over the counter medications, and prescribed medications can combine to create undesirable results and in some cases can have a toxic and dangerous effect on the patient.

After assessing the patient, the nurse considers a nursing diagnosis that is related to herbal therapies. These are:

- *Knowledge deficit*. The patient may be unaware of the impact herbal therapies have on the patient's health.
- *Altered nutrition*. The patient may be unaware of how herbal therapies alter the patient's nutritional balance.
- *Side effects*. The patient might be experiencing nausea, diarrhea, headache, fatigue, and other symptoms that are side effects of herbal therapies.
- *Toxicity*. The patient might be experiencing a toxic effect as a result of interactions of herbal therapies with prescribed medications.
- *Alteration in skin integrity*. The patient might have developed a reaction to the herbal therapy such as a rash.

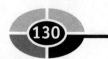

After choosing a nursing diagnosis that is related to herbal therapy, the nurse plans for the proper intervention. The goals are:

1. The patient will verbalize an understanding of the risks of herbal therapy.
2. The patient will verbalize an understanding of the interaction between herbal therapy and conventional therapy.

The nurse intervenes by:

- Monitoring the patient's response to conventional and herbal therapy looking for adverse side effects.
- Consulting with dietitians and other healthcare specialists to assure that the patient's nutrition remains balanced.
- Telling the patient to continue with the same brand of herbs and to notify the healthcare provider if there is a change in brand.
- Teaching the patient to
  - Understand the rationale for herbal therapy,
  - Notifying healthcare providers if he or she plans to substitute herbals for conventional therapies,
  - Read all labels,
  - Review the optimal storage for the herbal remedy,
  - Know what foods increase or decrease the action of the herbs,
  - Review the potential side effects, symptoms that require prompt reporting to healthcare provider, and the correct preparation for use of herbals.
- Evaluating the patient for the effectiveness of herbal remedies for alleviating symptoms and the patient's knowledge regarding the use of herbals.

The Do's and Don'ts About Herbs

- Don't take if pregnant or trying to become pregnant.
- Don't take if breast feeding.
- Don't give to babies or young children.
- Don't take large quantities.
- Buy herbs with the plant and quantities listed on the package.
- Don't stop taking prescribed medication before contacting the healthcare provider.

- Keep herbs away from children.
- Use fresh herbs.
- Don't delay seeking healthcare if you experience adverse symptoms.
- Herbs are not a miracle cure.

Make sure that the patient thinks of herbs as medicine that is less potent than conventional medication. However, adverse reactions can occur if conventional medication is taken with herbal therapy. For example, some conventional medication may act faster than expected when combined with herbal therapy.

The patient should not take any herbal where the following information is not included on the packaging:

- Scientific name of the product and the part of the plant used in the preparation
- Manufacturer's name and address
- Batch and lot number
- Date of manufacture and expiration.

Commonly Used Herbs

The following is a list of commonly used herbs.

ALOE VERA (ALOE BARBADENSIS)

Aloe Vera juice is used to treat minor burns, insect bites, and sunburn. It is also a powerful laxative when taken internally and can increase menstrual flow if given in small doses.

CHAMOMILE (MATRICARIA RECUTITA)

Chamomile is dried flower heads that are used in herbal tea for relief of digestive and GI disruptions such as irritable bowel syndrome and infant colic. Chamomile also has a sedative effect. It is also used in instances where the patient is allergic to daisy or ragweed-like plants. Chamomile can cause hives and bronchoconstriction.

DONG QUAI (ANGELICA SINESIS)

Dong Quai is used for menstrual cramps and to regulate the menstrual cycle. In rare instances, Dong Quai causes fever and excessive menstrual bleeding. Experts on herbal therapy recommend that patients avoid using Dong Quai.

ECHINACEA (ECHINACEA ANGUSTIFOLIA)

Echinacea enhances immunity by increasing white blood cells, cells in the spleen, and by activating granulocytes. The Echinacea leaf is used to combat respiratory and urinary infections. Native Americans use Echinacea to treat snake bites. Its root is used to treat symptoms of the flu. Patients with auto-immune disease and abnormal T-cell functions—such as those found in HIV, AIDS, and TB—should avoid Echinacea.

GARLIC (ALLIUM SATIVUM)

Garlic is a common herb used in food preparation and is reported to lower cholesterol and triglyceride levels and decrease blood pressure and reduce the clotting capability of blood. Garlic is also an antibiotic for internal and external treatment of infections and wounds. Warm garlic oil is used to treat ear aches. Garlic is also known as the herb of endurance.

GINGER (ZINGIBER)

Ginger increases the effectiveness of the immune system and is used to treat stomach and digestive disorders including motion sickness. Ginger is found to relieve nausea and relieves pain, swelling, and stiffness from osteoarthritis and rheumatoid arthritis.

GINKGO (GINKGO BILOBA)

Ginkgo is the most commonly used herbal therapy in the world and is used to increase the dilation of cerebral arteries and increase the uptake of oxygen and glucose. Ginkgo has been found useful for treating dementia syndromes, intermittent claudication (decreased circulation in the legs), vertigo (dizziness), and tinnitus (ringing in the ears). There is also evidence that Ginkgo improves cognition (thinking) and may be helpful in Alzheimer's disease, early stroke, and Raynaud's phenomenon (circulatory disorder). In rare instances, patients who take Ginkgo experience headache and GI disturbance.

GINSENG (PANAX GINSENG)

Ginseng is taken for short-term relief of stress and as an energy boost. Ginseng is also used to improve digestion. Red Korean and Chinese Ginseng are used for chronic inflammatory conditions such as arthritis.

KAVE KAVA (PIPER METHYSTICUM)

Kave Kava root promotes sleep and muscle relaxation. In tea, Kave Kava combats urinary tract infections. Some patients used Kave Kava with herbs such as valerian and St. John's Wort for anxiety.

LICORICE (GLYCYRRHIZA GLABRA)

Licorice seems to have physiologic effects similar to aldosterone (an anti-hypertensive) and corticosteroids (an anti-inflammatory) and is related to gly-cyrrhizin, which is a major ingredient.

PEPPERMINT (MENTHE PIPERITA)

Peppermint stimulates appetite and aids in digestion and treatment of bowel disorders when taken internally. Hot peppermint tea stimulates circulation, reduces fever, clears congestion, and helps restore energy. Peppermint is also an effective treatment for tension headache when rubbed on the forehead. Some research has shown peppermint to be as effective as Extra-strength Tylenol in relieving headache.

PSYLLIUM (PLANTAGO)

The psyllium seed is used as a laxative and for the treatment of hemorrhoids, colitis, Crohn's disease, and irritable bowel syndrome.

SAGE (SALVIA OFFICINALIS)

Dry sage leaves are used to heal wounds. Tea made from sage leaves soothes a sore throat when gargled. Sage also helps to dry mother's milk and reduce hot flashes. Sage is known as the herb of longevity.

ST. JOHN'S WORT (HYPERICUM PERFORATUM)

St. John's Wort is used to treat depression, anxiety, and psychogenic disturbances similar to the way monoamine oxidase (MAO) is used. However, unlike MAO, patients who use St. John's Wort do not have to avoid tyramine-rich foods. St. John's Wort is also known as "herbal prozac." Besides its psychological effect, St. John's Wort is also a dietary supplement in the United States, although it does not have FDA approval.

SAW PALMETTO (SERENOA REPENS)

Saw Palmetto relieves symptoms of benign prostatic hypertrophy (enlarged prostate) and other urinary conditions. Saw Palmetto is also used as an expectorant and treatment for colds, asthma, bronchitis, and thyroid deficiency.

VALERIAN (VALERIANA OFFICINALIS)

Valerian is a mild sedative and sleep-inducing agent that has an effect similar to benzodiazepines. It has been called herbal valium. However, Valerian has an odor of "dirty socks" making it a very low risk for overdose. There have been no reports that frequent use of Valerian leads to habituation and addiction.

YARROW (ACHILLEA MILLEFOLIUM)

Yarrow stops bleeding wounds and is used as a healing lotion and ointment. It also is used to reduce pain and heavy bleeding due to menstrual irregularities and helps to regulate the menstrual cycle. Yarrow enhances circulation, lowers blood pressure, and has an antispasmodic and anti-microbial effect. It also has an anti-inflammatory effect on skin and on mucous membranes. The most frequently reported side effect of Yarrow is dermatitis (skin rash). Yarrow should not be used for patients who have epilepsy or are pregnant.

Summary

Herbal therapy is the use of plants called herbs to treat symptoms and diseases. The government and the medical community do not regulate herbal therapies. This results in a lack of standards for the manufacture and sale of herbal therapies. The quality, purity, dosage, and side effects may be different for the same herb.

There are different forms of herbal therapies. These are oils, balms, creams, ointments, teas, tinctures, capsules, tablets, and syrups. Although herbs are available in these forms, some herbs should only be administered externally and not used internally.

While herbal therapies provide patients with a therapeutic effect, they can also leave the patient exposed to hazards. When combined with conventional therapies, herbal therapies can produce a toxic effect or an adverse reaction.

The nurse should ask if the patient is taking herbal therapies and, if so, for what condition. The patient should be taught about herbal therapies, the risks and benefits, and then given clear instructions on how to continue herbal therapies while undergoing conventional treatment—if approved by the patient's healthcare provider.

Quiz

1. Herbal therapies
    (a) require FDA approval.
    (b) are safe to use to self-medicate as long as the patient isn't undergoing conventional therapy.
    (c) are industry regulated.
    (d) are none of the above.

2. The "herbal prozac" is
    (a) sage.
    (b) St. John's Wort.
    (c) psyllium.
    (d) Kave Kava.

3. The patient should not take an herb unless which of the following information in on the package?
    (a) Scientific name
    (b) Manufacturer's name and address
    (c) Batch and lot number
    (d) All of the above

4. Chamomile should not be taken by a patient who is allergic to ragweed.
   (a) True
   (b) False

5. Peppermint relieves migraine headaches when rubbed on the forehead.
   (a) True
   (b) False

6. A patient who complains about palpitations and who is undergoing herbal therapy may be taking
   (a) comfrey.
   (b) chamomile.
   (c) ma huang.
   (d) ginkgo.

7. Patients should never use herbal therapies.
   (a) True
   (b) False

8. What herb has a therapeutic effect similar to Benadryl?
   (a) Ginseng
   (b) Zingiber
   (c) Valerian
   (d) None of the above

9. The nurse should instruct the patient on how to monitor for adverse side effects of herbal therapies.
   (a) True
   (b) False

10. Comfrey is an ointment used to relieve swelling associated with abrasions and sprains.
    (a) True
    (b) False

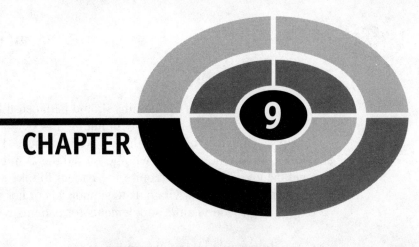

CHAPTER 9

Vitamins and Minerals

Growing up, you may have been told it is important to eat a well-balanced meal so that you get the vitamins and minerals needed to build a strong, healthy body. As kids, we probably consider this a ploy to finish our supper. We developed a respect for those words because vitamins and minerals are necessary to remain healthy.

Some patients may not eat a balanced diet for various reasons. Therefore, it is critical that you assess the patient for vitamin and mineral deficiencies and administer the prescribed therapy to restore the patient's nutritional balance.

In this chapter you'll learn about vitamins and minerals and how to assess patients for deficiencies. You'll also learn about vitamin therapy and mineral therapy and how to educate your patient about proper nutrition.

Vitamins

Vitamins are organic chemicals that are required for metabolic activities necessary for tissue growth and healing. Under normal conditions, only a small amount of vitamins—which are provided by eating a well balanced diet—are necessary.

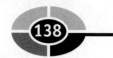
However, larger amounts of vitamins should be taken if the patient is pregnant, undergoing rapid growth or has a debilitating illness.

Likewise, patients who do not have a well-balanced diet (such as the elderly, alcoholics, children, and those who go on fad diets) might also develop a vitamin deficiency. That would require the patient to take vitamin supplements to assure there are sufficient vitamins to support his or her metabolism.

Expect to provide vitamin supplements for patients who have:

- Conditions that inhibit absorption of food.
- Diarrhea.
- Infection and fever.
- Inflammatory diseases.
- Cancer.
- Inability to use vitamins.
- Undergoing hemodialysis.
- Hyperthyroidism.
- GI surgery.
- Fad diets.
- Are pregnant.
- Growing children.

WELL-BALANCED DIET

Many patients realize the importance of having a well-balanced diet. Few however, know what constitutes a well-balanced diet. Patients can use the U.S. Department of Agriculture's (USDA) definition of a well-balanced diet as a guideline.

The USDA uses a food pyramid to illustrate the mixture of food groups that are necessary for us to receive the proper amount of vitamins and minerals for a healthy life. Recently the USDA revised its longstanding food pyramid to reflect the individual needs of people of a specific age, sex, and activity group. The previous food pyramid placed everyone in the same group, which is not realistic.

The revised food pyramid is organized into five color-coded groups, each with a general recommendation.

- *Grains.* Three ounces of whole grain bread, rice, cereal, crackers, or pasta every day (orange).
- *Vegetables.* Eat more dark green vegetables, orange vegetables, beans and peas (green).
- *Fruits.* Fresh frozen, dry, or canned fruit. Go easy on fruit juices (red).
- *Milk.* Calcium-rich foods. Choose lactose free products (blue).

- *Meat and beans.* Low-fat and lean meats and poultry. Bake it, broil it, grill it. More fish, beans, peas, nuts and seeds (purple).

However, the USDA has a web site (http://www.mypyramid.gov/pyramid/index.html) that will calculate the desired portions for each group based on a person's age, sex, and the amount of exercise the person performs daily.

In addition to the USDA, the National Academy of Sciences Food and Nutrition Board (http://www.iom.edu) publishes the U.S. Recommended Dietary Allowance (RDA) for daily dose requirements of each vitamin (Table 9-1).

Table 9-1.   RDA (recommended dietary allowances).

Vitamin	Food Sources	RDA
Fat Soluble A	Whole milk, butter, eggs, leafy green and yellow vegetables, fruits, liver	Male: 1000 µg or 5000 IU Female: 800 µg or 4000 IU Pregnancy: 1000 µg or 5000 IU Lactating: 1200 µg or 6000 IU
D	Fortified milk, egg yolk, tuna, salmon	Male and Female: 40–80 µg or 200–400 IU
E	Whole-grain cereals, wheat germ, vegetable oils, lettuce, sunflower seeds	Male: 10 mg/d; 15 IU Female: 8 mg/d; 12 IU Pregnancy: 10–12 mg/day
K	Leafy green vegetables, liver, cheese, egg yolk	Male: 70–80 µg/day Female: 60–65 µg/day Taking broad spectrum antibiotics: 140 µg/day Pregnancy: 65 µg/day
Water-Soluble C Ascorbic acid	Citrus fruits, tomatoes, leafy green vegetables, potatoes	Male and female: 60 mg/day Pregnancy: 70 mg/dL Lactating: 95 mg/dL
B_1 thiamine	Enriched breads and cereals, yeast, liver, pork, fish, milk	Male: 1.5 mg Female: 1.1 mg Pregnancy: 1.5 mg Lactating: 1.6 mg
B_2 riboflavin	Milk, enriched breads and cereals, liver, lean meats, eggs, leafy green vegetables	Male: 1.4–1.7 mg Female: 1.2–1.3 mg Pregnancy: 1.6 mg Lactating: 1.8 mg

Table 9-1. *(continued)*

B$_3$ niacin	Eggs, meat, liver, beans, peas, enriched bread and cereals	
B$_6$ pyridoxine	Lean meat, leafy green vegetables, whole-grain cereals, yeast, bananas	Male: 15–19 mg/day Female: 13–15 mg/day Pregnancy: 18 mg/day Lactating: 20 mg/day
B$_{12}$	Liver, kidney, fish, milk	Male and female: 3 µg/day Pregnancy: 4 µg/day
Folic Acid	Leafy green vegetables, yellow fruits and vegetables, yeast, meats	Male and female: 400 µg/day Pregnancy: 600–800 µg/day Lactating: 600–800 3 µg/day

TYPES OF VITAMINS

There are two groups of vitamins. These are fat-soluble vitamins and water-soluble vitamins.

Fat-soluble vitamins

Fat-soluble vitamins are absorbed by the intestinal tract following the same metabolism as used with fat. Any condition that interferes with the absorption of fats will also interfere with the absorption of fat-soluble vitamins. Fat-soluble vitamins are stored in the liver, fatty tissues and muscle and remain in the body longer than water-soluble vitamins. Fat-soluble vitamins are excreted slowly in urine. Hint to remember: ADEK = addicted to fat are fat soluble vitamins.

The following are fat-soluble vitamins.

Vitamin A

Vitamin A (Acon, Aquasol) helps to maintain epithelial tissue, eyes, hair and bone growth. It is also used for treatment of skin disorders such as acne. Vitamin A has a toxic effect if taken in excess. For example, birth defects can occur if the patient takes greater than 6000 international units (IU) during pregnancy. It is important to keep in mind that Vitamin A is stored in the liver for up to two years, which can result in inadvertent toxicity if the patient is administered large doses of Vitamin A.

Vitamin D

Vitamin D, absorbed in the small intestine with the assistance of bile salts, is necessary for the intestines to absorb calcium. Vitamin D plays a major role in

Vitamin A

Dose for treatment of deficiency	100,000–500,000 IU daily × 3 d; then 50,000 IU × 14 day
Maintenance	10,000–20,000 IU q.d. × 60 day
Pregnancy category	A; PB: UK; t$^{1}/_{2}$: weeks–months*
Deficiency conditions	Treats vitamin A deficiency, prevents night blindness, treats skin disorders, promotes bone development
Side effects	Headache, fatigue, drowsiness, irritability, anorexia, vomiting, diarrhea, dry skin, visual changes
Adverse reactions	Evident only with toxicity; leucopenia, aplastic anemia, papilledema, increased intracranial pressure, hypervitaminosis A (loss of hair and peeling skin). Excess dose during pregnancy can cause birth defects.
Contraindications	Mineral oil, cholestyramine, alcohol, and antilipemic drugs decrease the absorption of vitamin A. It is excreted through the kidneys and feces.

*PB = Protein Binding   UK = unknown   t½ = ½ life

Vitamin D

Dose for treatment of deficiency	Mild deficiency: 50–125 µg/dL Moderate to severe: 2.5–7.5 mg/d; 2500–7500 µg
Maintenance	Male and female: 40–80 µg; 200–400 IU
Pregnancy category	A
Deficiency conditions	Rickets, deficit of phosphorus and calcium in blood
Side effects	None significant
Adverse reactions	Excess of 40,000 international units (IU) results in hypervitaminosis D and may cause hypercalcemia (an elevated serum calcium level). Early symptoms of toxicity are anorexia, nausea, and vomiting.
Contraindications	Hypercalcemia, hypervitaminosis D, or renal osteodystrophy with hyperphosphatemia. Use with caution in patients with arteriosclerosis, hyperphosphatemia, hypersensitivity to vitamin D, and renal or cardiac impairment.

regulating the metabolism of calcium and phosphorus. There are two forms of Vitamin D: D_2, called ergocalciferol; and D_3, called cholecalciferol. D_2 is a synthetic fortified form of Vitamin D. D_3 is the natural form of Vitamin D that is produced in the skin by ultraviolet sunlight. Once absorbed, Vitamin D is converted into calcifediol in the liver and then converted to an activated form of calcifediol in the kidneys. The active form is a hormone that combines with parathyroid hormone (PTH) and calcitonin to regulate calcium and phosphorus metabolism in the body and stimulate the reabsorption of calcium and phosphorus by bone. When serum levels of calcium are low, more Vitamin D is used to create the active form of calcifediol. Low serum levels of calcium cause a decrease in the creation of the active form of calcifediol. Excess Vitamin D is then excreted in bile and a small amount is excreted in urine.

Vitamin E

Vitamin E protects the heart and arteries and cellular components from being oxidized and prevents red blood cells from hemolysis (rupture). If there is a sufficient balance of salts, pancreatic secretion, and fat, Vitamin E is absorbed from the GI tract and stored in all tissues, especially in the liver, muscle, and fatty tissues. Seventy-five percent of excess Vitamin E is excreted in the bile and the remainder is excreted in urine.

Vitamin E

Dose for treatment of deficiency	Malabsorption: 30–100 mg/day Severe deficit: 1–2 mg/kg/d or 50–200 IU/kg/day
Maintenance	Male: 10 mg/d; 15 IU Female: 8 mg/d; 12 IU Pregnancy: 10–12 mg/day
Pregnancy category	A (C if used in doses above RDA)
Deficiency conditions	Breakdown of red blood cells
Side effects	None significant
Adverse reactions	Large doses may cause fatigue, weakness, nausea, GI upset, headache, breast tenderness, and may prolong the prothrombin time (PT) (clotting time).
Contraindications	Patients taking warfarin (anticoagulant) should have their PT monitored closely. Iron and vitamin E should not be taken together because iron can interfere with the body's absorption and use of vitamin E.

Vitamin K

Dose for treatment of deficiency	5–15 mg/d (based on prothrombin time [PT] laboratory results)
Maintenance	Male: 70–80 µg/day Female: 60–65 µg/day If taking a broad-spectrum antibiotic: 140 µg/day Pregnancy: 65 µg/day
Pregnancy category	C
Deficiency conditions	Increased clotting time leading to increased bleeding and hemorrhage
Side effects	Occasional pain, soreness, and swelling at IM injection site; pruritic erythema (itchy redness) with repeated injections; flushed face, unusual taste.
Adverse reactions	Rare: severe reaction immediately following IV administration (cramplike pain, chest pain, dyspnea, facial flushing, dizziness, rapid/weak pulse, rash, profuse sweating, hypotension; may progress to shock, cardiac arrest)
Contraindications	Last few weeks of pregnancy and in neonates; Use with caution: asthma and impaired hepatic function

Vitamin K

Vitamin K comes from dietary sources such as leafy green vegetables, liver, cheese, and egg yolk and is synthesized by intestinal flora. Vitamin K is required to synthesize prothrombin and clotting factors VII, IX, and X and is an antidote for oral overdose of the anticoagulant Coumadin (Warfarin). There are four forms of Vitamin K: K_1 (phytonadione), which is the active form; K_2 (menaquinone), which is synthesized by intestinal flora, but not commercially available; K_3 (menadione) and K_4 (menadiol), both of which are produced synthetically. K_1 and K_2 are absorbed in the presence of bile salts. K_3 and K_4 are absorbed without bile salts. Vitamin K_1 prevents hemorrhage and is available as Mephyton, AquaMEPHYTON, and Konakion. Vitamin K_4 is available as Synkayvite. Vitamin K is absorbed in the intestines and is stored in the liver and in other tissues.

Water-soluble vitamins

Water-soluble vitamins are also known as the B Complex because it was originally considered as one vitamin. It was later discovered that these are separate vitamins. The following are water-soluble vitamins.

Vitamin C

Vitamin C may be found in citrus fruits, tomatoes, leafy green vegetables, and potatoes and used to metabolize carbohydrates and used for synthesis of protein, lipids, and collagen. Vitamin C is also required for capillary endothelium and repair of tissues. Vitamin C aids in the absorption of iron and the metabolism of folic acid. Unlike fat-soluble vitamins, vitamin C is not stored in the body and is excreted in urine. However, high serum levels of vitamin C can result from excessive doses and be excreted without any change. Vitamin C is commercially available as Ascorbicap, Cecon, Cevalin, Solucap C.

Vitamin C

Dose for treatment of deficiency	Adult per day is 50 to 100 mg. For severe deficit (scurvy) PO: IM: IV: 150–500 mg/d in 1 to 2 divided doses. 500 to 6000 mg/day for treatment of upper respiratory infections, cancer, or hypercholesterolemia.
Maintenance	45–60 mg/d
Pregnancy category	C
Deficiency conditions	Prevents and treats C deficiency (scurvy); increases wound healing; for burns; sickle cell crisis; deep vein thrombosis; Megavitamin therapy (massive doses) of vitamins are not recommended as it can cause toxicity.
Side effects	Headaches, fatigue, drowsiness, nausea, heartburn, vomiting, diarrhea. Vitamin C with aspirin or sulfonamides may cause crystal formation in the urine (crystalluria); it can also cause a false-negative occult (blood) stool result and false-positive sugar result in the urine when tested by the Clinitest method.
Adverse reactions	Kidney stones, crystalluria, hyperuricemia; Massive doses can cause diarrhea and GI upset.
Contraindications	Large doses can decrease the effect of oral anticoagulants; oral contraceptives can decrease C concentration in the body; smoking decreases serum levels of C, use with caution in renal calculi (kidney stones); gout, anemia, sickle cell, sideroblastic, thalassemia
Drug-lab-food interactions	Decrease ascorbic acid uptake taken with salicylates; may decrease effect of oral anticoagulants; may decrease elimination of aspirins

Vitamin B Complex

Vitamin B complex consists of four vitamins. These are B_1 (thiamine), B_2 (riboflavin), B_3 (niacin), and B_6 (pyridoxine). B_1 is used to treat peripheral neuritis from alcoholism or beriberi. B_2 is used to manage dermatologic problems, such as scaly dermatitis, cracked corners of the mouth, inflammation of the skin and tongue. B_3 is given in large doses to alleviate pellagra (dietary deficiency of niacin) and hyperlipidemia and may cause GI irritation and vasodilatation resulting in a flushing sensation. B_6 is given to correct B_6 deficiency and helps alleviate symptoms of neuritis causes by isoniazid (INH) therapy for tuberculosis.

Vitamin B Complex

Dose for treatment of deficiency	**Thiamine:** 30–60 mg/d
	Riboflavin: 5–25 mg/d Prophylactic: 3 mg/d
	Nicotinic acid or niacin: Prevention: 5–20 mg/d Deficit: 50–100 mg/d Pellagra: 300–500 mg in 3 divided doses Hyperlipidemia: 1–2 g/d in 3 divided doses
	Pyridoxine: 25–100 mg/d *Isoniazid therapy prophylaxis:* 20–25 mg/d *Peripheral neuritis:* 50–200 mg/d
Maintenance	**Thiamine:** Male 1.5 mg Female: 1.1 mg Pregnancy: 1.5 mg Lactating: 1.6 mg
	Riboflavin: Male: 1.4–1.7 mg Female: 1.2–1.3 mg Pregnancy: 1.6 mg Lactating: 1.8 mg
	Nicotinic acid or niacin: Male 15–19 mg/d Female: 13–15 mg/d Pregnancy:18 mg/d Lactating: 20 mg/d
	Pyridoxine: Male: 2.0 mg/d Female: 1.6 mg/d Pregnancy: 2.1 mg/d Lactating: 2.2 mg/d
Pregnancy category	A (C if dose is more than RDA)

Vitamin B Complex   *(continued)*

Deficiency conditions	**Thiamine:** sensory disturbances, retarded growth, fatigue, anorexia
	Riboflavin: visual defects such as blurred vision and photophobia, cheilosis, rash on nose; numbness of extremities
	Niacin or nicotinic acid: retarded growth, pellagra, headache, memory loss, anorexia, insomnia
	Pyridoxine: neuritis, convulsions, dermatitis, anemia, lymphopenia
Side effects	**Thiamine:** Raised skin rash, pruritus, or wheezing after a large IV dose;
	Riboflavin: orange-yellow discoloration in urine
	Niacin or nicotinic acid: flushing, pruritus, feelings of warmth; high doses: dizziness, arrhythmias, dry skin, hyperglycemia, myalgia, nausea, vomiting, diarrhea
	Pyridoxine: Occasional: Stinging at IM injection site; Rare: headache, nausea, somnolence; high doses cause sensory neuropathy (paresthesia, unstable gait, clumsiness of hands)
Adverse reactions	**Thiamine:** rare anaphylaxis after a large IV dose
	Riboflavin: none known
	Niacin or nicotinic acid: Cardiac arrythmias may occur rarely
	Pyridoxine: Long-term megadoses may produce sensory neuropathy
Contraindications	**Thiamine:** patients with renal dysfunction
	Riboflavin: patients with renal dysfunction
	Niacin or nicotinic acid: hypersensitivity to niacin or tartrazine; active peptic ulcer, severe hypotension, hepatic dysfunction, arterial hemorrhaging; Caution: diabetes mellitus, gallbladder disease, gout, history of jaundice or liver disease.
	Pyridoxine: IV therapy in cardiac patients; Caution: megadosage in pregnancy

Folic Acid (Folate, Vitamin B$_9$)

Folic acid is essential for body growth and is needed to synthesize DNA. Folic acid is found in leafy green vegetables, yellow fruits and vegetables, yeast, and meat and is absorbed in the small intestine. The active form of folic acid—called folate—circulates to all tissues in the body. A third of folate is stored in the liver and the remainder is stored in other tissues. Most folic acid is excreted in bile

Folic acid

Dose	1–2 mg/day
Maintenance	Male and female: 400 µg/day Pregnancy: 600–800 µg/day Lactating: 600–800 µg/day
Pregnancy category	A (C if more than RDA)
Deficiency conditions	Decreased WBC count and clotting factors, anemias, intestinal disturbances, depression
Side effects	None significant
Adverse reactions	High doses of folic acid can mask signs of B_{12} deficiency, which is a risk in the elderly. Patients taking phenytoin (Dilantin) for seizures should be cautious about taking folic acid because it can increase the risk of seizures. During the first trimester of pregnancy, folic acid deficiency can affect the development of the central nervous system (CNS) of the fetus; this can lead to neural tube defects such as spina bifida (a defective closure of the bony structure of the spinal cord) or anencephaly (lack of brain mass formation)
Contraindications	Pernicious, aplastic, normocytic, refractory anemias

and a small amount in urine. Chronic alcoholism, poor nutrition, pregnancy, and diseases that disrupts absorption by the small intestine can lead to an inadequate amount of folic acid. This can disrupt cellular division. A patient with low folic acid has nausea and diarrhea and is anorexic, fatigued, and has stomatitis, alopecia, and blood dyscrasias (megaloblastic anemia, leucopenia, and thrombocytopenia). Symptoms usually do not appear for 2 to 4 months after folic acid storage is depleted.

Vitamin B$_{12}$

Vitamin B_{12} may be found in liver, kidney, fish, and fortified milk and helps convert folic acid into its active form. Vitamin B_{12} is essential to synthesize DNA and promotes cellular division and is required for hematopoiesis (development of red blood cells in bone marrow) and to maintain the integrity of the nervous system. Vitamin B_{12} is absorbed in the intestine with the aid of an intrinsic factor produced by gastric parietal cells. Once absorbed, vitamin B_{12} binds to

Vitamin B$_{12}$

Dose	100 mg/dL 14 day Pernicious anemia: 40–100 µg/day or 1000 µg/wk x 3 wk
Maintenance	Male and female: 3 µg/day Pregnancy: 4 µg/day
Pregnancy category	A (C if use doses >RDA)
Deficiency conditions	Pernicious anemia, hemolytic anemia, hyperthyroidism, bowel and pancreatic malignancies, gastrectomy, GI lesions, neurologic damage, malabsorption syndrome, metabolic disorders, renal disease
Side effects	Occasional: diarrhea, itching
Adverse reactions	Rare allergic reaction; may produce peripheral vascular thrombosis, pulmonary edema, hypokalemia, CHF
Contraindications	History of allergy to cobalimin; folate deficient anemia, hereditary optic nerve atrophy

the transcobalamin II protein and is then transferred to tissues. Vitamin B$_{12}$ is stored in the liver for up to three years during which time it is slowly excreted in urine. Vitamin B$_{12}$ deficiency is common in patients who are strict vegetarians and in patients who have malaborption syndromes (cancer, celiac disease), gastrectomy, Crohn's disease, and liver and kidney diseases.

Vitamins and the Nursing Process

The nurse must assess the patient for signs and symptoms of vitamin deficiency before beginning vitamin therapy because vitamin therapy could result in a toxic effect if the patient does not have a vitamin deficiency.

In addition, the patient must be assessed for debilitating diseases and GI disorders that may disrupt the absorption, metabolism, and excretion of vitamins used to treat vitamin deficiency.

For some patients, vitamin deficiency is caused by inadequate nutrient intake. Therefore, it is critical that the patient's diet be assessed to determine if it is the

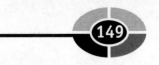
cause of the deficiency. If so, then the nurse should educate the patient on the importance of maintaining a balanced diet.

In many cases, the nurse may reach one of the following diagnoses:

- Altered nutrition; less than body requirements
- Lack of knowledge related to proper nutrition
- Lack of knowledge related to vitamin use

Based on these diagnoses, the nurse should develop a plan for having the patient eat a well-balanced diet and to take vitamin supplements as prescribed. The plan should also take into consideration the following interventions:

- Administer vitamins with food to promote absorption.
- Store vitamins in light-resistant container.
- Use a calibrated dropper for administration of liquid vitamins.
- Administer IM if patient is unable to take PO.

Teaching the patient is an important intervention because this gives the patient the knowledge to implement preemptive actions that lower the risk of vitamin deficiency in the future.

The nurse should teach the patient to:

- Take prescribed amount of vitamin.
- Read labels carefully.
- Not use megavitamins over a prolonged period of time.
- Check expiration dates on containers before purchasing or taking them (potency is reduced after the expiration date).
- Not take vitamin A with mineral oil because it interferes with the absorption of A.
- Not take megadoses of vitamin C (ascorbic acid) to "cure a cold."
- Not take megadoses of vitamin C with aspirin or sulfonamides.
- Avoid excessive intake of alcoholic beverages. (It can cause vitamin B-complex deficiencies.)

Refer the patient to the USDA web site (http://www.mypyramid.gov/pyramid/index.html) to calculate the desired portions for each food group based on age, sex, and the amount of exercise the patient performs daily. It is important that the patient understands that vitamin supplements are not necessary if he or she is healthy and eats properly.

Alert the patient to the signs and symptoms of hypervitaminosis. Hypervitaminosis A causes nausea, vomiting, headache, loss of hair, and cracked lips. Hypervitaminosis D causes anorexia, nausea, and vomiting.

The nurse should evaluate the patient for proper dietary intake and determine if vitamin therapy is having a therapeutic effect.

Minerals

Minerals are inorganic compounds that are required by the body for metabolism and to form bones and teeth. Minerals are extracted from ingested food such as meats, eggs, vegetables, and fruits. There are five minerals that are critical to maintain a healthy body.

Iron

Iron (ferrous sulfate, gluconate, or fumarate) is used for the regeneration of hemoglobin. Iron deficiency causes anemia. The patient requires 5 to 20 mg of iron each day from eating liver, lean meats, egg yolks, dried beans, green vegetables (such as spinach), and fruit.

Iron

Dose	Adult 50 mg/day
	Infant and child dose of iron, ages 6 months to 2 years old is 1.5/mg/kg
	Ferrous sulfate for therapeutic use 600 to 1200 mg/day in divided doses
Maintenance	Ferrous sulfate for prophylactic use is 300 to 325 mg/day
Pregnancy category	A; PB = UK t^1/2 : UK*
Treatment	Given to correct or control iron-deficiency anemia
Side effects	GI discomfort, nausea, vomiting, diarrhea, constipation, epigastric pain, elixir may stain teeth
Adverse reactions	Pallor, drowsiness. Life threatening: cardiovascular collapse, metabolic acidosis
Contraindications	Avoid a megadose in the first trimester because it might cause birth defects.

*PB = Protein-binding   UK = unknown   t½ = ½ life

Pregnant women require an increased an amount of iron, but they need to avoid a megadose in the first trimester because it might cause birth defects. Larger doses of iron are necessary in the second and third trimester. Iron is absorbed in the intestine where it enters plasma as heme or is stored as ferritin in the liver, spleen, and bone marrow. Food, the antibiotic tetracycline, and antacids decrease absorption up to 50% of iron. However, the patient should take iron with food to avoid GI discomfort. Vitamin C may slightly increase iron absorption. Iron toxicity is a serious cause of poisoning in children. Toxicity can develop with as few as 10 tablets of ferrous sulfate (3g) taken at one time—and can be fatal within 12 to 48 hours.

Copper

Copper is used in the formation of red blood cells and connective tissues. It is also a cofactor for many enzymes. Without copper enzymes are unable to initiate metabolic reactions in the body. Copper is also a component in the production of the neurotransmitters norepinephrine and dopamine. Foods rich in copper are shellfish (crabs and oysters), liver, nuts, seeds (sunflower, sesame), legumes, and cocoa. It is absorbed in the intestines. A prolonged copper deficiency can result in anemia and cause changes in the skin and blood including a decrease in the white blood count, intolerance to glucose, decrease in skin and hair pigmentation, and mental retardation if the patient is young. High levels of copper in serum can be an indication of Wilson's disease, which is an inborn error of metabolism that allows for large amounts of copper to accumulate in the liver, brain, cornea, or kidney.

Copper

Dose	1.5–3 mg/day
Maintenance	1.5–3mg/day
Pregnancy category	A (C if > RDA dose)
Deficiency conditions	Anemia, decreased WBCs, glucose intolerance, decrease in skin and hair pigmentation, and mental retardation in the young.
Side effects	None significant
Adverse reactions	Vomiting and diarrhea
Contraindications	None known

Zinc

Dose	12–19 mg/day
Maintenance	12–19 mg/day
Pregnancy category	A (C if taken in doses > RDA)
Deficiency conditions	Growth retardation, diarrhea, vomiting, delay in puberty, weakness, dry skin, delay in wound healing
Side effects	No known
Adverse reactions	Anemia, increased LDL cholesterol, muscle pain, fever, nausea, vomiting
Contraindications	Do not take with tetracycline.

Zinc

Zinc stimulates the activity of over 100 enzymes for important functions in the body which includes production of insulin and making of sperm and plays a key role in the immune system and DNA synthesis. Zinc helps wounds heal and helps the patient maintain a sense of taste and smell. A dose of zinc larger than 150 mg can cause copper deficiency, decrease high-density lipoprotein (HDL) cholesterol and weaken the patient's immune response. Zinc also inhibits tetracycline (antibiotic) absorption and therefore should not be taken with antibiotics. The patient should wait two hours after taking any antibiotic before taking zinc.

Chromium

Chromium is acquired from meats, whole-grain cereals, and brewer's yeast and plays a role in controlling non-insulin-dependent diabetes by normalizing blood glucose thereby increasing the effects of the body's insulin on cells. Chromium 50 to 200 µg/d is considered within the normal range for children older than 6 years old and adults.

Selenium

Selenium is a trace mineral that is a cofactor for antioxidant enzymes that protect protein and nucleic acids from damage caused by oxidation. Selenium is found in meats (especially liver), seafood, eggs, and dairy products. With a dose

Chromium

Dose	50 to 200 µg/d considered within the normal range for anyone > 6 years of age (There is no RDA.)
Maintenance	50 to 200 µg/d considered within the normal range for anyone > 6 years of age (There is no RDA.)
Pregnancy category	A
Deficiency conditions	Inability to properly use glucose
Side effects	None known
Adverse reactions	May cause hypoglycemic reaction in patients who are taking insulin or an oral hypoglycemic agent.
Contraindications	Although contraindicated for diabetic patients blood sugar levels should be monitored closely.

greater than 200 µg, selenium has a possible anticarcinogenic (anti-cancer) effect and may reduce the risk of lung, prostate, and colorectal cancer. However, such a dose might cause weakness, loss of hair, dermatitis, nausea, diarrhea, and abdominal pain.

Selenium

Dose	40 to 75 µg (high doses for males and lower dose for females)
Maintenance	40 to 75 µg (high doses for males and lower dose for females)
Pregnancy category	A
Deficiency conditions	Heart disease
Side effects	Causes a garlic-like odor from the skin and breath in large doses.
Adverse reactions	Disorders of nervous system and digestive system and loss of hair with doses greater than 200 µg
Contraindications	None known

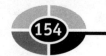

Summary

Vitamins and minerals are required for the body to function properly. Each day we need to eat a balanced diet that supplies us with the sufficient amount of vitamins and minerals to remain healthy. Our diet should contain grains, vegetables, fruits, milk, meat and beans. The portion of each varies depending on our age and gender. The USDA Web site publishes the Recommended Dietary Allowance (RDA) for daily dose requirement of each vitamin.

Vitamins are divided into two groups: fat-soluble and water-soluble. Fat-soluble vitamins can be stored in the body for up to two years. Water-soluble vitamins are used immediately and then excreted from the body in urine.

As part of the nursing process, assess the patient for vitamin deficiencies and determine what caused the deficiency. Some deficiencies are caused by changes in the body that affect absorption of vitamins. Other deficiencies are due to a poor or an unbalanced diet. After administering prescribed vitamin therapy, the patient should be educated about the importance of eating well-balanced meals and taking vitamin supplements if necessary.

Minerals are inorganic substances that the body uses for blood cells, tissues, and to stimulate enzymes to cause a catabolic reaction in the body.

In the next chapter, we'll examine the balancing act of fluids and electrolytes and how they maintain equilibrium. We'll also see how to use fluid and electrolyte therapies to restore the equilibrium if they become imbalanced.

Quiz

1. Vitamins that are stored in the body are called
   (a) water-soluble.
   (b) fat-soluble.
   (c) storage vitamins.
   (d) none of the above.

2. What vitamin is converted into calcifediol in the liver?
   (a) Vitamin A
   (b) Vitamin E
   (c) Vitamin D
   (d) Vitamin C

3. What vitamin protects the heart and arteries and cellular components from being oxidized?
    (a) Vitamin A
    (b) Vitamin E
    (c) Vitamin D
    (d) Vitamin C

4. Vitamin K is synthesized by intestinal flora.
    (a) True
    (b) False

5. Vitamin C is used to metabolize carbohydrates.
    (a) True
    (b) False

6. What vitamin is used to treat acne?
    (a) Vitamin A
    (b) Vitamin E
    (c) Vitamin D
    (d) Vitamin C

7. Fat-soluble vitamins are immediately excreted in urine shortly after they are absorbed.
    (a) True
    (b) False

8. What vitamin is given to help alleviate symptoms of neuritis caused by isoniazid therapy for tuberculosis?
    (a) Vitamin A
    (b) Vitamin E
    (c) Vitamin D
    (d) None of the above

9. Minerals are organic compounds synthesized in the liver.
    (a) True
    (b) False

10. Spinach is a source for iron.
    (a) True
    (b) False

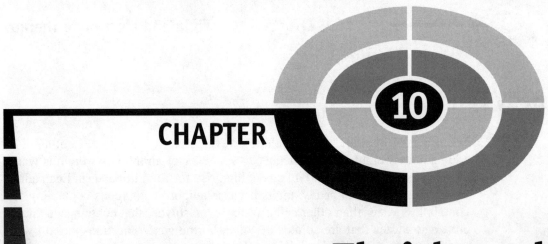

CHAPTER 10

Fluid and Electrolyte Therapy

What would happen if your muscles no longer contracted? You couldn't eat and digest food and water. You would be unable to move, talk, and eventually your brain would be unable to function. Most importantly, your heart is a muscle and it would just stop beating.

In order for muscles to contract, your body needs the proper balance between fluids and electrolytes inside and outside of cells. Electrolytes are salts whose positive and negative charges generate the electrical impulse to contract muscles in your body.

Diseases and treatment of disease can cause fluids and electrolytes to become imbalanced and require the patient to receive medication to restore the balance. In this chapter, you'll learn how to recognize the signs and symptoms of fluid and electrolyte imbalance and learn about therapeutic treatment that brings them back into balance.

Body Fluids

Water is 60% of adult body weight. However, water is 45% to 55% of an older adult's body weight and as much as 70% to 80% of an infant's weight is water. This makes older adults and infants at high risk for fluid imbalance. Lean adults have more water than heavy adults because adipose cells (cells containing fat) contain less water than other cells. Water is the solvent that contain salts, nutrients, and wastes that are solutes dissolved in the water and transported by the water throughout the body. Salts are electrolytes.

Body fluids are stored in compartments. These are intracellular and extracellular.

Intracellular fluid (ICF) is inside the cell and consists of 40% of body weight.

Extracellular fluid (ECF) is divided into smaller compartments. These spaces between the cells are called the interstitial space. The space is occupied by plasma and lymph, transcellular fluid, and fluid in the bone and connective tissues. This makes up 20% of body weight. About a third is plasma and two thirds of extracellular fluid is in the space between the cells. Transcellular fluid is also ECF but is found in the gastrointestinal (GI) tract, cerebrospinal space, aqueous humor, pleural space, synovial space, and the peritoneal space. Although fluid in the transcellular space is a small volume when compared with intracellular and extracellular compartments, the increase or decrease in volumes in transcellular spaces can have a dramatic effect on the fluid-electrolyte balance.

Electrolytes

An electrolyte is a substance that splits into ions when placed into water. An ion is an electrically charged particle that is either positively or negatively charged. A positively charged ion is called a cation and a negatively charged ion is called an anion.

- Sodium (Na^+), potassium (K^+), calcium (Ca^{2+}) , and Magnesium (Mg^{++}) are electrolytes that are cations.
- Chloride (Cl^-), Bicarbonate (HCO_3^-), Phosphate (PO_4^-), and Sulfate (SO_4^-) are electrolytes that are anions.

An electrolyte is measured as a millimole per liter (mmol/L). A millimole is the atomic weight of the electrolyte in milligrams. For example, the atomic weight of sodium is 23 milligrams. Therefore, 23 milligrams of sodium is measured as 1 mmol of sodium.

An electrolyte is stored either intracellularly (inside the cell) or extracellularly (outside the cell).

Intracellular electrolytes are mainly potassium, magnesium and some calcium.

Extracellular electrolytes are mainly sodium and some calcium.

Fluid Concentration

Electrolytes move between compartments based on the concentration of electrolytes, the gradients of the concentration, and the electrical charge. For example, there is a higher concentration of sodium outside the cell than inside the cell. Therefore, the gradient is towards the inside of the cell.

Fluids move through the body continuously. The heart pumps the blood, pressure is exerted on the vessels from outside the body, and muscles relax and contract to help the heart move the fluid through the vascular system. Fluid moves into and out of the cells and the extracellular spaces by osmotic pressure. This is the pressure exerted by the flow of water through a semipermeable membrane separating two solutions with different concentrations of solute. Osmotic pressure is determined by the concentration of the electrolytes and other solutes in water and is expressed as osmolarity or osmolality. However, the terms are used interchangeably.

Osmolality is the concentration of body fluids. Tonicity is the effect of fluid on cellular volume. Serum osmolality is a better indicator of the concentration of solutes in body fluids than tonicity; tonicity is primarily used as a measurement of the concentration of intravenous solutions.

There are three types of fluid concentration:

- *Iso-osmolar.* This is a fluid that has the same concentration of particles of solute as water.
- *Hypo-osmolar.* This is a fluid that has a lower concentration of particles of solute than water.
- *Hyper-osmolar.* This is a fluid that has a higher concentration of particles of solute than water.

Normal serum has an osmolality of between 275 and 295 mOsm/dg. Less than 275 mOsm/dg is hypo-osmolar and greater than 295 mOsm/dg is hyper-

osmolar. Hypo-osmolar might be caused by a fluid deficit. Hyper-osmolar might be caused by fluid excess.

The concentration of solutes is important when determining the proper replacement fluid for a patient whose fluids and electrolytes are imbalanced. Replacement fluids are replaced orally (by mouth or nasogastric tube) or parenterally with IV fluids (intravenously or subcutaneously).

IV Fluids

The osmolality of many IV fluids is similar to serum osmolality, which is 290 mOsm/kg H_2O. IV fluids are:

- *Isotonic.* This is in the iso-osmolar range (240 to 340 mOsm/L) where the concentration of the IV fluid is the same as concentration of intracellular fluid (NaCl 0.9%, normal saline).
- *Hypotonic.* This is in the hypo-osmolar range (< 240 mOsm/L) where the concentration of the IV fluid is less than the concentration of intracellular fluid (NaCl 0.45%, sodium chloride).
- *Hypertonic.* This is in the hyper-osmolar range (> 340 mOsm/L) where the concentration of the IV fluid is more than the concentration of intracellular fluid (Dextrose 5% in 0.45% saline).

IV solutions are classified as crystalloids, colloids, or lipids.

CRYSTALLOIDS

Crystalloids are used for replacement and maintenance of fluid balance therapy. These include dextrose, saline, and lactated Ringer's solution.

COLLOIDS

Colloids are volume expanders that increase the patient's fluid volume. These include Dextran, amino acids, hetastarch, and plasmanate.

- Dextran is not a substitute for whole blood because it does not have components that carry oxygen. Dextran 40 tends to interfere with platelet function resulting in prolonged bleeding times.

- Amino acids provide protein, calories, and fluid for the body. It is helpful for patients who are old and malnourished and for those with hypoproteinemia resulting from other causes.
- Hetastarch is a non-antigenic used to treat or prevent shock following serious injury, surgery, or for burn patients when blood is not available for transfusion. This too isn't a substitute for whole blood. In an isotonic solution (310 mOsm/L), hetastarch decreases platelet and hematocrit counts and must not be used for patients who have bleeding disorders, congestive heart failure (CHF), and renal dysfunction.
- Plasmanate is a protein-containing fluid that is derived from human plasma and is used to treat shock that results from burns, crushing injuries, abdominal emergencies, or any emergency where there is a loss of plasma, but not red blood cells. Plasmanate is non-antigenic and must not be given to patients who have anemia, increased blood volume, or congestive heart failure.

LIPIDS

Lipids are a fat emulsion that is given when IV therapy extends for longer than five days. This is used for prolonged parenteral nutrition to provide essential fatty acids.

Blood and Blood Products

Blood and blood products consist of whole blood, packed red blood cells, plasma, and albumin. Whole blood consists of all cellular and plasma components of blood. Whole blood should be used to treat severe cases of anemia—not mild cases of anemia—because one unit of whole blood elevates hemoglobin by 0.5 to 1.0 g. (By comparison, a unit of packed red bloods elevates the hematocrit—percentage of serum occupied by red blood cells—by three points.) Packed red blood cells are whole blood without plasma and are used to decrease circulatory overload and to decrease the risk of reaction to antigens contained in plasma.

Fluid Replacement

The amount of water a patient requires each day depends on the patient's age and the nature of the patient's medical condition. Water is 30 mL/kg of body weight.

A patient who weighs 70 kg has 2100 mL of water (70 kg × 30 mL/kg). In other words, a patient who weighs 150 lbs weighs 68 kg (150 lbs/2.2 lbs/kg) and has 2240 mL of water.

Each day the patient losses:

- 400 mL to 500 mL of water through evaporation from the skin.
- 400 mL to 500 mL of water through breathing.
- 100 mL to 200 mL of water in feces.
- 1000 mL to 1200 mL of water in urine.

This means that each day the patient must take in between 1900 mL and 2400 mL of fluid in order to maintain fluid-electrolyte balance. However, disease and the treatment of disease can increase the patient's output of water requiring that the patient increase the intake of water.

For example, a patient who has a fever loses as much as 15% more water than the normal daily water loss. That is, the patient loses between 2185 mL and 2760 mL of water each day when he or she has a fever.

FLUID REPLACEMENT AND THE NURSING PROCESS

When a patient is experiencing the loss of fluid, the nurse should:

- Establish baseline vital signs and weight.
- Review lab results and report elevations in the hematocrit and BUN. If both values are elevated this could indicate the patient is dehydrated. If the BUN is >60 mg/dL, renal impairment may be the cause.
- Measure urine output. Report if output is <30 mL/h or 600 mL/day. Normal urine output should be >35 mL/h or 1000 to 1200 mL/day.
- Review the lab results for urine specific gravity (SG). Normal range is 1.005 to 1.030. If the SG is greater than 1.030, dehydration may be the cause.
- Verify that the proper osmolality of the IV fluids are ordered. If there is continuous use of one type of IV fluid such as 5% dextrose in water (D_5W), hypo-osmolality of body fluid could occur.

Potential nursing diagnoses for a patient that is receiving fluid volume replacement therapy are:

- *Risk for fluid volume excess.* This can occur when the patient is given too much replacement fluid, fluid is infused too rapidly, or the volume is too much for the patient's physical size or condition.

- *Risk for fluid volume deficit related to inadequate fluid intake.*
- *Altered tissue perfusion, related to decreased blood circulation or inadequate fluid replacement.*

Before beginning fluid replacement therapy, goals should include:

- Patient will not develop fluid volume deficit or excess as a result of IV fluid replacement.
- Patient will remain hydrated.
- Vital signs and urine output will remain in normal ranges.

When fluid replacement therapy is underway, make sure to monitor:

- Vital signs.
- Fluid intake and output.
- Daily weight.
- Signs and symptoms of fluid volume excess (overload) which include cough, dyspnea (difficulty breathing), jugular vein distention (JVD) (neck vein engorgement), moist rales (abnormal breath sounds).
- Signs and symptoms of fluid volume deficit (dehydration) which include thirst, dry mucous membranes, poor skin turgor, decreased urine output, tachycardia, slight decrease in systolic blood pressure.
- Lab results especially BUN, hemoglobin and hematocrit.
- Types of IV fluids being infused.
- IV site for infiltration or phlebitis.

The patient should be taught:

- To recognize signs and symptoms of fluid volume excess and fluid volume deficit.
- How to measure fluid intake and output.
- How to weigh himself or herself.

The nurse must frequently evaluate the patient's

- Urine output (normal limits).
- Breath sounds (normal limits).
- Lab results (normal limits).
- Vital signs (normal limits).

- Weight (not increased).
- Skin turgor (normal).
- IV site (should not be red, swollen, hot or hard).
- IV patency (should be flowing as per the set drip rate).

Potassium

Potassium is an electrolyte cation that is more prevalent inside cells than it is in extracellular fluid. It is used to transmit and conduct neurological impulses and to maintain cardiac rhythms. Potassium is also used to contract skeletal and smooth muscles.

In order for a muscle to contract, the concentration of potassium inside the cell moves out and is replaced by sodium, which is the prevalent electrolyte outside the cell (see *Sodium*). These electrolytes reverse position when the muscle repolarizes. The concentration of potassium and sodium is maintained by the sodium-potassium pump found in cell membranes. The sodium-potassium pump uses adenosine triphosphate (ATP) to pump potassium back into the cell and sodium out of the cell.

Potassium regulates intracellular osmolality and promotes cell growth. It moves into cells as new tissues form and leaves cells when tissues break down. Patients receive potassium from their diet and excrete potassium in urine (90%) and feces (8%).

Serum potassium is measured to determine if the patient has a normal range of potassium. The normal serum potassium is between 3.5 to 5.3 milliequivalents per liter (mEq/L). Caution: Serum potassium less than 2.5 mEq/L or greater than 7.0 mEq/L can cause the patient to have a cardiac arrest. Diseases such as kidney disease can cause potassium to become imbalanced. When this happens, the patient will exhibit specific signs and symptoms and the serum potassium will be outside the normal range.

Hyperkalemia

Hyperkalemia occurs when a patient has a serum potassium level greater than 5.3 mEq/L. A number of factors can cause this condition including:

- Impaired renal excretion (most common).
- Massive intake of potassium.
- Medications such as potassium-sparing diuretics Aldactone and Dyrenium, angiotensin-converting enzyme (ACE) inhibitors Vasotec and Prinivil, which reduce the kidney's ability to secrete potassium.

The nurse should monitor a patient for the signs and symptoms of hyper-kalemia. The more common of these are:

- Nausea.
- Cold skin; grayish pallor.
- Hypotension.
- Mental confusion and irritability.
- Abdominal cramps.
- Oliguria (decreased urine output).
- Tachycardia (fast pulse) and later bradycardia (slow pulse).
- Muscle weakness to flaccid paralysis.
- Numbness or tingling in the extremities.
- Peaked T waves on the EKG.

The nurse must respond quickly once signs and symptoms of hyperkalemia develop as the patient is at risk for seizures, injury related to muscle weakness, and cardiac arrhythmias. Here is what needs to be done.

- Restrict intake of potassium rich foods.
- Administer diuretics and ion-exchange resins such as Kayexalate (retention enema) as directed to increase the elimination of potassium.
- Dialysis therapy may be ordered in critical cases to remove potassium.
- Administer insulin and glucose parenterally to force potassium back inside cells.
- Administer sodium bicarbonate intravenously to correct the acidosis (elevate pH).
- Administer calcium gluconate intravenously to decrease the irritability of the heart; it does not promote potassium loss.

Hypokalemia

Hypokalemia occurs when a patient has a serum potassium level of less than 3.5 mEq/L. A number of factors can cause this condition. These include:

- Diarrhea.
- Vomiting.
- Fistulas.
- Nasogastric suctionings.
- Diuretics.
- Hyperaldosteronism.
- Magnesium depletion.

- Diaphoresis.
- Dialysis.
- Increased insulin.
- Alkalosis.
- Stress (increases epinephrine).
- Starvation.
- Low potassium in diet.

The patient may have the following signs and symptoms when experiencing hypokalemia:

- Leg cramps.
- Muscle weakness.
- Vomiting.
- Fatigue.
- Decreased reflexes.
- Polyuria.
- Irregular pulse.
- Bradycardia.

The patient may also exhibit an abnormal EKG that shows:

- Depressed ST segment.
- Flattened T wave.
- Presence of U wave.
- Premature ventricular contractions.

The nurse must respond with the following interventions as the patient is a risk for injury related to muscle weakness and cardiac arrhythmias.

- Increase dietary intake of potassium.
- Teach the patient how to prevent hypokalemia by maintaining an adequate dietary intake of potassium. These include fruits, fruit juices, vegetables, or potassium supplements. Bananas and dried fruits are higher in potassium than oranges and fruit juices.
- Administer potassium chloride supplements (Table 10-1) orally (may take 30 minutes for onset) or IV. Use a central IV line for rapid infusion in critical conditions. Take with at least a half a glass of fluid (juice or water) because potassium is extremely irritating to the gastric and intestinal mucosa.
- Teach patients the signs and symptoms of hypokalemia and to call the healthcare provider if any of these are experienced.

Caution: This deficit cannot be corrected rapidly. The infusion should not exceed 10 to 20 mEq per hour or the patient may experience hyperkalemia and can experience cardiac arrest. Be alert that infusions containing potassium may cause pain at the IV insertion site. If urine output is <30 mL/hour notify prescriber. Infusions should not contain more than 60 mEq/L of potassium chloride (KCl). 40 mEq/L is the preferred amount to add to 1000 mL of intravenous solution.

Warning: NEVER give potassium as an intravenous push or intravenous bolus. This will cause immediate cardiac arrest which is not reversible with

Table 10-1. Potassium supplements.

Potassium Supplements	Description
10% potassium chloride	20 mEq/15 mL oral
20% potassium chloride	40 mEq/16 mL oral
10% Kaochlor	Oral
Potassium triplex (potassium actetate, bicarbonate, citrate)	Oral, rarely used
Kaon (potassium gluconate)	Enteric-coated tablet. Maintenance: 20 mEq in 1–2 divided dose
Kaon-Cl (potassium chloride)	Enteric-coated tablet. Maintenance: 20 mEq in 1–2 divided dose
Slow-K (potassium chloride)	Enteric-coated tablet. Maintenance: 8 mEq
Kaochlor (potassium chloride)	Correction: 40–80 mEq in 3–4 divided doses
K-Lyte (potassium bicarbonate)	Effervescent tablet. Correction: 40–80 mEq in 3–4 divided doses
K-Lyte/Cl (potassium chloride)	Effervescent tablet. Correction: 40–80 mEq in 3–4 divided doses
K-Dur (potassium chloride)	Effervescent tablet. Correction: 40–80 mEq in 3–4 divided doses
Micro-K (potassium chloride)	Effervescent tablet. Correction: 40–80 mEq in 3–4 divided doses
Potassium chloride	Clear liquid in multi-dose vial or ampule: 2 mEq/mL
Potassium chloride	IV: 20–40 mEq diluted in 1 L of IV solution

cardiopulmonary resuscitation. Potassium must be diluted in IV fluids as stated above. Don't give potassium if the patient suffers from renal insufficiency, renal failure, or Addison's disease. Do not give potassium if the patient has hyperkalemia, severe dehydration, acidosis, or takes potassium-sparing diuretics. Use with caution with patients who have cardiac disorders or burns.

Sodium

Sodium is the major cation in extracellular fluid found in tissue spaces and vessels. Sodium plays an important role in the regeneration and transmission of nerve impulses and affects water distribution inside and outside cells. It is part of the sodium/potassium pump that causes cellular activity. When it shifts into the cell, depolarization (contraction) occurs; when it shifts out of the cell, potassium goes back into the cell and repolarization (relaxation) occurs. Sodium also combines readily in the body with chloride (Cl) or bicarbonate (HCO_3) to promote acid-base balance (pH).

The patient receives sodium when food is absorbed in the GI tract. Typically, a patient takes in more sodium than the patient's daily requirement. The kidneys regulate the sodium balance by retaining urine when the sodium concentration is low and excreting urine when the sodium concentration is high. Most excess sodium is excreted in urine although sodium also leaves the patient as perspiration and in feces.

The serum sodium level, which is the ratio of sodium to water, is the indicator of the sodium level in a patient's body. Sodium is measured in milliequivalents per liter (mEq/L). The normal range of serum sodium is from 135 mEq/L to 145 mEq/L.

A patient's serum sodium level moves out of the normal range when the patient is retaining too much or too little water, has a high or low concentrations of sodium, or a combination of both. A patient is hypernatremic when there is a high concentration of sodium and hyponatremic when there is a low concentration of sodium.

Hypernatremia

Hypernatremia occurs when the patient's serum sodium is greater than 145 mEq/L. This happens for one of two reasons: The patient's sodium concentration has increased while the volume of water remains unchanged or the patient's water volume has decreased while the sodium concentration remains unchanged.

Regardless of what happened, the patient experiences hyperosmolality, which is a higher-than-normal concentration of sodium. This causes water to shift out of cells and into extracellular space resulting in cellular dehydration. A patient who is alert and can drink water to quench a thirst is at less risk for hypernatremia. However, a patient whose consciousness is impaired or who cannot swallow, such as a frail elderly patient, is at risk for hypernatremia.

Hypernatremia is caused by:

- Inadequate water intake.
- Inability of the hypothalamus gland to synthesize anti-diuretic hormone (ADH) (which the kidneys require to regulate sodium).
- Inability of the pituitary gland to release ADH.
- Inability of the kidneys to respond to ADH.
- Excess sodium (such as from a hypertonic IV solution).
- Inappropriate use of sodium-containing drugs.
- Ingestion of excessive amounts of sodium such as seawater.

The nurse can intervene by:

- Replacing water using an IV of 5% dextrose in water or a hypotonic saline solution as ordered.
- Lowering the serum sodium level slowly to avoid the risk of cerebral edema (brain swelling).
- Restricting sodium intake.
- Monitoring patient's weight.
- Assessing extremities for edema (swelling).
- Monitoring breath sounds and respiratory effort for signs of heart failure.

The nurse must be alert to recognize the signs and symptoms of hypernatremia. These are:

- Agitation
- Restlessness
- Weakness
- Seizures
- Twitching
- Coma
- Intense thirst
- Dry swollen tongue
- Edematous (swollen) extremities

The nurse should educate the patient to:

- Avoid foods rich in sodium such as canned foods, lunch meats, ham, pork, pickles, potato chips, and pretzels. Do not add salt to foods when cooking or at the table.

- Read all labels on food products.
- Monitor his weight if cardiac patient by weighing daily.
- Look for signs of swollen feet (tight shoes) and hands (tight rings).
- Notify healthcare provider if any respiratory distress occurs.

Hyponatremia

Hyponatremia occurs when the patient's serum sodium is less than 135 mEq/L. There are two reasons why this happens: the patient has increased the volume of water while the sodium concentration remains normal or the patient losses sodium while the water volume remains normal.

Hyponatremia is caused by:

- Profuse sweating on a hot day or after running a marathon,
- Inappropriate administration of a hypotonic IV solution (sodium loss),
- The result of major trauma or after surgery (sodium loss),
- Excessive ingestion of water (water gain),
- Syndrome of Inappropriate Anti-Diuretic Hormone (SIADH), which causes abnormal water retention (sodium loss) or Addison's Disease,
- Loss of sodium from the GI tract as a result of diarrhea and vomiting (sodium loss),
- The use of potent diuretics (lose water and salt together),
- Burns and wound drainage (sodium loss),
- Intake of too much water caused by polydipsia (excessive thirst).

The nurse must recognize the following symptoms of hyponatremia:

- Fatigue,
- Headache,
- Muscle cramps,
- Nausea,
- Seizures,
- Coma.

Hyponatremia is treated by:

- Treating the underlying cause.
- Administering hypertonic saline solution IV such as Dextrose 5% in saline to restore the serum sodium level.
- Replacing fluid loss with commercially available electrolytic fluids.

The nurse should monitor:

- Vital signs,
- Fluid intake and output,
- Serum sodium levels,
- Dietary sodium intake,
- Breath sounds and signs of respiratory distress.

The nurse should educate the patient to:

- Not drink excessive amounts of pure water on a hot day or after extreme exercise. Fluid replacement should be an electrolyte solution such as Gatorade or other commercial preparations that include sodium.
- Monitor for signs and symptoms of hyponatremia if the patient is taking a potent diuretic such as furosemide (Lasix) or a thiazide diuretic such as hydrochlorothiazide (HydroDiuril) .
- Report any signs of respiratory distress to healthcare provider.

Calcium

Calcium is found in equal proportion in intracellular fluid and extracellular fluid. It is combined with phosphate in bone and with protein (albumin) in the serum. A patient receives calcium from ingesting calcium-containing food. Calcium plays a critical role in transmission of nerve impulses, blood clotting, muscle contraction, and the formation of teeth and bone. There is also growing evidence that calcium can help with weight loss.

There are three forms of calcium in serum that can fluctuate among forms depending on changes to the serum pH and/or serum protein (albumin) levels.

1. Free ionized form, which is the biologically active form. Half of the patient's total calcium is in the free ionized form.
2. Protein bound, which binds primarily with albumin.
3. Complex form, which is where calcium is combined with phosphate, citrate, or carbonate.

The normal serum calcium ranges between 8.5 mg/dL to 10.5 mg/dL. This reflects the calcium level for all three forms of calcium. However, ionized calcium (iC) levels are sometimes reported separately (4–5 mg/dL).

There is a balance between calcium and phosphorus. As serum calcium increases, serum phosphorus decreases. Conversely, as serum calcium decreases, serum phosphorus increases. The level of calcium is regulated by the parathyroid hormone (PTH), calcitonin, and vitamin D.

Low serum calcium causes an increase in the production of PTH. PTH moves calcium out of bone and into the serum. It increases the absorption of calcium from the GI tract. PTH also increases reabsorption of calcium in the kidneys.

Calcitonin is produced by the thyroid gland. Production is increased when there is a high serum calcium level. Calcitonin reverses the action of PTH by increasing the absorption of calcium by bone, decreases calcium absorption in the GI tract, and causes an increase in urine to excrete calcium.

Table 10-2.   Medications that increase and decrease serum calcium.

Decreases Serum Calcium	Increases Serum Calcium
Magnesium sulfate	Calcium salts
Propylthiouracil (propacil)	Vitamin D
Colchicines	IV lipids
Pliamythin	Kayexalate androgens
Neomycin	Diuretics (Thiazides, Chlorthalidone, Hygroten)
Acetazolamide	
Aspirin	
Anticonvulsants	
Glutethimide	
Estrogens	
Aminoglycosides (gentamicin, amikacin, tobramycin)	
Phosphate preparations: oral, enema, and IV (sodium phosphate, potassium phosphate)	
Corticosteroids (cortisone, prednisone)	
Loop diuretics (furosemide [Lasix])	

Dairy products are the major source of dietary calcium. Eggs, green leafy vegetables, broccoli, legumes, nuts, and whole grains provide smaller amounts. Only about 10% to 30% of the calcium in foods is actually absorbed in the body. Calcium is absorbed in the small intestine. Absorption is influenced by the amount of vitamin D available and the levels of calcium already present in the body.

Hypercalcemia

Hypercalcemia is a condition when the serum calcium level is higher than 10.5 mg/dL indicating there is a higher than normal concentration of calcium. This usually produces a low serum phosphorus level.

Hypercalcemia can be caused by:

- Renal failure.
- Immobility.
- Cancer.
- Hyperparathyroidism.
- Excess intake of calcium supplements (such as in Tums and other medications to prevent and treat osteoporosis).
- Overuse of antacids for GI disturbances.
- Prolonged diarrhea.
- Excessive use of diuretics.

The nurse should be alert to identify the following signs and symptoms of hypercalcemia:

- Patients with mild hypercalcemia may have no signs and symptoms
- Nausea,
- Vomiting,
- Constipation,
- Anorexia,
- Abdominal pain,
- Polyuria (frequent urination),
- Polydipsia (extreme thirst),
- Decreased memory,
- Personality changes or mood swings,
- Confusion,
- Depressed reflexes,
- Muscular weakness,

- Bone pain,
- Fractures (occur when calcium leaves the bone due to cancer, osteoporosis, and other disorders),
- Kidney stones,
- Hypertension,
- Cardiac arrhythmias,
- Coma.

Treatment is based on the calcium level. The calcium level may need to be lowered quickly because severe hypercalcemia can be life threatening.
Treat the underlying cause if known.

- If kidney function is adequate:
  - ○ Administer isotonic saline IV to hydrate the patient.
  - ○ Make sure the patient drinks 3000 to 4000 ml of fluid to excrete the calcium in urine.
  - ○ Administer furosemide (Lasix) or ethcrynic acid (Edecrin) loop diuretics after adequate fluid intake is established.
- Administer synthetic calcitonin to lower serum calcium concentration
- Administer plicamycin (Mithracin) to increase absorption of calcium in bone.
- Provide a low-calcium diet.
- Make sure the patient performs weight-bearing activities.
- Take safety measure to protect the patient who experiences neuromuscular effects.

Hemodialysis is the most effective method to lower calcium levels in severe cases when kidney function is not normal.

Hypocalcemia

Hypocalcemia occurs when the serum calcium level is lower than 8.5 mg/dL indicating there is a lower than normal concentration of calcium. This usually produces a high serum phosphorus level. Too little calcium intake causes calcium to leave the bone to maintain a normal calcium level. Fractures (broken bones) may occur if a calcium deficit persists because of calcium loss from the bones (demineralization).
Hypocalcemia is caused by:

- Hypoparathyroidism.
- Thyroid or neck surgery where the parathyroid gland is removed or injured.

- Hypomagnesium caused by alcoholism.
- Ingestion of phosphates.
- Inadequate intake of dietary calcium and/or Vitamin D.

Patients who experience hypocalcemia may have the following symptoms:

- Depression.
- Memory loss.
- Confusion.
- Hallucinations.
- Numbness and tingling in the face, around the mouth, and in the hands and feet.
- Muscle spasms in the face, around the mouth, and in the hands and feet.
- Hyperreflexia.
- Ventricular tachycardia.

Patients with hypocalcemia can be treated as follows:

- Calcium preparations can be given PO in tablet, capsule, or powder form or IV. If given IV, then mix with 5% dextrose in water. Do not mix with a saline solution because sodium encourages the loss of calcium.
- Administer parenteral calcium. Caution: tissue infiltration leads to necrosis and sloughing. Calcium increases the action of digoxin and can result in cardiac arrest. Don't add calcium to bicarbonate or phosphorus because precipitates form.
- Administer the following medication intravenously if ordered:
  o Calcium chloride IV 10 mL
  o Calcium gluceptate 5 mL
  o Calcium gluconate 10 mL
- Administer the following medication PO if ordered:
  o Calcium carbonate (Os-cal, Tums, Caltrate, Megacal) 650–1500 mg tablets
  o Calcium gluconate (Kalcinate) 500–1000 mg tablets
  o Calcium lactate 325–650 mg tablets
  o Calcium citrate 950 mg tablet
- Take safety precautions because the patient is at risk for tetany and seizures.
- Tell the patient to refrain from alcohol and caffeine because they inhibit calcium absorption.
- Increase dietary calcium to 1500 mg/day by eating green leafy vegetables and fresh oysters and milk products.

- Administer vitamin D.
- Have the patient undergo regular exercises to decrease bone loss.

Patient education should include information about dietary sources of calcium, the need to maintain physical activity to avoid bone loss, avoid overuse of antacids, and chronic use of laxatives. Patients should be taught to use fruits and fiber for improving bowel elimination. Take oral supplements with meals or after meals to increase absorption.

Magnesium

Magnesium is a sister cation to potassium and is higher in intracellular fluid (ICF). If there is a loss of potassium there is also a loss of magnesium. Magnesium is the coenzyme that metabolizes carbohydrates and proteins and is involved in metabolizing nucleic acids within the cell. Magnesium also has a key role in neuromuscular excitability. The patient acquires magnesium by ingesting magnesium-rich food, where it is absorbed in the GI tract and then excreted in urine.

There is a close relationship between magnesium, potassium, and calcium. PTH (see calcium), which regulates calcium, also influences the magnesium balance. Typically, you'll assess serum magnesium, calcium, and potassium together. The normal serum magnesium level is between 1.5 mEq/L and 2.5 mEq/L.

Hypermagnesemia

Hypermagnesemia is a condition experienced by a patient whose serum magnesium level is greater than 2.5 mEq/L. The major cause of hypermagnesia is an excessive intake of magnesium salts in laxatives such as magnesium sulfate, milk of magnesia, and magnesium citrate. Antacids such as Maalox, Mylanta, and DiGel can also cause hypermagnesemia. Patients who take lithium (antipsychotic medication) are also at risk for hypermagnesemia.

The signs and symptoms of hypermagnesemia are:

- Lethargy.
- Drowsiness.
- Weakness.
- Paralysis.
- Cardiac (ventricular) arrhythmias.

- Heart block.
- Loss of deep tendon reflexes.
- Hypotension.

Hypomagnesemia

Hypomagnesemia happens when the serum magnesium level is less than 1.5 mEq/L. This can be caused by long-term administration of saline infusions which can result in the loss of magnesium and calcium. Diuretics, certain antibiotics, laxatives, and steroids are drug groups that promote magnesium loss. Hypomagnesemia also enhances the action of digitalis and can cause digitalis toxicity.

Patients who have hypomagnesemia may exhibit no signs and symptoms until the serum level approaches 1.0 mEq/L. Signs of severe hypomagnesemia include tetany-like symptoms caused by hyperexcitability (tremors, twitching of the face), ventricular tachycardia that leads to ventricular fibrillation, and hypertension.

Treatment for hypomagnesemia includes:

- Administering intravenous magnesium sulfate in solution slowly. Use an infusion pump to prevent rapid infusion that might result in cardiac arrest.
- Monitoring signs of magnesium toxicity such as hot flushed skin, anxiety, lethargy, hypotension and laryngeal stridor.
- Monitoring EKG and pulse.
- Taking safety precautions for patients who are at risk for seizures and mental confusion.
- Increasing the dietary sources of magnesium including nuts, whole grains, cornmeal, spinach, bananas, and oranges.

Keep calcium gluconate available for emergency reversal of hypermagnesemia as a result of overcorrecting hypomagnesemia.

Phosphorus

Phosphate is the primary anion inside the cell and plays a key role in the function of red blood cells, muscles, and the nervous system. Phosphate is also involved the acid–base buffering and is involved with metabolizing carbohydrates, proteins, and fats. Most of the body's phosphate (about 85%) is found in bones. The rest of it is stored in tissues throughout the body.

Phosphorus is acquired by eating phosphorus-rich foods. Phosphorus is absorbed in the GI tract and excreted in urine and a small amount in feces. It is converted to phosphate in the body.

Both phosphate and calcium levels are regulated by parathyroid hormone (PTH). The amount of phosphate in the blood effects the level of calcium in the blood. Both levels are usually measured at the same time. As the serum calcium concentration increases, the concentration of serum phosphorus decreases and conversely as serum phosphorus increases, serum calcium decreases. The normal range of serum phosphorus is between 2.5 mg/dL and 4.5 mg/dL.

The kidneys regulate the amount of phosphate in the blood. Abnormally high levels of serum phosphate are usually caused by kidney malfunction.

Hyperphosphatemia

Hyperphosphatemia is the condition exhibited by a patient whose serum phosphate is greater than 4.5 mg/dL, which is caused by:

- Kidney disease.
- Underactive parathyroid glands.
- Acromegaly.
- Rhabdomyolysis.
- Healing fractures.
- Untreated diabetic ketoacidosis.
- Certain bone diseases.
- Excessive ingestion of phosphate-containing laxatives.
- Excessive drinking of milk.
- Chemotherapy for neoplastic disease.
- Excessive intake of vitamin D.
- Decrease in magnesium levels as in alcoholism.
- Increased phosphate levels during the last trimester of pregnancy.

Unlike hyperkalemia and hypermagnesemia, acute hyperphosphatemia causes few sudden problems. The major effect is to cause hypocalcemia and tetany if serum phosphate rises too rapidly. Calcium can be deposited in the tissues in hyperphosphatemia.

The treatment for acute hyperphosphatemia is administration of phosphate binding salts, calcium, magnesium, and aluminum although aluminum is avoided in renal failure.

Patients who have hyperphosphatemia show the following signs and symptoms:

- Muscle problems.
- Hyperreflexia.
- Soft tissue calcification.
- Nausea.
- Vomiting.
- Hypocalcemia.
- Tachycardia.
- Anorexia.
- Tetany.

Treatment for hyperphosphatemia can include:

- Restricting foods and drinks (carbonated soda) high in phosphate.
- Treating the underlying cause.
- Institute seizure precautions.
- Administering sevelamer (Renagel).
- Administering calcium supplements.

Hypophosphatemia

Hypophosphatemia occurs in a patient's whose serum phosphate is less than 2.5 mg/dL and is caused by:

- Inadequate intake.
- Diuresis.
- Dialysis.
- Alcoholism.
- Steroids.
- Overuse of phosphate-binding antacids.

The nurse should monitor the patient for the following signs and symptoms of hypophosphatemia:

- Bone and muscle pain.
- Muscle weakness.
- Rhabdomyolysis.

- Confusion.
- Osteomalacia.
- Coma.

Hypophosphatemia can be treated by:

- Administering phosphate supplements such as Neutra-Phos PO.
- Administering sodium phosphate IV.
- Administering potassium phosphate IV.

Nursing interventions should include:

- Assessing vital signs.
- Assessing changes in metal status.
- Institute seizure precautions.
- Monitor blood levels.

Summary

Our body contains fluids (water) and salts called electrolytes. Electrolytes are positive and negatively charged particles that generate electrical impulses that, among other things, cause our muscles to contract.

Fluids and electrolytes are stored in two compartments: intracellular (inside the cell) and extracellular (outside the cell). The amount of electrolytes in fluid is called a concentration. There are three types of fluid concentrations: iso-osmolar (same concentration), hypo-osmolar (low concentration), and hyperosmolar (high concentration). These concentrations are used to describe IV solutions as isotonic (iso-osmolar), hypotonic (hypo-osmolar), and hypertonic (hyper-osmolar).

There are five key electrolytes: potassium, sodium, calcium, magnesium, and phosphorus. Collectively, they must remain in balance for our body to function properly. Diseases and treatment of diseases are two factors that can cause fluids and electrolytes to become imbalanced. The healthcare professional must quickly identify the signs and symptoms of the imbalance and then take steps to restore the balance between electrolytes and fluids.

Quiz

1. A decrease in serum potassium is called
   (a) hyperkalemia.
   (b) hypokalemia.
   (c) hypernatremia.
   (d) none of the above.

2. What is determined by the concentration of electrolytes and other solutes in water?
   (a) osmotic pressure
   (b) protein fluid
   (c) potassium fluid
   (d) calcium fluid

3. Electrolytes are found in
   (a) intracellular fluid.
   (b) interstitial fluid.
   (c) intravascular fluid.
   (d) all of the above.

4. Sodium and chloride are most prevalent outside the cell.
   (a) True
   (b) False

5. The concentration of a hypotonic intravenous solution has the same concentration as intracellular fluid.
   (a) True
   (b) False

6. Which of the following is a volume expander?
   (a) Blood and blood products
   (b) Lipids
   (c) Colloids
   (d) All of the above.

7. Potassium is necessary for conduction of nerve impulses:
   (a) True
   (b) False

8. Insulin and glucose administered parenterally
    (a) forces potassium out of the cell.
    (b) forces potassium into the cell.
    (c) corrects the acidosis balance.
    (d) None of the above.

9. Vitamin D increases absorption of calcium in the GI tract.
    (a) True
    (b) False

10. The calcium balance can be affected by medications taken by the patient.
    (a) True
    (b) False

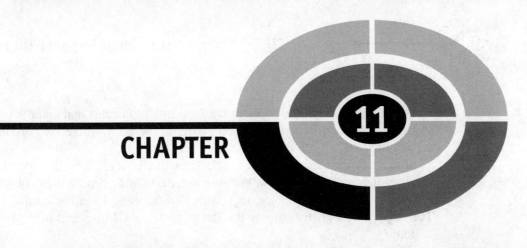

CHAPTER 11

Nutritional Support Therapies

You probably ignored your mom when she told you to eat your veggies so you can grow big and strong. Yet today you're probably eating more nutritional foods—foods you wouldn't touch when you were a kid—because you've learned that healthy foods provide the balanced nutrition needed to fend off diseases.

You might wonder how a chapter on nutrition slipped into a book on pharmacology. Nutrients are given to patients who are at risk for malnutrition caused by disease and caused by treatments given to cure diseases. Nutrients are also given to strengthen the patient following a trauma such as surgery.

In this chapter, you'll learn about nutritional support therapies, how to prepare them, how to administer them, and how to avoid any complications that might arise.

Nutrition

Nutrition is a three-step process that gives the body materials needed to make the body grow and function. The process begins when food is ingested. Chemical reactions in the body then break down food into molecules that enter the bloodstream and are distributed to different parts of the body where they are used to sustain life.

Some nutrients are used for cell growth and cellular functions. Other nutrients become involved in enzyme activities and carbohydrate-fat-protein synthesis. Nutrients are used to contract muscles and help wounds to heal. They also play a critical role in the integrity of the GI tract and in the immune system.

Think of nutrients as fuel for your car. Fuel is used as you drive your car. The same is true about your body. Your body uses nutrients to go about daily activities. And just like your car, your body can continue to operate without a full complement of nutrients—that is, without a full tank of gas. A healthy, well-nourished person has a nutritional level to last 14 days before they begin to show signs of malnutrition. That is, your full tank of gas will last 14 days.

However, there comes a point when your performance sputters—the level of nutrients fall below the level needed to sustain your daily activity. You simply run out of fuel and become fatigued, irritable, and exhibit an abnormal appearance.

This is referred to as a *nutritional deficit.* A nutritional deficit can occur from a number of situations. The most obvious is not eating a balanced, nutritional diet. However, there are less apparent reasons that cause a nutritional deficit. These are surgery, trauma, malignancy, and other illnesses that break down (catabolize) the body.

The effect of a nutritional deficit can be dramatic. The body needs nutrients to recover from trauma and disease. A nutritional deficit prolongs healing and severe cases can prevent total recovery. Critically ill patients have sufficient nutrients to sustain them for a few days to a week before they begin to show signs of nutritional deficit.

Healthcare professionals provide nutritional support therapy for patients who are at risk for nutritional deficit. Nutritional support therapy replaces nutrients that the patient has lost and thereby provide the patient with the fuel needed for a full recovery.

A nutritional deficit is called a negative nitrogen balance, which means that the patient lacks sufficient nitrogen to fight infectious disease. Healthcare professionals treat patients who are at risk for negative nitrogen balance by providing the patient with nutrients before the imbalance occurs. The patient is then able to fight infectious diseases.

A common misnomer is that dextrose 5% in water (D5W), normal saline, and lactated Ringer's solution provide nutrients to the patient. However, these intravenous fluids are not forms of nutrients. These are electrolytes and fluids.

NUTRITIONAL SUPPORT

Nutrients are given to a patient via an enteral or parenteral route. Using the enteral route, food is administered by mouth or by a feeding tube that is directly inserted into the GI tract—usually into the stomach or small intestine. A feeding tube is used whenever the patient cannot swallow.

The parenteral route is the use of high caloric nutrients administered through large veins such as the subclavian vein in a process called total parenteral nutrition (TPN) or hyperalimentation. The parenteral route is the least preferred because the process is three times more expensive than enteral without a significantly improved benefit. Furthermore, the parenteral route has a high rate of infection and does not promote GI function, liver function, or weight gain.

Enteral nutrition

Enteral feeding is the preferred method of providing nutritional support to a patient. However, the patient must have adequate GI tract function to enable food to be digested, absorbed, and waste eliminated.

It is important to determine if the patient has GI motility and small bowel function. Otherwise, the patient may experience uncontrolled vomiting and become at high risk for aspiration should the intestine be obstructed. Decreased bowel sounds are common in critically ill patients. They may also have a decrease or absence of gastric emptying.

There are several methods used for enteral feeding. These are:

- *Oral.* This is ingesting food naturally.
- *Nasogastric tube.* This is the most common method. It consists of a tube passed through the nose and down the esophagus ending shortly below the xiphoid process. This is used for short-term therapy.
- *Gastrostomy.* A feeding tube placed in a hole in the abdomen leading to the stomach. This is used for long-term therapy.
- *Nasoduodenal.* A tube is passed through the nose and down the esophagus ending in the duodenum.
- *Nasojejunal.* A tube is passed through the nose and down the esophagus ending in the small intestine.
- *Jejunostomy.* A feeding tube is placed in a hole in the abdomen leading to the small intestine.

There are various mixtures that are given to patients who are receiving nutritional support therapy based on the nutrient, caloric values, and osmolality that the patient requires. These mixtures belong to one of the following groups:

- *Blenderized.* This consists of liquids that are individually prepared based on the nutritional needs of the patient and can include baby food with added liquid.
- *Polymeric.* This is divided into two subgroups:
  1. Milk-based. Powder mixed with milk or water is given in large amounts to provide complete nutritional requirements and can be used as a nutritional supplement in smaller amounts.
  2. Lactose-free. Liquid is used for replacement feedings and consists of 50% carbohydrates, 15% protein, 15% fat, and 20% other nutrients in an isotonic solution (300 to 340 mOsm/kg H_2O). This provides 1 calorie per milliliter of feeding. This includes Ensure, Isocal, and Osmolite.
- *Elemental.* Also know as monomeric, this is the more expensive enteral solution. It is useful for partial GI tract dysfunction and is available in both liquid and powder. Elemental nutrients are rapidly absorbed in the small intestines.

Regardless of the group, these solutions consists of

- Carbohydrates in the form of dextrose, sucrose, and lactose. These are simple sugars that are absorbed quickly. Starch and dextrin are also carbohydrates that the solution may contain.
- Protein in the form of intact proteins, hydrolyzed proteins, or free amino acids.
- Fat in the form of corn oil, soybean oil, or safflower oil.

Enteral feedings are administered as:

- Bolus, 250–400 mL 4 to 6 times each day. Each bolus may take about 10 minutes to administer. The patient may experience nausea, vomiting, aspiration, abdominal cramping, and diarrhea if he or she cannot tolerate the large amount of solution given in a short timeframe. This method is if the patient is ambulatory and relatively healthy.
- Intermittent drip or infusion, 300–400 mL given 3 to 6 hours over 30–60 minutes by gravity drip or infusion pump.

- Continuous drip or cyclic infusion, 50–125 mL infused per hour at a slow rate over a 24-hour period using an infusion pump such as a Kangaroo set. This method is used for treating critically ill patients and for patients who have a feeding tube in their small intestine or in the stomach.

Enteral feedings expose the patient to complications. These are:

- Dehydration. An insufficient amount of water is given to the patient or a hyperosmolar solution is given, which draws water from the cells to maintain serum iso-omolality.
- Aspiration. The patient is fed while in a supine position or is unresponsive. Prevent this by raising the head of the bed 30° and check for gastric residuals by gently aspirating the stomach contents before the next feeding.
- Diarrhea. A major complication due to rapid administration of feeding, the high caloric solution, malnutrition, GI bacteria (*Colstridium difficile*), and medications such as antibiotics and magnesium containing drugs such as antacids and sorbitol. Sorbitol is a used as a filler for certain drugs. Drugs in the form of oral liquids are hypersomolar and pull water from the cells and into the GI tract resulting in diarrhea. Decreasing the infusion rate, diluting the solution, changing the solution, discontinuing the medication, or increasing daily water intake helps to manage diarrhea.

Table 11-1 contains commonly used preparations for enteral feeding.

Table 11-1. Commonly used preparations for enteral feeding.

Category	Supplement	Comment
Blenderized	Compleat B (Sandox) Formula 2 (Cutter) Vitaneed (Sherwood)	Blended natural foods Ready to use
Polymeric milk-based	Meritene (Sandox) Instant Breakfast (Carnation) Sustacal Power (Mead Johnson)	Provides nutrients that are intact Pleasant tasting oral supplement

Table 11-1. *(continued)*

Category	Supplement	Comment
Lactose-free	Ensure, Jevity, Osmolite (Ross) Sustacal Liquid, Isocal, Ultracal (Mead Johnson) Fibersource, Resource (Sandox) Entrition, Nutren (Clintec) Attain, Comply (Sherwood)	Used as oral supplement, tube feeding, or meal replacement Ready to use Meets daily intake of vitamins and minerals.
Elemental (monomeric) formulas	Vital HN (Ross) Vivonex T.E.N. (Sandox) Criticare HN (Mead Johnson) Trayasorb (Clintec) Peptamen (Clintec) Reabilan (O'Brian)	Partially digested nutrients for feeding tube Required reconstitution except for Peptamen, Reabilan, and Criticare.

Administering medications through the NG tube is discussed in Chapter 6; the drug must be in liquid form or dissolved into a liquid and must be properly diluted—it is usually given as a bolus and followed by water—liquid medications should be diluted with water to reduce the osmolality to 500 mOsm/kg H_2O (mildly hypertonic) to decrease GI intolerance

Calculation for dilution of enteral medications:

1. Calculate the drug order to determine the volume of the drug:

   $\dfrac{D \times V}{H}$ or H:V::D:x

   D: Desired dose: dose ordered
   H: Have (on-hand dose; dose on label of container
       [bottle, vial or ampule])
   V: Vehicle: form and amount in which the drug is available
       (tablet, capsule, liquid)

2. Determine the osmolality of the drug (drug literature or pharmacist) and liquid dilution. Use 500 mOsm as a constant for the desired osmolality:

   $\dfrac{\text{known mOsm} \times \text{volume of drug}}{\text{desired mOsm}} = \text{total volume of liquid}$

3. Determine the volume of water for dilution:

   total volume of liquid − volume of drug = volume of water for dilution

   Example: acetaminophen 650 mg, q6h, PRN for pain

   Have (on hand): Acetaminophen elixir 65 mg/mL.
   Average mOsm/kg = 5400

1. $D \times V = \dfrac{650 \text{ mg} \times 1 \text{ mL}}{65 \text{ mg}} = 10 \text{ mL}$

   $$
   \begin{array}{ccccc}
   H & : & V & D & :x \\
   65 \text{ mg} & : & 1\text{mL} & :: \ 650 \text{ mg}: & :x\text{mL}
   \end{array}
   $$
   $$65x = 650$$
   $$x = 10 \text{ mL of acetaminophen}$$

2. known mOsm (5400) × volume of drug (10) = $\dfrac{5400 \times 10}{500}$ = 108 mL of
   liquid desired mOsm (500)

3. total volume of liquid (108 mL) × volume of drug (10 mL0 = 98 mL of
   water for dilution

Nursing Process

Assessment
- Assess the tape around the nasogastric tube
- Assess sign and symptoms of intolerance to feedings
- Intake and output
- Bowel sounds
- Baseline laboratory values

Nursing Diagnoses
- Risk for fluid volume deficit
- Risk for diarrhea related to tube feedings

- Potential for loss of skin integrity related to diarrhea
- Risk for aspiration

Planning

- Patient will receive adequate nutritional support
- Side effects will be managed
- No skin breakdown will occur
- Patient will not aspirate

Interventions

- Check tube placement
- Check for gastric residual before intermittent or bolus feedings
- Check continues feedings for residual every 2 to 4 hours
- Feeding should be at room temperature
- Flush feeding tube based on method of delivery
- Monitor side effects such as diarrhea
- Dilute drug solutions appropriately
- Monitor vital signs
- Monitor hydration
- Weigh patient daily
- Change feeding bag daily

Education

- Patient should report diarrhea, sore throat, and abdominal cramping

Evaluation

- Patient will not lose weight
- Patient will not have skin break down
- Patient will not experience diarrhea, abdominal cramping or distention
- Patient will remain in a positive nitrogen balance
- Patient will not become dehydrated

PARENTERAL NUTRITION

Parenteral nutrition support is used for patients who have severe burns, disorders of the GI tract, acquired immunodeficiency syndrome (AIDS), or a debilitating disease such as metastatic cancer.

These patients receive an infusion of a solution that contains hyperosmolar glucose, amino acids, vitamins, electrolytes, minerals, and trace elements. In addition, the patient might be given fat emulsion supplemental therapy to increase the number of calories and to receive fat-soluble vitamins. The infusion is given through a central venous line such as the subclavian or internal jugular vein to prevent irritation to the peripheral veins.

The nurse must monitor the patient for signs of complications as a result of inserting the catheter and the infusion of the feeding.

Catheter insertion can cause

- Pneumothorax.
- Hemothorax.
- Hydrothorax.

Parental nutrition infusion can cause:

- Air embolism.
- Infection.
- Hyperglycemia.
- Hypoglycemia.
- Fluid overload.

It is important that strict asepsis (gloves and masks) be used when changing the IV tubing and the dressing at the infusion site because parenteral nutrition solutions are an excellent medium for yeast and bacteria to grow. The pharmacy uses a laminar airflow hood when preparing parenteral nutritional solutions to reduce this risk.

Monitor the patient carefully for hyperglycemia when you initiate parenteral nutrition support because the pancreas needs time to adjust to the hypertonic dextrose solution, which is high in glucose. Sometimes hyperglycemia is temporary and dissipates once the pancreas makes the necessary adjustments.

However, hyperglycemia might persist if the infusion rate is too fast. To prevent this from occurring, begin with 1 liter of solution for the first 24 hours. Increase this by 500 to 1000 mL each day until you reach a daily volume of 2500 mL to 3000 mL.

Change the solution and tubing every 24 hours. Change the dressing every 48 to 72 hours or according to the agency policy.

Caution: Don't suddenly interrupt parenteral nutrition support because the patient can experience hypoglycemia. Discontinue gradually by decreasing the infusion rate. However, hypoglycemia may occur in spite these precautions.

The Nursing Process and Parenteral Nutritional Therapy

When administering parenteral nutritional therapy, the nurse should use the following nursing process:

Assessment
- Assess:
    - vital signs.
    - patient'sweight
    - lab values.
    - patient's intake and output.

Nursing Diagnoses
- Risk for:
    - fluid volume excess.
    - fluid volume deficit.
    - infection.
    - respiratory complications.
    - altered nutrition.

Planning
- Patient will:
    - meet nutritional needs.
    - maintain body weight.
    - maintain fluid volume balance.
- Patient will not:
    - develop infection at the insertion site or a systemic infection.

Interventions
- Maintain sepsis when changing the solution and dressing.
- Weigh the patient each day.
- Refrigerate the solution until time for use.
- Do not use the parenteral nutritional line to draw blood, give medication, or check central venous pressure
- Monitor:
    - vital signs.

- o patient weight.
- o lab values.
  - intake and output.
  - catheter insertion site.
- o signs of hyperglycemia when therapy is started.
- o signs for hypoglycemia after therapy is discontinued.
- Change:
  - o the solution as ordered.
  - o the tubing per agency policy
  - o the dressing per agency policy.

Education

- Teach the patient:
  - o signs of complications.
  - o to report complications.
  - o the difference between a parenteral nutritional infusion and an intravenous infusion.

Evaluation

- The patient will not:
  - o lose body weight.
  - o develop fluid volume overload.
  - o develop hyperglycemia.
  - o develop dehydration.
  - o develop an infection.
- The patient will:
  - o maintain positive nitrogen balance.

Summary

The body requires nutrients for cell growth, cellular functions, muscle contraction, wound healing, and other vital activities. Nutrients enter the body as food and are absorbed as chemical reactions break down food into molecules that enter the bloodstream where they are distributed throughout the body.

Surgery, trauma, malignancy, and other catabolic illnesses cause a nutritional imbalance that, if prolonged, can have a dramatic impact on the patient that could ultimately lead to death.

Healthcare professionals can restore or maintain the patient's nutritional balance by administering nutritional support therapy to replace nutrients that the patient lost. There are two types of nutritional support therapies: enteral and parenteral.

Enteral nutritional support therapy introduces nutrition into the patient by mouth or a feeding tube that is directly inserted in the stomach or small intestine. Parenteral nutritional support therapy administers high caloric nutrients through large veins such as the subclavian vein.

Quiz

1. Hyperalimentation is
    (a) parenteral nutrition.
    (b) enternal nutrition.
    (c) a high saline concentration for parenteral nutrition therapy.
    (d) none of the above.

2. Blenderized
    (a) is a lactose-free liquid.
    (b) consists of liquids that are individually prepared based on the nutritional needs of the patient.
    (c) is powder mixed with milk.
    (d) is powder mixed with water.

3. Nausea and vomiting may occur during enteral therapy if which of the following occurs?
    (a) Large amounts of solution are infused too rapidly.
    (b) The solution is infused directly onto the patient's stomach.
    (c) The solution is infused very slowly.
    (d) The solution is mixed with water.

4. Monomeric is the least expensive enteral solution.
    (a) True
    (b) False

5. Parenteral nutrition therapy is used for a severely burned patient.
    (a) True
    (b) False

6. Catheter insertion can cause
   (a) pneumothorax.
   (b) hemothorax.
   (c) hydrothorax.
   (d) all of the above.

7. It is dangerous to suddenly interrupt parenteral nutrition therapy.
   (a) True
   (b) False

8. Nutrients play a role in
   (a) carbohydrate-fat-protein synthesis.
   (b) enzyme activities.
   (c) the GI tract.
   (d) All of the above

9. A healthy, well-nourished person has a nutritional level to last 14 days before they begin to show signs of malnutrition.
   (a) True
   (b) False

10. A nutritional deficit is called a negative nitrogen balance
    (a) True
    (b) False

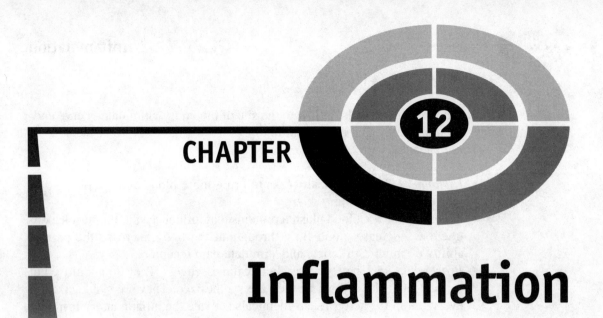

CHAPTER 12

Inflammation

Scratch your arm and within minutes the site turns red and hurts. This is your body's inflammatory response to tissue injury. Fortunately, most times the pain goes away and the inflammation subsides relatively quickly and doesn't interfere with daily activities.

However, this isn't always the case—especially when the injury is severe such as arthritis, gout, toothache, or other painful conditions including menstrual cramps. For these conditions, medication is needed to decrease the inflammation so your daily activities are not interrupted.

In this chapter, you'll learn about inflammation and the medications that are prescribed to reduce the redness, swelling, warmth, and pain that is associated with inflammation.

An Inside Look at Inflammation

Inflammation is the body's protective response to injury to tissues. Injury causes the release of three chemicals that stimulate a vascular response that force fluid and white blood cells to flow to the site of the injury. Stimulated nerve endings signal the brain that there is an injury.

These chemicals are

- *Histamines.* This chemical works to bring more blood and lymph fluid to the site of the invasion.
- *Kinins.* These are blood plasma proteins that influence smooth muscle contractions, increase blood flow throughout the body, increase the permeability of small capillaries, and stimulate pain receptors.
- *Prostaglandins.* They work as chemical messengers. They do not move but work right in the cell where they are synthesized. They are synthesized in every cell in the body. These chemicals activate the inflammatory response and produce pain and fever. They are produced in response to the white blood cells that flow to the area of injured tissue.

The injured tissue becomes red, swollen, warm and loses its normal function. These, along with pain, are the five cardinal signs of inflammation. It is important not to confuse inflammation and infection because they are not the same.

Only a small percentage of inflammation is caused by infection from microorganisms. Trauma, surgery, extreme heat or cold, electricity, and caustic chemicals cause most inflammation.

Inflammation occurs in two phases.

VASCULAR PHASE

The vascular phase occurs 10 to 15 minutes after the tissue is injured. It is during this phase that blood vessels dilate (vasodilation) and become more permeable, enabling fluid and white blood cells to leave the plasma and flow to the injured tissue.

DELAYED PHASE

The delayed phase occurs when the injured tissue is infiltrated by white blood cells. White blood cells (also called leukocytes or immune cells) are components found in the blood. They are also found in the spleen, the lymphatic system, and other tissues. They help defend the body against infectious disease and foreign material as part of the immune system. The three main types of leukocytes (white blood cells) are granulocytes (neutrophils, basophils, and eosinophils), lymphocytes (B-cells, T-cells, and natural killer cells), and monocytes.

Combating Inflammation

Although inflammation is a natural response to injury, this process can be uncomfortable for a patient, especially when there is fever, pain, and swelling. Anti-inflammatory medication can be given to reduce the inflammatory process and bring comfort to the patient.

Anti-inflammatory medication stops the production of prostaglandins resulting in a decrease in the inflammatory process. There are three categories of anti-inflammatory medication.

1. Analgesic. Pain relieving medication
2. Antipyretic. Fever reducing medication
3. Anticoagulant. Inhibits platelet aggregation (grouping to form clot)

Many anti-inflammatory medications fall within all three categories. Aspirin is one of them, which is the oldest and least expensive anti-inflammatory medication available and, along with acetaminophen and ibuprofen, is the choice for relieving headaches.

Corticosteroids, such as prednisone, are frequently used as anti-inflammatory agents. This group of drugs can control inflammation by suppressing or preventing many of the components of the inflammatory process at the injured site.

There are other anti-inflammatory medications that are not chemically the same as corticosteroid medication. These are referred to as nonsteroidal anti-inflammatory drugs (NSAIDs). NSAIDs are appropriate for reducing swelling, pain, and stiffness.

There are eight groups of NSAIDs.

1. Salicylates (related to aspirin)
2. Parachlorobenzoic acid derivatives or indoles
3. Pyrazolone derivatives
4. Propionic acid derivatives
5. Fenamates
6. Oxicams
7. Phenylacetic acids
8. Selective COX-2 inhibitors

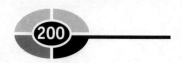
COMMON TYPES OF ARTHRITIS

Osteoarthritis or degenerative joint disease affects 86% of persons over 70 years of age, although symptoms may start in the fifth or sixth decade of life. This common form of arthritis is the result of deformation or mismatched joint surfaces, rather than an inflammatory disease. Symptoms include joint stiffness that usually lasts only a few minutes after initiating movement and perhaps an aching pain in weight-bearing joints. Early disease stages may respond to local heat and nonprescription analgesics. Later stages may require orthopedic or other interventions.

Rheumatoid arthritis usually occurs between 30 to 70 years of age and occurs more often in women than in men. Early symptoms may include feelings of fatigue and weakness, joint pain and stiffness, and, joint swelling several weeks later. Joints are inflamed (warm, red, swollen) and often are limited in range of motion. This is a progressive disease that leads to joint deformity. Aspirin and aspirin-type products (NSAIDs) and Disease Modifying Anti-Rheumatic Drugs (DEMARDs) are usually necessary to reduce the inflammation around the joints and inhibit the progression of the disease. Heat therapy, weight control, and exercise may also be helpful.

A list of drugs utilized in the treatment of arthritis is provided in the Appendix. Detailed tables show doses, recommendations, expectations, side effects, contraindications, and more; available on the book's Web site (see URL in Appendix).

Gout has been called the "disease of Kings" because in the past, royalty ate rich foods and drank wine and alcohol and suffered from gout. However, it is not just for the "rich and famous." Gout is an inflammatory condition that attacks joints, tendons, and other tissues. The most common site of acute gouty inflammation is at the joint of the big toe. It may also be referred to as gouty arthritis. It is characterized by a uric acid metabolism disorder and a defect in purine (products of certain proteins) metabolism, resulting in an increase in urates (uric acid salts) and an accumulation of uric acid (hyperuricemia) or an ineffective clearance of uric acid in the kidneys. Uric acid solubility is poor in acid urine and urate crystals may form, causing urate calculi (stones). Gout may appear as bumps or "tophi" in the subcutaneous tissue of earlobes, elbows, hands, and the base of the large toe. The complications of untreated or prolonged periods of gout include tophi, gouty arthritis, urinary calculi, and gouty nephropathy.

Fluid intake should be increased while taking antigout drugs and the urine should be alkaline. Foods rich in purine, including wine, alcohol, organ meats, sardines, salmon, and gravy should be avoided.

A list of drugs utilized in the treatment of gout is provided in the Appendix. Detailed tables show doses, recommendations, expectations, side effects, contraindications, and more; available on the book's Web site (see URL in Appendix).

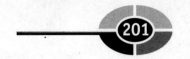

Summary

Inflammation is the body's response to tissue injuries. The body releases histamines, kinins, and prostaglandins that force fluid and white blood cells to the site of the injury to stimulate nerve endings and clean the area so it can heal.

The site of the injury becomes red, swollen, and warm and loses its normal function. This happens in two phases. The vascular phase is where blood vessels dilate and become permeable so fluid and white blood cells can leave the vessel. The delayed phase is where white blood cells infiltrate the tissue.

Anti-inflammatory medication reduces the inflammatory process which may allow the patient to go about normal daily activities while the tissue heals. There are three categories of anti-inflammatory medications: analgesic, to relieve pain; antipyretic, to reduce fever; and anticoagulants, to inhibit blood clotting.

Aspirin and other anti-inflammatory medications are called NSAIDs (non-steroidal anti-inflammatory drugs). These are eight groups of NSAIDs: salicylates, parachlorobenzoic acid derivatives, pyrazolone derivatives, propionic acid derivatives, fenamates, oxicams, phenylacetic acids, and selective COX-2 inhibitors. Corticosteroids are also used as anti-inflammatory medication.

You learned in this chapter that inflammation is not an infection although inflammation frequently occurs when a patient becomes infected with a microorganism. Inflammation occurs in response to tissue injury whether it is from an injury or an acute or chronic disease such as rheumatoid arthritis or gout. You'll learn about infection and fever and antimicrobial medication in the next chapter.

Quiz

1. What stimulates nerve endings at the site of an injury?
   (a) hypothermic response
   (b) infection response
   (c) inflammatory response
   (d) None of the above

2. During what phase of the inflammation response does WBC infiltrate the injured tissue?
   (a) anti-inflammatory phase
   (b) vascular phase
   (c) delayed phase
   (d) All of the above

3. Which of the following relieves pain?
   (a) analgesic
   (b) antipyretic
   (c) anticoagulant
   (d) All of the above

4. Anti-inflammatory medication stops the production of prostaglandins resulting in a decrease in the inflammatory process.
   (a) True
   (b) False

5. Tinnitus is a side effect of salicylates
   (a) True
   (b) False

6. The vascular phase occurs
   (a) 10 to 15 minutes before the tissue is injured.
   (b) 10 to 15 minutes after the tissue is injured.
   (c) 10 to 15 minutes before the tissue heals.
   (d) None of the above

7. DMARDs may arrest the progression of rheumatoid arthritis.
   (a) True
   (b) False

8. Which of the following is a sign of inflammation?
   (a) redness
   (b) warmth
   (c) swelling (edema)
   (d) All of the above

9. A large percentage of inflammation is caused by infection.
   (a) True
   (b) False

10. The choice of medications for relieving headaches are aspirin, acetaminophen, and ibuprofen.
    (a) True
    (b) False

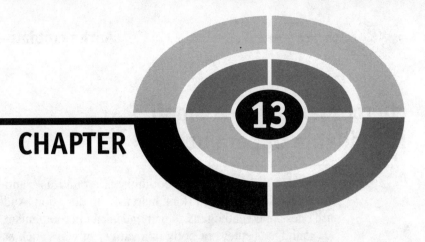

CHAPTER

Antimicrobials— Fighting Infection

Pharmacology conjures images of the magic pill a prescriber gives you to relieve your runny nose, headache, fever, and other symptoms that make it unbearable to go about daily activities. Sometimes those symptoms are from your body adjusting to irritants like pollen. Other times, symptoms are caused by malfunctioning parts of your body such as the pancreas in the case of diabetes.

There is a third cause of symptoms—invading microbials. You'll remember from your courses on anatomy and physiology and microbiology that a microbial is a tiny organism—such as bacteria and viruses—that can enter the body and make you sick.

The immune system produces antibodies that seek out, attack, and kill microbials. However, this natural defense isn't sufficient for some patients who need to call in the cavalry. The cavalry is medication that kills the invading microbial. You'll learn about antimicrobial medication in this chapter.

Microorganisms—A Small Formidable Opponent

There are millions of microorganisms around us—and in our body. Some are harmless. Others, called flora, help us with digestion. And then there are the harmful ones called pathogens. A pathogen is a microorganism that causes an infection.

Pathogens enter our body in a variety of ways such as a cut or in food that we ingest. Once inside, a race begins between the invading organism and the body's defenses. Our body reacts with an inflammatory response that dilates blood vessels so they become permeable. This allows fluid containing white blood cells to infiltrate the infected area. Nerve endings are stimulated and send a message to your brain that there is something wrong.

You know when this happens because the infected area turns red, swollen, and it hurts. The infection might be a patch of tissue referred to as a local infection. Other infections affect an organ or entire system of your body, which is referred to as a systemic infection or septecemia. An infection can also affect multiple organs and systems. This is called sepsis.

You can learn more about microbials by reading *Microbiology Demystified*.

Medication—A Formidable Defender

Your natural defense against bacteria is a phagocytic response. Cells in your body engulf a pathogen, basically eat it and remove the injured tissue. Many times your body needs help from medication that can kill microbials. These are called antimicrobials. An antimicrobial is a medication that kills a microorganism. There are many types of antimicrobials. Each is designed to kill specific microorganisms. The most familiar is an antibiotic, which kills bacteria. Antibiotics kill microbials—the good and the bad. For example, an antibiotic used to kill bacteria that causes a urinary tract infection will also kill the flora in your intestine that are used to help digest food.

Patients are also treated with medication that eases the symptoms of inflammation but doesn't kill microbials. These are prostaglandin inhibitors.

Prostaglandins are chemical mediators that bring about the inflammatory response by vasodilatation, relaxing smooth muscle, making capillaries permeable, and sensitizing nerve cells within the affected area to pain. A prostaglandin inhibitor reduces the production of prostaglandins and thereby reduces the symptoms of inflammation.

Nonsteroidal anti-inflammatory drugs (NSAIDs) are aspirin and "aspirin-like drugs." Aspirin is the most commonly used prostaglandin inhibitor because it is an analgesic to relieve pain. It is also an antipyretic to lower body temperature and it is an anticoagulant that inhibits the formation of platelets.

Other nonsteriodal anti-inflammatory drugs (NSAIDs) are also prostaglandin inhibitors. Other NSAIDs require a lower dose than aspirin to have the same analgesic effect. However, most NSAIDs have a lower anti-inflammatory effect than aspirin.

ANTIMICROBIALS—STUFF MICROORGANISMS DIE FOR

Two of the first antimicrobials developed were sulfonamides and penicillin (PCN). Sulfonamides are bacteriostatic, which means they stop the growth of bacteria, but do not kill bacteria. Penicillin, the first antibiotic, is a bacteriocidal and kills bacteria using lysis, which explodes the bacteria into parts.

Tip: A static means stops growth while cidal (homicide) means kills.

Today there are many synthetic and semi-synthetic antimicrobials on the market that stop some bacteria from growing and kill other bacteria. For example, chloramphenicol is bacteriostatic and stops most bacteria from growing while it is bacteriocidal and kills *S pneumoniae and H influenza* in cerebral spinal fluid. Tetracycline is also bacteriostatic and bacteriocidal; in small concentrations it stops the growth of bacteria and in high concentration it kills bacteria.

Sulfonamides and penicillin are administered orally, topically as an ointment or cream, or parenterally and are absorbed into the body and distributed by the circulatory system. In severe infections, they can be administered directly at the site of the infection such as in the eye or rubbed on the skin.

There are four ways in which these medications work.

1. They inhibit the bacteria from growing a cell wall (cell wall synthesis).
2. They disrupt or alter the permeability of the bacteria's membrane. The membrane is within the cell wall and is used to let nutrients into the cell and send waste out of the cell.
3. They inhibit the bacteria's ability to make protein (protein synthesis). Medications that stop the growth of bacteria interrupt steps in protein synthesis. Those that kill bacteria cause the bacteria to form defective proteins.

4. They inhibit the bacteria's capability to make (synthesize) essential metabolites. A metabolite is a component necessary for bacteria's metabolism to function properly.

Medication used to stop the growth of microbials or kill them outright have side effects, some of which can adversely affect the patient. Some cause an allergic reaction while others lead to an exaggerated immune response. Here are a few common ones that you probably recognize:

- Rash
- Fever
- Urticaria (hives) with pruritis (itching)
- Chills, general erythema (redness)
- Anaphylaxis (circulatory collapse)

These side effects are usually treatable by using other medication such as:

- Antihistamines (Benadryl)
- Epinephrine (adrenalin)
- Steroids for anti-inflammatory response

Superinfections

Antibiotics are a good thing—and a not so good thing. The benefit is obvious. Antibiotics kill bacteria, however, problems can arise. The normal microbial flora die along with the bacteria. This flora can be replaced by resistant bacteria and superinfection can occur. This is a greater risk when large doses of antibiotics are used, when more than one antibiotic is used at a time, or when broad-spectrum drugs are used. For example, the overuse of cephalosporins may cause *pseudomonas* and the overuse of tetracycline may cause *candida albicans*. *Pseudomonas* and *candida albicans* are then considered to be a superinfection in response to the use of cephalosporins and tetracycline.

Resistance to the antibiotic is another problem that can occur. Culture and sensitivity studies should be performed on all infections in order to determine which antibiotics will work for the microorganism that is causing the infection. The test can be performed on blood or wound drainage to identify the bacteria and help identify which antibiotic will be effective.

Some patients stop taking medication as soon as the symptoms of infection dissipate, however the bacterium is still alive and actively growing. As a result, the patient has a relapse and is again prescribed the antibiotic.

Other times, the prescriber may underprescribe an antibiotic by giving the patient a lower-than-effective dose or order the antibiotic for a short period of time. At first this seems like a logical way to prevent the bacterium from becoming resistant to the antibiotic. However, a low dose may not completely kill the bacterium resulting in a recurrence of symptoms that requires additional doses of antibiotics. It is very important to choose the right antibiotic, in the right dose, for the right amount of time.

Preparing to Administer Antimicrobial Medication

Antimicrobial medication requires the nurse to follow the same general administration procedures that are required for any type of medication. The most critical step is to determine if the patient has allergies to drugs, food, environmental stimuli, and a family history of allergies to antibiotics. There is also a high incidence of cross sensitivity between some antibiotics such as penicillin and cephalasporins. Always display allergies in red and clearly write them on the patient's record. Even if the patient's record indicates that the patient doesn't have allergies, always ask the patient each time you administer the antimicrobial medication.

Always have emergency medications such as epinephrine, Benadryl, and steroids handy so they can be given to counteract any adverse side effect of the antimicrobial medication. Be sure to carefully monitor the patient for a half hour after the medication is given to determine if the patient experiences an adverse reaction.

During treatment, you'll need to monitor the therapeutic effect of the medication by monitoring the signs and symptoms of the disease and by obtaining the patient's white blood cell count. Although you can monitor the antimicrobial serum level to determine if the medication has achieved a therapeutic level, this is only done in cases where the therapeutic range is narrow resulting in possible toxicities (i.e., vancomycin ototoxicity).

It is important to administer antimicrobials at the times described in the prescriber's order in order to maintain a therapeutic blood level of the medication.

Otherwise, this can lead to undertreatment or ineffective treatment if not maintained. Sometimes a double dose of an antibiotic is administered as the first dose to quickly achieve a therapeutic level. This is called a loading dose.

Intramuscular injections of antibiotics should be given deep into the muscle and sites should be rotated if more than one injection is prescribed. Stop orders and the need for renewal orders will depend on the healthcare agency policy. However, it is common that antibiotic orders are for 72 hours only until the results of a culture and sensitivity test can be obtained. Antibiotic prescriptions are usually not renewed. This is an effort to limit the opportunity for the microbial to become resistant to the medication.

In severe cases, aggressive treatment is necessary to control the growth and destroy the microbial quickly. To do this, the medication is administered parenterally in an IV dose that is diluted in a neutral solution (pH 7.0 to 7.2) such as normal saline (N.S.) or isotonic sodium chloride or 5% dextrose and water (D5W). Antibiotics should not be mixed together or administered at the same time. They can be administered as a piggyback infusion. Information about how long an interval should occur between the infusion of different antibiotics should be obtained from the pharmacy or the drug insert.

The following nursing diagnoses can be used for patients who are taking antibiotics:

- Risk of infection related to treatment failure or superinfection.
- Risk of fever related to treatment failure or superinfection.
- Risk of fluid volume deficit related to adverse GI reaction such as anorexia, nausea/vomiting/diarrhea, and complications of allergic reaction.

They are also at risk for having the following collaborative problems:

- Sepsis
- Ototoxicity (ears)
- Blood dyscrasias
- Nephrotoxicity (kidney)

It is critical that the patient be given information on the management of his or her condition. These instructions include:

- Take all the medication even after the symptoms subside.
- Do not take medication that is left over from a previous illness. (The medication may not treat the patient's condition or may have lost its therapeutic capabilities.)

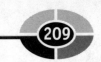

- Do not share drinks, food, and utensils with others until the healthcare provider determines that the patient is no longer infected by the microbial. Sharing may enable the microbial to spread to other people.
- Recognize the expected effects, side effects, and adverse reactions that might occur as a result of taking the medication. Also provide the patient with a telephone number to call if the patient has questions about these effects.
- Wear a Med-alert bracelet if the patient has allergies to medication.

PENICILLIN

Penicillin (PCN) is derived from molds that you sometimes see on bread and fruit. It was discovered in 1940 and remains the most effective—and least toxic—antimicrobial drug. Penicillin weakens the cell wall of a bacteria resulting in the rupture and destruction of a cell, which is called lysis.

Penicillin is most active against gram-positive bacteria and some gram-negative bacteria. However, it isn't active against bacteria that contain enzymes that destroy penicillin.

There are four types of penicillin:

1. Basic (natural)
2. Penicillinase-resistant (resistant to beta-lactamase inactivation)
3. Aminopenicillins (broad spectrum)
4. Extended-spectrum

Besides route, dose, and time, drugs are also characterized by pregnancy category, protein-binding, and half-life. Pregnancy category indicates if the drug has been tested using pregnant women and how safe the drug might be if used during pregnancy. Penicillin is categorized by its usefulness against bacterial enzymes capable of destroying the drug. Four different classifications of antibiotics exist that contain the beta-lactam ring and are more active against gram-negative cell wall organisms and decrease its susceptibility to enzymes that inactivate the antibiotic. Protein-binding is when a drug binds to plasma proteins. When a drug is bound to a protein it is not available for therapeutic use. The percent of protein binding is the amount of drug that can't be used until it is released when the free drug or the amount not bound to protein is excreted from the body. Half-life is the amount of time for half the drug to be eliminated from the body.

The category appears at the top of the table if the value of the category applies to all the drugs in a table, otherwise the category appears beneath the name of the drug in the table.

There are several precautions that must be taken when administering penicillin. If penicillin is given PO, avoid giving this medication an hour before and an hour after the patient has eaten. However, food doesn't have any effect on amoxicillin, amoxicillin and clavulanate, and bacampicillin. Give penicillin with a full glass of water and not with acidic fruit juices.

If penicillin is administered IV, give it slowly because penicillin contains a large amount of potassium that can cause heart failure in patients with renal insufficiency.

Before penicillin is administered, the patient must be assessed for a number of conditions. One of the most important is allergies. An allergic reaction to penicillin can be anywhere from a mild rash to anaphylactic shock and death.

Furthermore, don't administer penicillin to patients who have:

- A tendency to bleed.
- Ulcerative colitis and other GI diseases.
- Mononucleosis (a skin rash may develop with use of ampicillin or bacampicillin).
- A low-salt diet (parenteral carbenicillin and ticarcillin have high sodium content
- Impaired renal function (a lower dose may be given in such cases).

After penicillin is administered, monitor the patient for:

- Serum electrolytes for hyperkalemia (elevated potassium) and/or hypernatremia (elevated sodium)
- Unusual weight loss (especially in the elderly)
- Vital signs
- WBC
- Cultures
- Prothrombin Time (PT) (bleeding times)

Descriptions of medication throughout this chapter use the following abbreviations:

PB	protein-binding	IV	intravenous
t½	half-life	IM	intramuscular
UK	unknown	A	adult
PO	by mouth	C	child

Basic (Natural) Penicillin
Pregnancy Category: B
Protein-Binding: 65%
Half-Life: ¹/₂ hour

Route	Dose	Time
Penicillin G		
PO	200,000–500,000	Every 4 to 6 hours
IV	1–5 mu	Every 4 to 6 hours
IM	1.2–2.4 micro units	Single dose
Penicillin V (take on empty stomach)		
PO	125–500 mg	Every 8 hours

Penicillinase-Resistant Penicillin
Pregnancy Category: B
Half-Life: ¹/₂–1 hour

Route	Dose	Time
cloxacillin (Tegopen) Protein-Binding: 90%		
PO		Every 6 hours
IV	250–500 mg	Every 4 to 6 hours
dicloxacillin (Dynapen) Protein-Binding: 90%		
PO	125–250 mg	Every 6 hours
methicillin (Staphcillin) Protein-Binding: 25%–40%		
IV	1 g	Every 6 hours
IM	1 g	Every 4 to 6 hours
nafcillin (Unipen) Protein-Binding: 90%		
PO	250 mg–1 g	Every 4 to 6 hours
IV	0.5–1.5 g	Every 4 hours
IM	500 mg	Every 4 to 6 hours

Penicillinase-Resistant Penicillin *(continued)*
oxacillin (Prostaphlin)
Protein-Binding: 95%

PO	0.5–1 g	Every 4 to 6 hours
IV	250–1 g	Every 6 hours
IM	250–1 g	Every 4 to 6 hours

Aminopenicillins (Broad Spectrum) Penicillin
Pregnancy Category: B

Route	Dose	Time
amoxicillin (Amoxil) Protein-Binding: 20% Half-Life: 1–1.3 hours		
PO	250–500 mg	Every 8 hours
amoxicillin + potassium clavulanate (Augmentin, Clavulin) Protein-Binding: 25% Half-Life: 1–1^1/$_2$ hours		
PO	5000 mg	Every 8 hours
ampicillin (Polycillin, Omnipen) Protein-Binding: 15%–28% Half-Life: 1–2 hours		
PO	250–500 mg	Every 6 hours
IV	250–500 mg	Every 8 hours
IM	250–500 mg	Every 8 hours
ampicillin and sulbactam (Unasyn) Protein-Binding: 28%–38% Half-Life: 1–2 hours		
IV	1.5–3 g	Every 6 hours
IM	1.5–3 g	Every 6 hours
bacampicillin (Spectrobid) Protein-Binding: 17%–20% Half-Life: 1 hour		
PO	499–800 mg	Every 12 hours

Extended-spectrum Penicillin Pregnancy Category: B		
Route	**Dose**	**Time**
carbenicillin (Geocillin) Protein-Binding: 50% Half-Life: 1–1½ hours		
PO	0.5–1 g	Every 6 hours
IV	50–83.3 mg/kg	Every 4 hours
IM	50–83.3 mg/kg	Every 4 hours
mezlocillin (Mezlin) Protein-Binding: 30%–40% Half-Life: ½–1 hour		
IV	33.3–58.3 mg/kg	Every 4 hours
IM	33.3–58.3 mg/kg	Every 4 hours
piperacillin (Pipracil) Protein-Binding: 16%–22% Half-Life: 0.6–1.5 hours		
IV	3–4 g	Every 4 to 6 hours
IM	3–4 g	Every 4 to 6 hours
piperacillin + tazobactam (Zosyn, Tazocin) Protein-Binding: Unknown Half-Life: 0.7–1.2 hours		
IV	3.375–4 .5 g	Every 6 to 8 hours
ticarcillin (Ticar) Pregnancy Category: C Protein-Binding: 45%–65% Half-Life: ½–1½ hours		
IV	1–4 g	Every 6 hours
IM	1 g	Every 6 hours
ticarcillin + clavulanate (timentin) Protein-Binding: 45%–65% Half-Life: 1–1½ hours		
IV	33.3–50 mg	Every 4 hours

PENICILLIN AND DRUG-DRUG INTERACTIONS

Penicillin can produce adverse effects if it is administered in conjunction with other drugs. This is the situation with giving penicillin with an anti-hypertensive such as Captopril (angiotensin-converting enzyme [ACE] inhibitors), potassium-sparing diuretics such as Aldactone, potassium-containing drugs, or potassium supplements such as Kay Ciel. The combination of drugs may increase the patient's potassium level (hyperkalemia) and therefore require that the patient's serum potassium levels be carefully monitored while the patient receives penicillin.

There is an increased risk of bleeding when administering high doses of parenteral carbenicillin or ticarcillin as these drugs inhibit platelet aggregation. These penicillins also increase the risk for severe bleeding if given with thrombolytic agents such as streptokinase.

The absorption of penicillin G when taken PO may be decreased if taken with cholestyramine (Questran) or colestipol (Colestid). Similarly, the use of penicillin might decrease the effectiveness of estrogen contained in contraceptives.

Two other drugs affected by penicillin are methotrexate (Folex) and probenecid (Benemid). There is a decrease in the body's ability to clear methotrexate when penicillin is present. There can be a build up of methotrexate resulting in toxicity.

Probenecid decreases renal secretion of penicillin resulting in an increase of the serum level of penicillin.

Penicillin, Nursing Diagnosis, and Collaborative Problems

A patient who is receiving penicillin may experience one or more conditions that require intervention. Here are the common nursing diagnoses that are related to a patient who is receiving penicillin.

- Altered protection against infection related to reduction in normal flora (superinfection)
- Altered bowel elimination pattern related to antibiotic-associated pseudo-membranous colitis
- Fluid volume deficit related to nausea, vomiting, and/or diarrhea

- Impaired skin integrity related to side effects or allergic reaction
- Allergic response
- Hepatotoxicity (toxicity affecting the liver)
- Leukopenia (A decrease in the number of circulating white cells in the blood)
- Neutropenia (abnormal decrease in the number of neutrophils, which are the most common type of white blood cells in the blood)
- Thrombocytopenia (decreased number of platelets in the blood)
- Mental disturbances
- Seizures
- Cross-sensitivity to cephalosporins, cephamycins, griseofulvin, or penicillamine
- Abdominal cramps
- Diarrhea
- Darkened or discolored tongue
- Sore mouth

Penicillin and Patient Education

The patient must be instructed to monitor his or her temperature to be sure that the infection is subsiding. Generally, healthy patients can expect to see some improvement in the infection within 48 hours. They should be instructed to return to or contact the prescriber if symptoms worsen or do not improve somewhat in 48 hours. Patients with diabetes, immunosuppressed conditions such as AIDS, or some cancers might not respond as quickly to antibiotic therapy.

In addition to information described for generic antibiotics, female patients should be informed that penicillin can interfere with the effectiveness of birth control pills that contain estrogen. It is recommended that females use alternative forms of birth control while being treated with penicillin.

CEPHALOSPORINS

The cephalosporin family of medications is a chemically modified version of penicillin that stops growth and kills a broad spectrum of bacteria by making it impossible for bacteria to create a cell wall. There are four generations of cephalosporins.

Cephalosporin can be prescribed for patients who are allergic to penicillin. However, about 10% of those patients might also be allergic to cephalosporins. Do not administer cephalosporins to patients who have had a serious reaction to penicillin such as anaphylaxis.

Prescribers use cephalosporins to combat a wide variety of infections and typically use it as a prophylaxis to prevent a bacterial infection to occur during or after surgery.

Cephalosporins also have side effects which include diarrhea, abdominal cramps or distress, oral and/or vaginal candidiasis, rash, pruritis, redness, or edema. There is also an increase of bleeding and bruising with four commonly prescribed cephalosporins: cefamandole, cefmetazole, cefoperazone, and cefotetan.

The patient assessment for cephalosporins is the same as for penicillin. However, pay particular attention to any previous bleeding disorder reported by the patient because cephalosporins can exacerbate this condition.

Before administering cephalosporins, assess for allergies, vital signs, and urine output. Check laboratory results, especially those that indicate renal and liver function such as BUN, serum creatinine, AST, ALT, ALP, and bilirubin. Also monitor bleeding time (PT and PTT) and white blood cell count. Obtain a tissue or blood specimen for a culture and sensitivity if possible to determine if cephalosporins are the right antibiotic.

Administer cephalosporins using the same methods as used for penicillin. If given IM, it should be injected deeply into a large muscle mass. This decreases pain, induration (becoming hard), and a sterile abscess.

The patient should be provided with the same instructions as is given to a patient who is receiving penicillin (see Penicillin and Patient Education).

CEPHALOSPORINS AND DRUG-DRUG INTERACTIONS

Alcohol should be avoided when taking certain cephalosporins (cefamandole, cefoperazone, or moxalactam) because patients might experience adverse side effects that include:

- Stomach pain
- Nausea
- Vomiting
- Headaches

- Hypotension
- Tachycardia (fast heart rate)
- Difficulty breathing
- Sweating
- Flushed face

Some medications include alcohol and the patient should be advised to check the labels carefully if taking one of these cephalosporins.

Besides alcohol, some cephalosporins (cefamandole, cefmetazole, cefoperazone, or cefotetan) expose the patient to an increased risk of hemorrhaging if administered with anticoagulants such as coumarin or indanedione, heparin, and with clot-busting drugs such as thrombolytics. The same adverse reaction might occur if the patient takes NSAIDs, especially aspirin, or sulfinpyrazone (Anturane) while on cephalosporins.

Probenecid (Benemid) may extend the half-life of cephalosporins and can result in toxicity. However, cephalosporins and probenecid are sometimes given together to treat sexually transmitted diseases when a high serum level and prolonged level of cephalosporins are desirable.

A patient who is undergoing treatment with cephalosporins might experience other problems. These are a fever and rash brought about by hypersensivity, an allergic reaction such as anaphylaxis, Stevens-Johnson syndrome, renal dysfunction, serum sickness-like reaction, or seizures.

Cephalosporins, Nursing Diagnosis, and Collaborative Problems

Here are the common nursing diagnoses that are related to a patient who is receiving cephalosporins.

- Altered bowel elimination pattern related to antibiotic-associated pseudo-membranous colitis
- Risk for superinfection
- Altered protection related to hypoprothrombinemia and superinfection

First Generation: Effective against gram-positive bacteria
Pregnancy Category: B

Route	Dose	Time
Cefadroxil (Duricef) Protein-Binding: 20% Half-Life: $1/2$–2 hours		
PO	500 mg	Every 12 hours
Cefazolin (Ancef, Kefzol) Protein-Binding: 75%–85% Half-Life: $1/2$–$2^{1}/2$ hours		
IV	0.25–1.5 g	Every 6-8 hours
IM	1 g	Presurgery
Cephalexin (Keflex) Protein-Binding: 65%–80% Half-Life: 0.5–1 hour		
PO	250–500 mg	Every 6 hours
Cephalothin (Keflin) Protein-Binding: 10%–15% Half-Life: 0.5–1.2 hours		
IM/IV	0.5–1 g	Every 4 to 6 hours
Cephapirin (Cefadyl) Protein-Binding 40%–50% Half-Life: 0.5–1 hour		
IM /IV	0.5–1 g	Every 4 to 6 hours
Cephradine (Velosef, Anspor) Protein-Binding: 20% Half-Life: 1–2 hours		
PO	250–500 mg	Every 8 hours
IM/IV	0.5–1 g	Every 6 hours

Second Generation: Increased activity against gram (−) microorganisms Pregnancy Category: B		
Route	**Dose**	**Time**
Cefaclor (Ceclor) Protein-Binding: 25% Half-Life 0.5–2 hours		
PO	250–500 mg	Every 8 hours
IM/IV	500 g	Every 6 hours
Cefamandole (Mandol) Protein-Binding: 60%–75% Half-Life: 0.5–1 hour		
IM/IV	500 mg	Every 6–8 hours
Cefmetazole (Zefazone) Protein-Binding: 68% Half-Life: 2.5–3 hours		
IV	2g	Every 12 hours
Cefonicid (Monocid) Protein-Binding: 98% Half-Life: 0.5–1.2 hours		
IM/IV	0.5–1 g	Every 24 hours
Cefotetan (Cefotan) Protein-Binding: 85% Half-Life: 3–5 hours		
IM /IV	102 g	Every 12 hours
Cefoxitin (Mefoxin) Protein-Binding: 70% Half-Life: 45 minutes–1 hour		
IV	102 g	Every 6 to 8 hours
Cefprozil (Cefzil) Protein-Binding: 99% Half-Life: 1–2 hours		
PO	500 mg	Every 12 hours

Second Generation: Increased activity against gram (−) microorganisms *(continued)*
Pregnancy Category: B

Route	Dose	Time
Cefurozine (Ceftin, Zinacef) Protein-Binding: 50% Half-Life: 1.5–2 hours		
PO	250–500 mg	Every 12 hours
IM/IV	0.75–1.5 g	Every 8 hours
Loracarbef (Lorabid) Protein-Binding: Unknown Half-Life: 1 hour		
PO	200–400 mg	Every 12 hours

Third Generation: More active against gram (−); ceftazidime and cefoperazone are also effective against *Pseudomonas aeruginosa* (gram −) and β-lactamase-producing microbial strains; less effective against gram (+) cocci
Pregnancy Category: B

Route	Dose	Time
Cefixime (Suprax) Protein-Binding: 65% Half-Life: 2.5–4 hours		
PO	200 mg	Every 12 hours
Cefoperazone (Cefobid) Protein-Binding: 70%–80% Half-Life: 2.5 hours		
IV	1–2 g	Every 12 hours
Cefotaxime (claforan) Protein-Binding: 30%–40% Half-Life: 1–1.5–3 hours		
IV	1–2 g	Every 12 hours

Third Generation *(continued)*
Pregnancy Category: B

Route	Dose	Time
Cefpodoxime (Vantin, Proxetil) Protein-Binding: 20%–40% Half-Life: 2–3 hours		
PO	200 mg	Every 12 hours
Ceftazidime (Fortaz) Protein-Binding: 10%–17% Half-Life: 1–2 hours		
IM /IV	0.5–2 g	Every 8 to 12 hours
Ceftibuten (Cedax) Protein-Binding: Unknown Half-Life: 1.5–3 hours		
PO	400 mg	Once per day
Ceftriaxone (Recephin) Protein-Binding: 85–95% Half-Life: 8 hours		
IV	1–2 g	Every 24 hours
Ceftizoxime (Cefizox) Protein-Binding: 30%–60% Half-Life: 2 hours		
IM/IV	500 mg	Every 8 to 12 hours
Cefdinir (Omnicef) Protein-Binding: Unknown Half-Life: 1.7 hours		
PO	300 mg or 600 mg/d	Every 12 hours

Fourth Generation: Cefipime same as third generation + more resistant to β-lactamases Pregnancy Category: B		
Route	**Dose**	**Time**
Cefepine (Maxipime) Protein-Binding: Unknown Half-Life 0.5–2 hours		
IM.IV	0.5–1 g	Every 12 hours

MACROLIDE ANTIBIOTICS

Macrolide antibiotics are used to combat gram-positive and gram-negative bacteria. As you'll recall from microbiology, the gram stain is used as a method to identify a bacteria. If after staining, the bacteria it appears purple, then the bacteria are said to be gram positive. If it is pink, then the bacteria are gram-negative. There is one exception: If the bacteria are either purple or pink, then a macrobide antibiotic is effective against the bacteria.

The exception is with troleandomycin, which is a macrolide antibiotic. Troleandomycin is used to fight *Streptococcus pneumoniae* and *Streptococcuus pyogenes*.

Macrolide antibiotics are bacteriostatic. That is, they inhibit reproduction of bacteria, but do not kill the bacteria. By inhibiting reproduction, macrolide antibiotics control the bacterial growth giving the body's own immune system— or other medication—time to kill the bacteria.

Prescribers give patients macrolide antibiotics to fight soft tissue infections, skin infections, and infections of the respiratory and gastrointestinal tract.

Macrolides antibiotics have some side effects that adversely affect the patient. The most common side effects are nausea, vomiting, stomach pain, and cramps. These occur with azithromycin, clarithromycin, erythromycin, and dirithromycin. Troleandomycin causes stomach cramps and discomfort.

Before administering macrolides, the patient is assessed using the same techniques as described for other antibiotics. However, caution must be used when prescribing macrolides to patients who have liver disease. Those with a history of cardiac arrhythmias should not take erythromycin.

The patient should be advised to take macrolides with a full glass of water either an hour before meals or two hours after meals to avoid gastric distress. Some patients are intolerant to some marcrolides when taken orally. In these cases, enteric-coated or delayed-release capsules are appropriate to prescribe.

If marcolides are administered IV, they must be diluted in 100 to 200 mL of 0.9% NS solution or 5% dextrose solution (D5W) and infused over a period of 20 to 60 minutes.

The patient should be provided with the same instructions as those given to a patient who is receiving penicillin (see Penicillin and Patient Education).

Route	Dose	Time
Macrolide Antibiotics Pregnancy Category: B		
Erythromycin (E-Mycin, Erythrocin, Erythrocin Lactobionate) Protein-Binding: 65% Half-Life: PO 1–2 hours; IV 3–5 hours		
PO	250–500 mg	Every 6 hours
IV	1–4 g/d	Divided doses
Azithromyzin (Zithromax) Protein-Binding: 50% Half-Life: 11–55 hours		
PO	500 mg	First Day
	250 mg	Daily thereafter
Clarithromycin (Biaxin) Protein-Binding: 65%–75% Half-Life: 3–6 hours Pregnancy Category: C		
PO	250–500 mg	Every 12 hours
Erythromycin, dirithromycin (Dynabac) Protein-Binding: Unknown Half-Life: 20–50 hours Pregnancy Category: C		
PO	250 mg (Erythromycin)	Every 6 hours
	500 mg (dirithromycin)	Once a day
IV	250–500 mg	Every 6 hours

Macrolides and Drug-Drug Interactions

Macrolides have various effects on other medications. Therefore, the nursing assessment should include obtaining a history of all drugs (OTC or prescribed) or herbals the patient may be taking. Macrolides can increase the therapeutic levels of alfentanil (Alfenta), carbamezepine (Tegretol), and cyclosporine (Sandimmune), resulting in the patient experiencing a toxic effect.

Terfenadine (Seldane) or astemizole (Hismanal) given with macrolides might cause toxicity to the heart. The patient is also at risk for hemorrhage if the patient takes both warfarin (Coumadin) and marolides within the same time period. The patient may also experience increased theophylline levels which can lead to toxicity when theophylline is given along with zanthines such as aminophylline and caffeine.

Macrolides, Nursing Diagnosis, and Collaborative Problems

Here are the common nursing diagnoses that are related to a patient who is receiving marolides.

- Altered bowel elimination pattern
- Impaired tissue integrity related to inflammation or phlebitis at the injection site
- Fluid volume deficit related to nausea and vomiting
- Alteration in comfort related to abdominal cramping
- Sensory-perceptual disturbance related to hearing loss
- Altered protection related to loss of normal flora

LINCOSAMIDES

Lincomycin (Lincocin) has been used in the past to treat serious streptococci, pneumococci, and staphylococci infections but has generally been replaced by safer and more effective antibiotics. Clindamycin (Cleocin) is a semisynthetic derivative of lincomycin and has a similar mechanism but is more effective. It is indicated for the treatment of bone and joint infections, pelvic (female) and intraabdominal infections, bacterial septicemia, pneumonia, and skin and soft tissue infections. In a normal dose, lincosamides prevent the growth of bacteria (bacteriostatic). In larger doses, it kills bacteria (bacteriocidal).

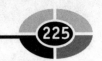

The use of lincomycin is avoided because there is a significant occurrence of pseudomembranous colitis. Clindamycin is the drug of choice because it is safer and more effective than lincomycin.

Patient assessment before administering lincosamides is the same as for all antibiotics. In addition, determine if the patient has a history of GI diseases, liver or kidney problems.

Administer lincosamides with a full glass of water or with meals to prevent esophageal ulceration. After lincosamides are administered, request additional white blood count studies to determine the effectiveness of the medication. Monitor the patient for:

- Abdominal cramps.
- Diarrhea.
- Weight loss.
- Weakness.

The patient should be provided with the same instructions as is given to a patient who is receiving penicillin (see Penicillin and Patient Education).

Clindamycins and Drug-Drug Interactions

Besides being associated with pseudomembranous colitis, clindamycin can also cause an adverse interaction with antidiarrheals, chloramphenicol (Chloromycetin), and erythromycin.

Clindamycin is known to enhance the neuromuscular blockage caused by anesthetic agents. This might result in the patient experiencing skeletal muscle weakness, respiratory depression, and even paralysis if used during or immediately after surgery.

Lincosamides, Nursing Diagnosis, and Collaborative Problems

Patients who receive clindamycin may also experience hypersensitivity. Therefore, you must be prepared to identify the signs and symptoms of hypersensitivity and treat them if conditions become intolerable for the patient.

Lincosamides Pregnancy Category: B		
Route	**Dose**	**Time**
Clindamycin (Cleocin, Dalacin) semisynthetic Protein-Binding: 94% Half-Life: 2–3 hours		
PO/IM/IV	150–300 mg	Every 6 hours
Lincomycin (Lincorex) Protein-Binding: 70–75% Half-Life: 4-6 hours		
PO	500 mg	Every 6 to 8 hours Max 8g/d
IM	600 mg	Every day
IV	Dilute in 100 cc fluid	Every day

Here are the common nursing diagnoses that are related to a patient who is receiving lincosamides.

- Altered bowel elimination patterns
- Fluid volume deficits related to nausea and vomiting
- Altered protection related to neutropenia (infection), thrombocytopenia (bleeding), and loss of normal flora (superinfection)

VANCOMYCIN

Vancomycin is a bactericidal agent used for infections of the bone and joints and bacterial septicemia caused by *Staphylococcus*. It is also used to treat *Staphylococcus*-causing endocarditis including the methicillin-resistant strains. Prescribers commonly prescribe vancomycin to patients who are susceptible to endocarditis in an effort to prevent the infection.

Vancomycin is also used for the treatment of *Clostridium difficile* and staphylococcal enterocolitis, which are treated orally or parenterally. However, parenteral vancomycin is not recommended for treating antibiotic-associated pseudomenbranous colitis.

Before administering vancomycin, use the same assessment criteria used for all antibiotic therapy described throughout this chapter. In addition, determine if the patient has hearing loss, kidney problems, or an inflammatory intestinal disorder. Use of vancomycin should be avoided or used with caution for patients who have a hearing loss. A lower dose of vancomycin should be used for patients who have kidney problems. Carefully monitor patients who have inflammatory intestinal disorders as they are at a higher risk for toxicity. Make sure the patient has adequate renal function.

When administering vancomycin, don't give it as an IV bolus. Vancomycin should be infused over a 24-hour period or infused intermittently over 60 minutes. If given continuously for 24 hours, dilute 1–2 grams of vancomycin in a sufficient amount of .09% sodium chloride (normal saline) or D5W. If infused intermittently for 60 minutes, dilute the dose in 100 ml of .09% sodium chloride (normal saline) or dilute in 100 mL of 5% dextrose solution (D5W). Rotation of the IV sites will help prevent local irritation.

After administering vancomycin, monitor the patient's renal function to assure there is adequate volume to excrete vancomycin. Also monitor the patient's white blood cell count to determine if the drug is effective.

The patient should be provided with the same instructions as is given to a patient who is receiving penicillin (see Penicillin and Patient Education).

Vancomycin and Drug-Drug Interactions

Vancomycin has adverse reactions when used with some medications. You must wait several hours before giving vancomycin to a patient who has received oral cholestyramine (Questran) or colestipol (Colestid) because these medications lower the therapeutic effect of vancomycin.

Also avoid giving vancomycin if the patient has taken any aminoglycosides because they increase the potential for ototoxicity (ear) and nephrotoxicity (kidney). If the patient receives vancomycin and aminoglycosides, then you must closely monitor vancomycin serum levels to determine that it remains within the safe range. Drug-drug interaction may occur if administering Vancomycin with:

- Amphotericin B
- Aspirin
- Bacitracin
- Parenteral bumetanide [Bumex]
- Capreomycin [Capastat]
- Cisplatin [Platinol]
- Cyclosporine [Sandimmune]

- Ethacrynate parenteral [Edecrin]
- Furosemide parenteral [Lasix]
- Paromomycin [Humatin]
- Polymyxins
- Streptozocin [Zanosar]

Vancomycin, Nursing Diagnosis, and Collaborative Problems

Patients who receive vancomycin may also experience nephrotoxicty (kidney). Monitor urine output for kidney function.

Here are the common nursing diagnoses that are related to a patient who is receiving vancomycin.

- Risk for injury related to histamine release if administered too rapidly
- Fluid volume deficit related to nausea and vomiting
- Impaired tissue integrity
- Sensory-perceptual disturbance related to ototoxicity (loss of hearing and tinnitus [ringing in the ears])

AMINOGLYCOSIDES

Aminogylcosides are potent antibiotics used to kill bacteria that cause serious or life-threatening infections. They are very effective against many bacteria (gram-positive and gram-negative) but are generally used for gram-negative infections.

Vancomycin Pregnancy Category: C		
Route	**Dose**	**Time**
Vancomycin (Vancocin) Protein-Binding: 10% Half-Life: 5–11 hours		
IV	500 mg	Every 6 hours

Safer and less toxic agents are available to treat the majority of gram-positive infections. Since the patient is experiencing a life-threatening infection, pre- scribers combine animoglycosides with penicillin, cephalosporins, or ancomycin to give a one-two punch knockout to the bacteria.

There are significant side effects to using aminogylcosides. These are nephro- toxicity, neurotoxicity, hyersensitivity, and ototoxicity (problems with hearing and balance).

Assess the patient according to the guidelines for all antibiotics as described previously in this chapter for penicillin. Infants with botulism and patients with myasthenia gravis or Parkinsonism will experience more muscle weakness than other patients who are treated with animoglycosides. You must also assess if the patient has hearing or kidney problems or allergies.

Before administering aminoglycosides, obtain a baseline assessment for the patient including audiogram, renal function, and vestibular function studies.

When administering aminoglycosides intravenously, dilute the medication in solution as per the package insert and infuse it over a 30- to 60-minute period. Use a smaller than normal dose for elderly patients who are at greater risk for kidney toxicity and ototoxicity.

If aminoglycides are given IM, then give the injection deep into the upper outer quadrant of the gluteal muscle.

After administering aminoglycides, keep the patient well hydrated and mon- itor the patient's intake and output to determine if there is nephrotoxicity. Monitor the patient's temperature, cultures, and WBC to determine if the infection is resolving. A daily urinalysis should be obtained for signs of kidney irritation.

The patient should be provided with the same instructions as those given to a patient who is receiving penicillin (see Penicillin and Patient Education). Advise the patient to report any hearing problem including ringing or buzzing in the ears as well as dizziness, numbness, tingling, twitching, or changes in urinary pat- terns especially blood in the urine.

Aminoglycosides and Drug-Drug Interactions

Aminoglycosides can have undesirable interactions with other medications. When taken with other aminoglycosides or capremycin (Capastat) the patient has an increased potential for hearing, kidney, and neuromuscular problems. Hearing loss can lead to total deafness long after the patient stops treatment with aminoglycosides.

Neuromuscular blockage may increase when aminoglycosides are given to patients who have received anesthetics (halogenated hydrocarbon) or citrate-anticoagulated blood through massive transfusions. Methoxyflurane (Penthrane) and polymyxins, given parenterally also increase the possibility for neuromuscular blockage as well as kidney toxicity.

In addition, patients who are treated with aminoglycides can have interactions with the following medications:

- Amphotericin B parenteral (Fungizone)
- Aspirin
- Bacitracin parenteral
- Bumetanide parenteral aspirin
- Bacitracin
- Parenteral bumetanide (Bumex)
- Cephalothin (Keflin)
- Cisplatin (Platinol)
- Cyclosporine (Sandimmune)
- Ethacrynate parenteral (Edecrin)
- Furosemide parenteral (Lasix)
- Paromomycin (Humatin)
- Polymyxins
- Streptozocin (Zanosar)
- Vancomycin (Cancocin)

Aminoglycosides, Nursing Diagnosis, and Collaborative Problems

Patients who receive aminoglycosides may also experience nephrotoxicty (kidney), neurotoxicity (muscle twitching, numbness or seizures), and hypersensitivity.

Here are the common nursing diagnosis related to a patient who is receiving aminoglycosides.

- Sensory-perceptual alterations: auditory ototoxicity (loss of hearing and tinnitus), vestibular ototoxicity (dizziness and loss of balance) and peripheral neuritis (tingling of the fingers and toes)

Aminoglycosides
Pregnancy Category: C

Route	Dose	Time

Amikacin (Amikin)
Protein-Binding: 4%–11%
Half-Life: 2–3 hours

Route	Dose	Time
IM/IV	5 mg/kg	Every 8 hours

Gentamicin (Garamycin)
Protein-Binding: Unknown
Half-Life: 2 hours

Route	Dose	Time
IM/IV	1–1.7 mg/kg	Infusion every 8 hours

Kanamycin (Kantrex)
Protein-Binding: 10%
Half-Life: 2–3 hours
Pregnancy Category: D

Route	Dose	Time
IM	3.75 mg/kg	Every 6 hours

Neomycin SO$_4$ (Myclfradin)
Protein-Binding: 10%
Half-Life: 2–3 hours

Route	Dose	Time
PO (GI Surgery)	1 g	Every hour for 4 doses
	1 g	Every 4 hours thereafter for 24 hours or other regimens
(Hepatic Coma)	4–12 g/d	Divided doses
IM	15mg/kg/d	Every 6 h for 4 doses Max 1 g/d

Netilmicin (Netromycin)
Protein-Binding: 10%
Half-Life: 2–3 hours
Pregnancy Category: D

Route	Dose	Time
IM/IV	1.3–2.2 mg/kg	Every 8 hours

Aminoglycosides *(continued)* Pregnancy Category: C		
Streptomycin S O$_4$ Protein-Binding: 30% Half-Life: 2–3 hours		
Route	**Dose**	**Time**
IM (tuberculosis)	1 gm	Every day with antimycobacterials
(Endocarditis)	1 g	Every 12 hours for 1 week. Dose may be decreased
Tobramycin SO$_4$ (Nebcin) Protein-Binding: 10% Half-Life: 2–3 hours		
IM/IV	0.75 mg to 1.25 mg/kg	Every 6 hours

TETRACYCLINES

Tetracyclines are the first broad-spectrum antibiotic that was used to halt the growth of many gram-positive and gram-negative bacteria. It is used to treat a variety of infections including acne vulgaris, actinomycosis, anthrax, bronchitis, and other systemic bacterial infections including bacterial urinary tract infections.

Demeclocycline, a member of the tetracycline family, is also used to treat conditions that are associated with inappropriate diuretic hormone since demeclocycline inhibits water-induced reabsorption in the kidneys.

Assess the patient the same way as described previously in this chapter for a patient taking penicillin. Do not use tetracyclines if the patient is pregnant or breastfeeding. Furthermore, tetracyclines should not be given to children under 8 years of age because tetracyclines can permanently mottle and discolor the teeth and decrease linear skeletal growth in both children and the fetus.

Patients who have a hypersenitivity to caine medication such as lidocaine and procaine may be intolerant to tetracyclines because caine medication is mixed in the tetracycline intramuscular injection.

Only doxycycline and minocycline, which are members of the tetracyclines family, can be used with patients who have renal problems. Other members of the tetracycline family should not be prescribed for those patients.

Tetracyclines should be taken with a full glass of water on an empty stomach. It should not be administered an hour before meals or two hours after meals except for doxycycline and minocycline.

The patient should not be given antacids containing aluminum, calcium, or magnesium, laxatives, iron products, food, or milk or other dairy products for 1 hour before or 2 hours after tetracycline is administered.

Doxycycline and oxytetracycline can be administered IV. Doxycycline may be given in concentrations not less than 100μg or > than 1 mg/mL. Don't administer doxycycline IM or SQ. Oxytetracycline needs to be diluted in at least 100 mL of appropriate IV solution. Don't infuse rapidly.

Tetracycline may be administered IM not exceeding 2 ml at each injection site. Don't administer tetracycline IV or SQ.

The patient should be provided with the same instructions as those given to a patient who is receiving penicillin (see Penicillin and Patient Education). However, also advise the patient to avoid direct sunlight and ultraviolet light because tetracyclines might cause the patient to become sensitive to sunlight. The patient should use sunscreen in the sun.

Advise the patient to discard unused tetracycline because tetracyline becomes toxic as it decomposes. Tetracycline should be taken on an empty stomach as food affects absorption of the drug.

Tetracyclines and Drug-Drug Interactions

Tetracyclines can interact with other medications. Avoid giving tetracyclines two hours before or after the patient receives colestipol (Colestid) or cholestyramine (Questran) because these medications decrease the absorption of tetracycline.

Give tetracycline 1–3 hours before or after giving the patient antacids, calcium supplements, choline and magnesium salicylates, iron supplements, magnesium salicylate, or magnesium laxatives, foods containing milk and milk products. These lower the absorption of tetracycline.

Don't give tetracycline if the patient is taking estrogen-containing oral contraceptives since this reduces the contraceptive effectiveness and may result in breakthrough bleeding. Female patients should be advised to use alternative methods of birth control while on antibiotics.

Tetracyclines, Nursing Diagnosis, and Collaborative Problems

Patients who receive tetracycline may also experience nephrogenic diabetes insipidus, hepatotoxicity, pancreatitis, dizziness, syncope, and their skin might be increasingly sensitive to sunlight.

Here are the common nursing diagnoses that are the related to a patient who is receiving tetracyclines.

- Altered comfort (heartburn and abdominal cramping)
- Fluid volume deficit related to anorexia, nausea, and vomiting
- Altered bowel elimination (diarrhea)
- Altered protection related to loss of normal florae (fungal overgrowth)

Tetracyclines Pregnancy Category: D		
Route	**Dose**	**Time**
Tetracycline—Short Acting Protein-Binding: 20%–60% Half-Life: 6–12 hours		
PO	250–500 mg	Every 6 hours
IM	150 mg	Every 12 hours
Oxytetracycline (Terramycin)—Short Acting Protein-Binding: 20%–40% Half-Life: 6–10 hours		
PO	250–500 mg	Every 6 hours
IV	250–500 mg	Infusion every 12 hours
Democlocycline (Declomycin)—Intermediate Acting Protein-Binding: 35%–90% Half-Life: 10–17 hours		
PO	150 mg	Every 6 hours
	300 mg	Every 12 hours

Tetracyclines *(continued)* Pregnancy Category: D		
Route	**Dose**	**Time**
Doxycycline (Vibramycin)—Long Acting Protein-Binding: 25%–92% Half-Life: 20 hours		
PO	100 mg	Twice the first day
	100 to 200 mg	Once a day there after
Minocycline (Minocin)—Long Acting Protein-Binding: 55%–88% Half-Life: 11–20 hours		
PO	200 mg	First dose
	100 mg	Every 12 hours

CHLORAMPHENICOL (CHLOROMYCETIN)

Chloramphenicol is a broad-spectrum antibiotic that slows the growth of a wide variety of gram-positive and gram-negative bacteria. In high doses, chloramphenicol can kill bacteria. Chloramphenicol is given for treatment of meningitis (*H influenzae, S pneumoniae,* and *N meningitides*), parathyroid fever, Q fever, Rocky Mountain spotted fever, typhoid fever, typhus infections, brain abscesses, and bacterial septicemia.

Chloramphenicol should not be used for a patient who is pregnant or is breastfeeding. Neonates may develop gray syndrome, which is blue-gray skin, hypothermia, irregular breathing, coma, and cardiovascular collapse.

Chloramphenicol is not recommended for use with a patient who is undergoing radiation therapy or who has bone marrow depression.

Monitor the chloramphenicol serum level to assure that chloramphenicol stays within therapeutic limits. Chloramphenicol does have a seriously toxic effect on bone marrow.

Patients have infrequently reported experiencing diarrhea, nausea, or vomiting. Serious adverse effects include blood dyscrasias, optic neuritis, and possibly irreversible bone marrow depression that may lead to aplastic anemia.

Chloramphenicol and Drug-Drug Interactions

Chloramphenicol can have an adverse interaction with alfentanil (Alfenta) by increasing alfentanil levels in the patient. Chloramphenicol is known to increase bone marrow depression when given with anticonvulsants.

Patients who are taking antidiabetic medication may see an increase in the level of that medication when taken with chloramphenicol resulting in hypoglycemia. Therefore, diabetics who take chloramphenicol must closely monitor their blood glucose level.

Chloramphenicol also causes a decrease in the therapeutic effect of clindamycin, erythromycin, or lincomycin. Chloramphenicol increases the drug serum levels of phenobarbital (Luminal), phenytoin (Dilantin), or warfarin (Coumadin) which can lead to toxicity.

Chloramphenicol, Nursing Diagnosis, and Collaborative Problems

Patients who take chloramphenicol may also experience rash, fever, and dyspnea. Neonates experience gray syndrome.

Here are the common nursing diagnoses that are related to a patient who is taking chloramphenicol.

- Fluid volume deficit related to anorexia, nausea, and vomiting
- Altered protection related to dose-related bone marrow depression
- Altered bowel elimination (diarrhea)
- Altered thought processes (confusion, delirium) related to neurotoxic reactions; sensory-perceptual disturbances related to optic neuritis (blurred vision, loss of vision, eye pain); and to peripheral neuritis (tingling, numbness, and burning pain of the hands and feet)

FLUOROQUINOLONES

Fluoroquinolones are a broad spectrum, synthetic antibiotic that stop bacterial growth in bone and joint infections, bronchitis, gastroenteritis, gonorrhea, pneu-

Chloramphenicol (Chloromycetin) Pregnancy Category: C		
Route	**Dose**	**Time**
Chloramphenicol (Chloromycetin) Protein-Binding: 50%–60% Half-Life: 4 hours		
PO/IV	12.5 mg/kg	Every 6 hours

monia, urinary tract infection, and many others diseases. However, fluoroquinolones should not be prescribed for infants or children.

Make sure that the patient doesn't have an allergic reaction to any fluoroquinolone. If they are allergic to one drug within the fluoroquinolone family, then they are highly likely to be allergic to other fluoroquinolone medications.

Patients who take fluoroquinolones can, in rare cases, experience dizziness, drowsiness, restlessness, stomach distress, diarrhea, nausea and vomiting, psychosis, confusion, hallucinations, tremors, hypersensitivity, and interstitial nephritis (kidney).

The dose of fluoroquinolones should be lowered in patients with hepatic (liver) or renal (kidney) problems. Carefully monitor the serum level of fluoroquinolones for patients who have CNS disorders such as cerebral arteriosclerosis (hardening of the arteries in the brain), epilepsy (seizures), or alcoholism because they are at risk for CNS toxicity.

Administer fluoroquinolones with a full glass of water to minimize the possibility of crystalluria. Fluoroquinolones should be infused slowly. Ofloxacin, a member of the fluoroquinolones family, must be infused into a large vein over 60 minutes to minimize discomfort and venous irritation.

After administering fluoroquinolones, monitor the patient's urinary output. The patient should void at least 1200 to 1500 mL daily. Also monitor the pH of the urine; it should remain at 7.0 or less.

The patient should be provided with the same instructions as those given to a patient who is receiving penicillin (see Penicillin and Patient Education). Tell the patient to report blurry or double vision, sensitivity to light, dizziness, lightheadedness, or depression. These are signs of CNS toxicity.

If fluoroquinolones are self administered, tell the patient to avoid taking the drug within two hours of taking an antacid. The patient should also avoid exposure to sunlight and sunlamps. The patient must wear sunglasses and avoid bright lights.

Fluoroquinolones and Drug-Drug Interactions

If ciprofloxacin, a member of the fluoroquinolones family, is prescribed, then it should be given two hours before the patient is given antacids, ferrous sulfate, or sucralfate because these medications lower the absorption of ciprofloxacin.

Patients who are taking theophylline or other xanthines with fluoroquinolones should be aware that the theophylline plasma levels can rise leading to toxicity.

If the patient takes fluoroquinolones while also taking warfarin, the anticoagulant effect of warfarin increases and could result in bleeding. The prothrombin time (PT) should be monitored if both are administered together.

Fluoroquinolones, Nursing Diagnosis, and Collaborative Problems

Patients who receive fluoroquinolones may also experience rash, fever, dyspnea, nephritis, blood in the urine, lower back pain, rash, edema, and photosensitivity (increased sensitivity of skin to sunlight). In addition they might have CNS toxicity (dizziness, headache, insomnia).

Here are the common nursing diagnoses that are the related to a patient who is receiving fluoroquinolones.

- Fluid volume deficit related to anorexia, nausea and vomiting
- Altered comfort related to arthralgia (joint discomfort and stiffness)
- Impaired tissue integrity related to phlebitis (IV cipro and ofloxacin only)
- Altered bowel elimination (diarrhea)
- Altered thought processes related to CNS stimulation (confusion, hallucinations)

Route	Dose	Time

Fluoroquinolones
Pregnancy Category: C

Route	Dose	Time
Ciprofloxacin (Cipro) Protein-Binding: 20% Half-Life: 3–4 hours		
PO Fluroquinoline Severe Infections	250–500 mg 500–750 mg	Every 12 hours Every 12 hours
IV Mild to Moderate Infections	400 mg	Every 12 hours
Enoxacin (Penetrex) Protein-Binding: 40% Half-Life: 3–6 hours		
PO	200-400mg	Every 12 hours 1–2 weeks
Levofloxacin (Levaquin) Protein-Binding: 50% Half-Life: 6 hours		
PO	250-750mg	
IV	500 mg/d	7–14 days
Lomefloxacin (Maxaquin) Protein-Binding: Unknown Half-Life: 6–8 hours		
PO	400 mg	10–14 days
Norfloxacin (Noroxin) Protein-Binding: 10%–11% Half-Life: 3–4 hours		
PO	400 mg	Every 12 hours for 72 hours
Ofloxacin (Floxin) Protein-Binding: 20% Half-Life: 5–8 hours		
PO/IV	300–400 mg	Every 12 hours for 10 days

MISCELLANEOUS ANTIBIOTICS

The following shows other antibiotics that are likely to be prescribed to treat microbial infections.

Antibiotic	Description
Aztreonam (Azactam)	Synthetic bactericidal activity similar to PCN
	Use: treats urinary tract, bronchitis, intraabdominal, gynecologic, and skin infections
	Route: IV
	Dose: 0.5 to 2g
	Time: q8–12 h
	Protein-Binding: 56%
	Half-Life: 1.7–2.1 h
	Pregnancy Category: B
	Side Effects: Gastric distress, diarrhea, nausea, vomiting, hypersensitivity, and thrombophlebitis at the site of injection
	Drug interaction: None
Imipenem-cilastatin (Primaxin IM, Primaxin IV)	Use: treats bone, joint, skin, and soft tissue infections, bacterial endocarditis, intraabdominal bacteria infections, pneumonia, and gram-+, gram- –aerobic and anerobic organisms
	Route: IV, IM
	Dose: IV 250–500 mg q6h for mild infections to 500 mg for moderate to severe infections. Maximum dose is 50 mg/kg daily IM 500–750 mg up to a maximum of 1500 mg/day.
	Time: IV q6–8h IM q12h
	Protein-Binding: 20%
	Half-Life: 1 h
	Pregnancy Category: C
	Side Effects: gastric distress, diarrhea, nausea, vomiting, allergic type reactions, confusion, lightheadedness, convulsions, and tremor

Antibiotic	Description
Imipenem-cilastatin (Primaxin IM, Primaxin IV) *(continued)*	Drug interaction: None Contraindication: not for use in children under 12 years old
Meropenem (Merrem IV)	Use: treats susceptible intraabdominal infections (complicated appendicitis and peritonitis) and bacterial meningitis Route: IV, IM Dose: IV 1 g over 40–60 minutes. Time: q8h Protein-Binding: 20% Half-Life: 1 h Pregnancy Category: C Side Effects: pseudomembranous colitis, hypersensitivity, diarrhea, nausea, vomiting, headache, and rash Drug interaction: None Contraindications: Use with caution with clients with allergy to imipenem, cilastin or other beta-lactams. Kidney problems require a reduced dosage. More than 2 g daily increase the risk for seizures

Sulfonamides

Urinary tract infections (UTI) are the most commonly reported bacterial infection in the United State. *E coli* causes 90% of them, some of which are hospital acquired. Hospital acquired UTI are difficult to treat. Other UTI are caused by *Pseudomonas aeruginosa, Serratia,* and *Enterobacter.*

A family of antibiotics called sulfonamides, that stops the growth of bacteria, is used to treat UTI. These include trimethoprim-sulfamethoxazole (TMP-SMX) and cephalasporins. Aztreonam and fluoroquinolones are used as urinary tract antiseptics. Phenazopyridine (Pyridium) is used to treat pain from a UTI.

Patients who are prescribed sulfonamides should avoid coffee, tea, and juices. These are high in citric acid. They also should abstain from cola, alcohol, chocolate, and spices which irritate the bladder.

Avoid using sulfonamides if the patient is allergic to one member of the sulfonamide family of medication. Sulfonamides should not be administered to neonates.

Sulfonamides may adversely affect the level of some medications causing a toxic effect. Avoid using sulfonamides with anticoagulants such as coumarin or indanedione derivatives and anticonvulsants (hydantoin) as well as oral antidiabetic agents and methotrexate.

Patients need at least 3000 mL of fluid each day in order to flush the urinary tract and follow good hygiene to reduce the likelihood of acquiring the infection again. The patient should be instructed to drink at least three quarts of water

Sulfonamides Pregnancy Category: C		
Route	**Dose**	**Time**
Sulfadiazine Protein-Binding: 20–30% Half-Life: 8–12 hours		
PO Drink 250 mL H$_2$O with each dose	2–4 mg first dose 2–4 g subsequent	7–10 days
Sulfisoxazole (Gantrisin): Protein-Binding: 60–70% (TMP-SMX) Half-Life: 7–12 hours		
PO	2–3 g/d in 2–3 divided doses	7–10 days
Trimethoprim-sulfamethoxazole Protein-Binding: 50–65% (TMP-SMX) Half-Life: 8–12 hours Most widely used antibacterial agent in the world		
PO	160/800 mg	q12h
Sulfamethoxazole (co trimoxazole) (TMP) Protein-Binding: 99% Half-Life: 5.5 hours		
PO IV	160 mg TMP BID 20 mg/kg	 q6hr

daily and take sulfonamides on an empty stomach. Patients should avoid the use of antacids while taking sulfonamides because antacids decrease the absorption of sulfonamides.

Tuberculosis

Tuberculosis is caused by acid-fast bacillus *Mycobacterium tuberculosis*. It is a major health problem and kills more than any other infectious disease. One and one-half billion people have TB. There are 8 million new cases each year. The incidence had decreased in the United States but increased again in the 1980s. This has been attributed in part to the numbers of persons with AIDS which compromises the immune system.

First-line drugs used to treat tuberculosis are

- Isoniazid (INH, Nydrazid, Laniazid) PO/IM: 5–10 mg/kg/d in a single dose; max: 300 mg/d; Prophylaxis: 300 mg/d
  - Pregnancy Category: C; PB: 10%; t½: 104 h
  - Side effects: drowsiness, tremors, rash, blurred vision, photosensitivity;
  - Adverse reactions: psychotic behavior, peripheral neuropathy, vitamin B$_6$ deficiency
  - Life threatening: blood dyscrasias, thrombocytopenia, seizures, agranulocytosis, hepatotoxicity

Antitubular Drugs				
Phase	**Example 1**	**Example 2**	**Example 3**	**Example 4**
First phase (2 mo)	Isoniazid, rifampin	Isoniazid, rifampin, Pyrazinamide	Isoniazid, rifampin, streptomycin	Isoniazid, rifampin, phrazinamide, kanamycin or ciprofloxacin
Second phase (4–7 mo)	Isoniazid, rifampin	Isoniazid, rifampin, ethambutol	Isoniazid, rifampin, capreomycin or cycloserine	Isoniazid, rifampin, ethambutol, streptomycin or kanamycin or ciprofloxacin or clarithromycin or capreomycin

- Ethambutol HCL (Myambutol) PO: 15 mg/kg as a single dose; retreatment PO: 25 mg/kg as a single dose for 2 mo; then decrease to 15 mg/kg/d
  - Pregnancy category: C; PB:10–20%; t½: 3–4 h (8 h with renal dysfunction)

- Pyrazinamide (Tebrazid): PO: 20–35 mg/kg/d in 3–4 divided doses; max: 3 g/d
  - Pregnancy category: C; PB: 10–20%; t½: 9.5 h—Promote fluid intake

- Rifampin (Rifadin, Rimactane): PO: 600 mg/d as a single dose
  - Pregnancy category: C; PB 85%–90%; t½: 3 h—monitor liver enzymes

- Streptomycin SO_4: IM: 1 g daily or 7–15 mg/kg/d for 2–3 mo, then 2–3 × wk
  - Pregnancy category: C; PB: 30%; t½: 2–3 h

Second-Line Drugs are:

- Aminosalicylate sodium, P.A.S. sodium: PO: 14–16 g/d in 2–3 divided doses
  - Pregnancy category: C; PB: 15%; t½: 1 h—take after meals to reduce gastric irritation

- Capreomycin (Capastat): IM: 1 g/d for 2–4 mo. Then 1 g 2–3 × per week
  - Pregnancy category: C; PB: UK; t½: 3–6 h—hearing loss is an adverse reaction; patients should take pyridoxine (to avoid peripheral neuropathy)

- Cycloserine (Seromycin): PO: 200 mg q12 h for 2 wks; max: 1 g/d
  - Pregnancy category: C; PB: UK; t½: 10 h

- Ethionamide (Treacator-SC): PO: 250 mg, q8–12h
  - Pregnancy category: C; PB: UK; t½: 2–3h—side effects include GI discomfort. Use with caution in patients with diabetes mellitus, alcoholism, and hepatic disorder

- Rifabutin (Mycobutin) PO: 300 mg/d in 1 or 2 divided doses
  - Pregnancy category: B; PB: 85%; t½: 16–69 h

Side effects and adverse reactions differ according to the drug prescribed. The nursing assessment should include:

- History of past TB; PPD tests and reactions, chest xray and results, and previous allergy to any antitubercular drugs.
- Medical history; most are contraindicated with severe hepatic disease (liver).
- Assess for sign and symptoms of peripheral neuropathy.

Check for hearing changes because some of the drugs are ototoxic. Nursing diagnoses related to drug therapy for TB are:

- Risk for infection
- Risk for impaired tissue integrity
- Risk for hearing loss

Nursing interventions for patients being treated for tuberculosis are:

- Administer 1 h before or 2 h after meals.
- Administer pyridoxine as prescribed.
- Monitor serum liver enzymes.
- Collect sputum specimens in early morning (usually 3 consecutive mornings).
- Arrange for eye examinations.
- Emphasize importance of complying with drug regimen.

Patient education:

- Take before meals or 2 h after for better absorption.
- Take as prescribed.
- Do not to take antacids because they decrease TB drug absorption.
- Keep medical appointments and have sputum tested.
- Check with healthcare provider before becoming pregnant.
- Report numbness, tingling, or burning of the hands and feet.
- Avoid direct sunlight—use sunblock.
- Rifampin (urine, feces, saliva, sputum, sweat, and tears may be a harmless red-orange color; soft contact lenses may be permanently stained.

Evaluation: Evaluate effectiveness with sputum specimens.

Antifungal Drugs (antimycotic drugs)

These drugs are used to treat two types of fungal infections

1. Superficial fungal infections of skin or mucous membrane.
2. Systemic fungal infections of the lung or central nervous system.

The conditions may be mild such as tinea pedis (ahtlete's foot), or severe as in pulmonary conditions or meningitis.

Fungi, such as *Candida* spp. (yeast), are normal flora of mouth, skin, intestine, and vagina. Candidiasis might be an opportunistic infection when the defense mechanisms are impaired. Antibiotics, oral contraceptives, and immunosuppressives may alter the body's defense mechanisms. Infections can be mild (vaginal yeast infection) or severe (systemic fungal infection).

There are four groups of anti-fungal medications. They are:

1. Polyenes, including amphotericin B and nystatin.
2. Imidazoles which include ketoconazole, miconazole, and clotrimazole.
3. Antimetabolic antifungal flucytosine.
4. Antiprotozoal agents.

Polyenes such as amphotericin B are the drug of choice for treating severe systemic infections. It is effective against numerous diseases including histoplasmosis, cryptococcosis, coccidioidomycosis, aspergillosis, blastomycosis, and candidiasis (system infection), however, it is very toxic. It is not absorbed from the GI tract so it cannot be given by mouth.

It is usually prescribed as Amphotericin B (Fungizone). A test dose is given IV: 0.25–1.0 mg in 20 mL of D5W infused over 20–30 min; IV: 0.25–1.0 mg/kg/d in D5W or 1.5 mg/kg qod; max; 1.5 mg/kg/d. The drug is pregnancy category: B; PB: 95%; t½: 24 h.

Side effects and adverse reactions include flushing, fever, chills, nausea, vomiting, hypotension, paresthesias, and thrombophlebitis. It is **highly toxic,** causes nephrotoxicity and electrolyte imbalance, especially hypokalemia (low potassium) and hypomagnesemia (low serum magnesium). Urinary output, BUN, and serum creatinine levels should be closely monitored.

Nystatin (Mycostatin) can be given orally or topically to treat candidal infection. It is available in suspensions, cream, ointment, and vaginal tablets. It is poorly absorbed via the GI tract but the oral tablet form is used for intestinal candidiasis. It is more commonly used as an oral suspension for candidal infection in the mouth as a swish and swallow.

Side effects include anorexia, nausea, vomiting, diarrhea (large doses), stomach cramps, rash; vaginal: rash, burning sensation. There are no reported adverse reactions.

It is used topically and PO at doses of 500,000–1,000,000 U tid or q8h. This drug has a Pregnancy category: C; PB: UK; t½: UK.

The Imidazole group is effective against candidiasis (superficial and systemic), coccidioidomycosis, cryptococcosis, histoplasmosis, and paracoccidioidomycosis.

Antimalarial

Malaria is still one of the most prevalent protozoan diseases in the world. The mosquito infects the human and the parasite passes through two phases. The tissue phase causes no clinical symptoms in the human and the erythrocytic phase invades red blood cells and causes chills, fever, and sweating, In the United States the 1000 cases reported annually are almost all from international travel. Quinine was the only antimalarial drug from 1820 to the early 1940s when synthetic antimalarial drugs were developed. Chloroquine is commonly prescribed. If drug resistance develops quinine is used in combination with an antibiotic such as tetracycline.

Nursing process related to treating patients who have malaria.

- Assessment
  - Assess patient's hearing (drugs may affect 8th cranial nerve)
  - Assess for visual changes (should have frequent ophthalmic examinations)

- Nursing diagnoses
  - Risk of infection
  - Risk for impaired tissue integrity
  - Risk for sensory disturbances (auditory and visual)

- Planning
  - Patient will be free of malarial symptoms

- Nursing interventions
  - Monitor urinary output (600 mL/d) and liver function (liver enzymes)
  - Report if serum liver enzymes are elevated

- Client teaching
  - Advise patients traveling to malaria-infested countries to take prophylactic doses of antimalarial drugs before leaving, during the visit, and upon return.
  - Instruct patient to take oral antimalarial drugs with food or at mealtime if GI upset occurs.
  - Monitor patients returning from international travel for malarial symptoms.
  - Instruct the client to report vision or hearing changes immediately.
  - Advise the patient to avoid consuming large quantities of alcohol.

- Evaluation
  - Evaluate effectiveness of drug by determining the patient is free of symptoms

- Side effects and adverse reactions
  - General side effects include GI upset, 8th cranial nerve involvement (quinine and chloroquine), renal impairment (quinine) and cardiovascular effects (quinine)

Anthelmintic

Helminths are large organisms (parasitic worms) that feed on host tissue. The most common site is the intestine. Other sites are the lymphatic system, blood vessels, and liver.

There are four groups of helminths:

1. Cestodes (tapeworms) (enter via contaminated food [pork (trichinosis), fish, dwarf])
2. Trematodes (flukes)
3. Intestinal nematodes (roundworms)
4. Tissue-invading nematodes (tissue roundworms and filariae)

The nursing process related to treatment of patients who are taking antihelmiths is:

- Assessment
  - History of foods eaten, especially meat and fish and how it was prepared
  - Note if other persons in household have been checked for worms
  - Obtain baseline vital signs and collect a stool specimen

- Nursing diagnoses
  - Altered comfort
  - Activity intolerance related to dizziness, headache, drowsiness
  - Altered nutrition
  - Alteration in skin integrity

- Planning
  - Patient will be free of helminths
  - Patient/family will understand how to prepare foods to avoid recurrence

- Interventions
  - Collect stool specimen
  - Administer the prescribed anthelmintics after meals
  - Report side effects to the health care provider

- Patient teaching:
  - Explain importance of hand washing
  - Instruct to take daily showers, NOT baths
  - Instruct to change sheets, bedclothes, towels, and underwear daily
  - If problem persists, a second course of therapy may be necessary
  - Take prescribed drug at the designated time and keep health care appointments
  - Alert that drowsiness may occur; avoid operating a car or machinery if drowsiness occurs
  - Report side effects to health care provider

- Evaluation
  - Evaluate effect of the anthelmintics and absence of side effects
  - Determine if patient is using proper hygiene to avoid spread of parasitic worms

- Side effects and adverse reactions:
  - ○ Common side effects include GI upset such as anorexia, nausea, vomiting, and occasionally diarrhea and stomach cramps; neurological problems include dizziness, weakness, headache, and drowsiness; Adverse reactions do not occur frequently

Examples of anti-helmiths include:

- Diethylcarbamzine (Hetrazan); Used for nematode-filariae; PO: 2–3 mg/kg/tid
- Ivermectin (Mectizan) broad-spectrum antiparasitic drug; PO: 200 ug/kg/1dose
- Mebandazole (Vermox); used for giant roundworm, hookworm, pinworm, whipworm. PO: 100 mg. bid × 3 d; repeat in 2–3 wk if necessary
- Niclosamide (Niclocide) used for beef and fish tapeworms: PO 2 g, single dose; treatment of dwarf tapeworms PO: 2 g/d × 1 wk
- Oxamniquine (Vansil) treatment against mature and immature worms; PO: 15 mg/kg/bid for 1–2 d
- Piperazine citrate (Antepar, Vermizine); treatment of roundworms and pinworms; Roundworms: PO: 3.5 g/d × 2 d; Pinworms: 65 mg/kg/d × 7 d max: 2.5 g/d
- Praziquantel (Biltricide) treatment for beef, pork, fish tapeworms; PO: 10–20 mg/kg single dose; Blood flukes: PO 20 mg/kg, tid × 1 d; liver, lung, and intestinal flukes; 25 mg/kg tid 1–2 d
- Pyrantel pamoate (Antiminth) treatment of giant roundworm, hookworm, pinworm; PO: 11 mg/kg single dose; repeat in 2 weeks if necessary
- Thiabendazole (Mintezol, Minzolum) treatment of threadworm and pork worm; PO 25 mg/kg 2–5 d; repeat in 2 d if necessary

Summary

When microbials invade, the body's defenses go into action to surround and kill microbials. The inflammatory response is the first line of attack bringing white blood cells to the site of the infection in an attempt to stifle the spread of the microbial. Microbials that cause infections are called pathogens.

Symptoms of inflammation can disrupt the patient's normal daily activities. Anti-inflammatory medication is administered to patients to reduce the inflammatory response enabling the patient to return to normal activities.

Sometimes the microbial attack overwhelms the body's defenses. In these cases the patient requires medication to help the body destroy the microbial. The most commonly prescribed medication to combat microbials is an antibiotic.

There are two types of antibiotics: bacteriostatic and bacteriocidal. Bacteriostatic antibiotics stop bacteria from growing inside the body. Bacteriocidal antibiotics kill bacteria.

In this chapter, you learned about the most commonly prescribed antibiotics. You learned how they work, how to administer them, their side effects, and when they should not be administered to a patient.

In the next chapter you will learn about respiratory diseases and about the medications that are prescribed to treat those diseases.

Quiz

1. A new infection caused by a bacterium that is resistant to the present antibiotics being given is called a
   (a) communicable infection.
   (b) superinfection.
   (c) a hospital acquired infection.
   (d) None of the above

2. A patient should always be asked if he or she is allergic to any medications, foods, or herbals or who has a family history of allergies to antibiotics. This is because
   (a) patients who have a family member who is allergic to an antibiotic might also have an allergy to some antibiotics.
   (b) shell fish contain bacteria.
   (c) patients can contract drug resistant bacteria from shellfish.
   (d) All of the above

3. Antibiotics fight off bacteria by
   (a) inhibiting the bacteria's ability to make protein called protein synthesis.
   (b) inhibiting the bacteria from growing a cell wall.
   (c) disrupting or altering the permeability of the bacteria's membrane.
   (d) All of the above

4. All antibiotics kill bacteria.
   (a) True
   (b) False

5. Some antibiotics kill only specific bacteria
   (a) True
   (b) False

6. What chemical mediators bring about the inflammatory reaction by vaso-dilatation, relaxing smooth muscles, making capillaries permeable, and sensitizing nerve cells within the affected area to pain?
   (a) PCN
   (b) Sulfonamides
   (c) Prostaglandins inhibitors
   (d) Prostaglandins

7. Bacteriocidal antibiotics can only stop the growth of bacteria.
   (a) True
   (b) False

8. Which of the following symptoms are possible side effects of an antibiotic?
   (a) Rash
   (b) Fever
   (c) Hives and itching
   (d) All of the above

9. The patient's white blood count should be studied after the patient is given an antibiotic.
   (a) True
   (b) False

10. Penicillin is the most effective and least toxic antibiotic.
    (a) True
    (b) False

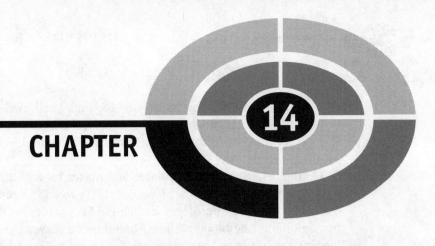

CHAPTER

14

Respiratory Diseases

No one looks forward to the cold season when many of us come down with a sore throat, the sniffles, and a cough and feel utterly dreadful. A lot of chicken soup and TLC usually is the cure. Chicken soup is not a drug but it does contain a mucous-thinning amino acid called cysteine and is considered "grandma's remedy" for the common cold. Actually, time is the best cure and most people feel better in 7 to 10 days with or without chicken soup.

The common cold is one of a number of respiratory diseases that can infect our body. The common cold can be annoying. However, some respiratory diseases—such as emphysema—are debilitating and can slowly choke the life out of a person.

In this chapter, we'll explore the more common respiratory diseases and learn about the medications that are used to either destroy the disease-causing microorganism or to manage the symptoms of the disease.

A Brief Look at Respiration

Before learning about respiratory diseases and the medications used to treat them, let's take a few moments to briefly review the anatomy and physiology of the respiratory tract. This review will help you better understand the disease and treatment.

The respiratory tract is divided into the upper and the lower tracts. The upper respiratory tract contains the nares, nasal cavity, pharynx, and larynx and the lower tract consists of the trachea, bronchi, bronchioles, alveoli, and alveolar-capillary membrane.

During respiration, air is inhaled and makes its way through the upper respiratory tract and travels to the alveoli capillary membrane in the lower respiratory tract, which is the site of gas exchange. Oxygen from the air attaches to the hemoglobin of the blood while carbon dioxide leaves the blood and is expelled through the lower and upper respiratory tracts during expiration.

RESPIRATION

There are three phases of respiration:

Ventilation

Ventilation is the process by which oxygenated air passes through the respiratory tract during inspiration.

Perfusion

Perfusion is when blood from the pulmonary circulation is sufficient at the alveolar-capillary bed to conduct diffusion. In order for perfusion to occur, the alveolar pressure must be matched by adequate ventilation. The presence of mucosal edema, secretions and bronchospasm increase resistance to the airflow, which results in decreased ventilation. Decreased ventilation causes a decrease in diffusion.

Diffusion

Diffusion is the process where oxygen moves into the capillary bed and carbon dioxide leaves the capillary bed.

COMPLIANCE AND THE LUNGS

There are two lungs inside the chest cavity. Each is surrounded by a membrane called the pleura. Each lung is divided into parts called lobes. The right lung has three lobes and the left lung has two lobes.

You'll frequently hear the term "lung compliance" used when measuring the functionality of the lungs. Compliance is the ability of the lungs to be distended and is expressed as a change in volume per unit change in pressure. That is, a measurement of how well the lungs can stretch when filling with air.

There are two factors that affect compliance. These are the connective tissue that consists of collagen and elastin and surface tension in the alveoli, which is controlled by surfactant. Surfactant is a substance that lowers surface tension in the alveoli, thereby preventing interstitial fluid from entering the alveoli.

Compliance is increased in patients who have chronic obstructive pulmonary disease (COPD). Compliance is decreased with patients who have restrictive pulmonary disease. A decrease in compliance results in a decreased lung volume. That is, the lungs become stiff requiring more-than-normal pressure to expand the lungs. This is typically caused by an increase in connective tissue or an increase in surface tension in the alveoli.

CONTROLLING RESPIRATION

Respiration is controlled by three factors that sense the need for the body's increased or decreased requirement for oxygen. These are the concentration of oxygen (O_2), carbon dioxide (CO_2), and hydrogen (H^+) ion concentration in the blood.

Throughout the body chemoreceptors sense the concentration of oxygen, carbon, and carbon dioxide and then send a message to the central chemoreceptors located in the medulla near the respiratory center of the brain and through cerebrospinal fluid to respond to changes.

When an increase in carbon dioxide is detected and there is an increase in hydrogen ions, the message goes out to increase ventilation. Hydrogen ions are measured using the pH scale. The pH of normal blood is between 7.35 and 7.45. A pH lower than 7.35 means the blood is acidic and a pH higher than 7.45 means pH is alkaline. The chemoreceptors respond to an increase in CO_2 and a decrease in pH by increasing ventilation. If the CO_2 level remains elevated, the stimulus to increase ventilation is lost.

There are chemoreceptors located in carotid arteries and aortic arteries that monitor changes in oxygen pressure (PO_2) levels in the arteries. These are called peripheral chemoreceptors. Once the oxygen pressure falls below <60 mmHg, the peripheral chemoreceptors send a message to the respiratory center in the medulla to increase ventilation.

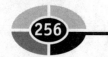

TRACHEOBRONCHIAL TUBE

The tracheobronchial tube connects the pharynx to the bronchial tree that extends into the terminal bronchioles in the lungs providing an unobstructed pathway for air to enter the body and carbon dioxide to leave the body.

The tracheobronchial tube is a fibrous spiral of smooth muscles that become more closely spaced as they near the terminal bronchioles. The size of the airway can be increased or decreased by relaxing or contracting the bronchial smooth muscle. This is controlled by the parasympathetic nervous system—particularly the vagus nerve.

The vagus nerve releases acetylcholine when it is stimulated, which causes the tracheobronchial tube to contract. This is referred to as bronchoconstriction. The opposite effect is created when the sympathetic nervous system releases epinephrine that stimulates the beta$_2$ receptor in the bronchial smooth muscle. This causes the tracheobronchial tube to dilate. This is called bronchodilation. In a healthy patient the sympathetic and parasympathetic nervous systems counterbalance each other to maintain homeostasis.

Upper Respiratory Tract Disorders

Respiratory disorders are divided into two groups: upper respiratory tract disorders and lower respiratory tract disorders. Upper respiratory tract disorders are called upper respiratory infections (URIs). These include the common cold, acute rhinitis (not the same as allergic rhinitis), sinusitis, acute tonsillitis, and acute laryngitis.

THE COMMON COLD

The common cold is caused by the rhinovirus invading the nasopharyngeal tract. The rhinovirus is frequently accompanied by acute inflammation of the mucous membranes of the nose and increased nasal secretions. This is known as acute rhinitis.

Adults have between two and four colds per year. Children are more susceptible to colds. The average child has between 4 and 12 colds each year. The rhinovirus is seasonable: 50% of the infections occur in the winter and 25% during the summer. The other 25% occur anytime throughout the year. Although no one has directly died from the common cold, it does create both physical and mental discomfort for the person and leads to a loss of work and school.

The rhinovirus is contagious one to four days before the patient notices the symptoms of the cold. This is referred to as the incubation period. During this time, the rhinovirus can be transmitted by touching contaminated surfaces and from contact with droplets from an infected patient who sneezes and coughs. After the incubation period, the patient experiences a watery nasal discharge called rhinorrhea, nasal congestion, cough, and an increasing amount of mucosal secretions.

Many patients try home remedies to battle the rhinovirus, however these don't affect the virus. Instead, they may help ease the symptoms of the cold. Home remedies include rest, vitamin C, mega doses of other vitamins, and, of course, chicken soup. Vitamin C and mega doses of other vitamins have not been proven effective against the common cold.

When home remedies fail, patients turn to both prescription and over-the-counter medication. Cold medications fall into the following drug groups. Charts throughout these pages provide information about specific drugs in each group.

Antihistamines (H₁ blocker)

Many cold symptoms are caused by the body's overproduction of histamines. Histamines are potent vasodilators that react to a foreign substance in the body such as the rhinovirus. They cause redness, itching, and swelling. They are part of the body's defense mechanism. Antihistamines are drugs that compete for the same receptor sites as histamines. Once they latch onto the site, there is no room for the histamine. Therefore, the reaction caused by the histamine doesn't occur. It is this reaction that produces many cold symptoms.

There are two types of histamine receptors: H_1 and H_2. H_2 receptors cause an increase in gastric secretions and are not involved in this response. The differences are illustrated in the charts. (See Antihistamine (H_1 blocker) chart and Antihistamine Use to Treat Allergic Rhinitis chart.)

Decongestants (sympathomimetic amines)

Patients have a runny nose when they get a cold. This is referred to as nasal congestion and is caused when the nasal mucous membranes swell in response to the rhinovirus. A decongestant is a drug that stimulates the alpha-adrenergic receptors to tell the brain to constrict the capillaries within the nasal mucosa. The result is that the nasal mucous membranes shrink, reducing the amount of fluid that is secreted from the nose. That is, a decongestant stops a runny nose.

Decongestants are available in nasal spray, drops, tablets, capsules, or in liquid form. Although decongestants address the congestion, frequent use of decongestants—especially nasal spray and drops—can lose its effectiveness because the patient becomes tolerant to the medication. In some cases, the patient may even experience nasal congestion again. This is referred to as rebound nasal congestion. Therefore, decongestants should not be used longer than five days.

There are three types of decongestants. These are nasal decongestants that provide quick relief to the patient; systemic decongestants that provide a longer lasting relief from congestion; and intranasal glucocorticoids that are used to treat seasonal and perennial rhinitis.

Cough Preparations

A cough is a common symptom of a cold brought about by the body's effort to remove nasal mucous that might drain into the respiratory tract. Antitussives are the ingredients used in cough medicine to suppress the cough center in the medulla. Although the cough reflex is useful to clear the air passages, suppression of the cough reflex can provide some rest for the patient. There are non-narcotic and narcotic antitussives.

Expectorants

When an individual has a cold or other respiratory infection, it is common to have rather thick mucous that is difficult to expectorate. Expectorants are medications that loosen the secretions making it easier for the patient to cough up and expel the mucous. They work by increasing the fluid output of the respiratory tract and decrease the adhesiveness and surface tension to promote removal of viscous mucus.

A list of drugs utilized in the treatment of upper respiratory tract disorders is provided in the Appendix. Detailed tables show doses, recommendations, expectations, side effects, contraindications, and more; available on the book's Web site (see URL in Appendix).

Antihistamine Used to Treat Allergic Rhinitis	
Phenothiazines (anti-histamine action) promethazine HCl (Phenergan)	PO/IM: 12.5–25 mg q4–6h PRN Maximum dose: 150 mg/d Before meals and bedtime Pregnancy category: C Protein bound: Unknown Half-life: Unknown

Antihistamine Used to Treat Allergic Rhinitis *(continued)*	
Piperazine Derivative—hydroxyzine (Atarax, Vistaril)	PO: 25–100 mg tid/qid Pregnancy category: C Protein bound: Unknown Half-life: 3 hours
Butyrophenone Derivative (terfenadine (Seldane)	PO: 60 md bid Pregnancy category: C Protein bound: 97% Half-life: 20 hours
Ethanolamine Derivative—carbinoxamine and pseudoephedrine (Rondec)	PO: 5 mL qid or 1 tab qid Pregnancy category: C Protein bound: Unknown Half-life: Unknown
Clemastine fumarate (Tavist)	PO: 1.34–2.68 mg bid, tid Maximum dose 8 mg/d Pregnancy category: C Protein bound: Unknown Half-life: Unknown
Propylamine Derivatives—brompheniramine maleate (Bromphen, Dimetane, Histaject, Hasahist B, Oraminic II)	PO: 4 mg q4 h–6h or SR: 8 mg q8–12h maximum dose 24 mg/d IM/IV/SC: 10 mg q8–12h; max: 40 mg/d Pregnancy category: C Protein bound: Unknown Half-life: 25–36 hours
Triprolidine and pseudoephedrine (Actifed)	PO: 2.5 mg q6–8h; max: 10 mg/d Pregnancy category: B Protein bound: Unknown Half-life: 3 hours

SINUSITIS

Sinusitis is the inflammation of the mucous membranes of the maxillary, frontal, ethmoid, or sphenoid sinuses. Patients may take systemic or nasal decongestants to reduce the congestion that frequently accompanies sinusitis. Patients are told to drink plenty of fluids, to rest, and to take acetaminophen (Tylenol) or ibuprofen for discomfort. In some cases, antibiotics are prescribed if the condition is severe or long lasting and an infection is suspected.

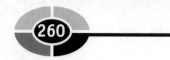

ACUTE PHARYNGITIS

Acute pharyngitis is inflammation of the throat. It is more commonly known as a sore throat. The patient may have an elevated temperature, a cough, and pain when swallowing.

Pharyngitis is caused by a virus (viral pharyngitis) or by bacteria (bacteria pharyngitis) such as the beta-hemolytic streptococci. Patients know this as strep throat. A throat culture is taken to rule out beta-hemolytic streptococcal infection. Sometimes patients experience acute pharyngitis along with other upper respiratory tract disease such as a cold, rhinitis, or acute sinusitis.

Patients who have a viral pharyngitis are given medications that treat the symptoms rather than attacking the underlying virus. Acetaminophen or ibuprofen is given to reduce the patient's temperature and discomfort. Saline gargles, lozenges, and increased fluid are usually helpful to soothe the sore throat.

Patients who have bacterial pharyngitis are given antibiotics to destroy the beta-hemolytic streptococci bacteria. However, antibiotics are only prescribed if the result of the throat culture is positive for bacteria. Patients are also given the same treatments for viral pharyngitis to address the symptoms of pharyngitis.

ACUTE TONSILLITIS

Acute tonsillitis is the inflammation of the tonsils which can be caused by a streptococcus microorganism. Patients who come down with acute tonsillitis experience a sore throat, chills, fever, aching muscles, and pain when they swallow.

A throat culture is taken to determine the cause of the infection before an appropriate antibiotic is prescribed to the patient. The patient is also given acetaminophen or ibuprofen to reduce the fever and the aches and pains associated with acute tonsillitis. The patient is also encouraged to use saline gargles, lozenges, and increased fluid to soothe the soreness brought on by infected tonsils. Antibiotics are only used if a bacterial infection is suspected.

ACUTE LARYNGITIS

Acute laryngitis is an infection that causes swelling (edema) of the vocal cords. This results in the patient having a weak or hoarse voice. Acute laryngitis can be caused by a viral infection. Other times it is caused by stress or overuse of the vocal cords—a common occurrence for fans whose team wins the Super Bowl.

Refraining from speaking and avoiding exposure to substances that can irritate the vocal cords, such as smoking, is the preferred treatment for acute laryngitis.

Lower Respiratory Disorders

Lower respiratory disorders are conditions that obstruct or restrict tracheo-bronchial tubes and prevent the exchange of gas within the lungs. These conditions are referred to as chronic obstructive pulmonary disease (COPD) and include chronic bronchitis, bronchiectasis, emphysema, and asthma.

COPD obstructs the patient's airway by increasing resistance of the airflow during inspiration and expiration. The result is an impairment of oxygen reaching lung tissues that can in some cases irreversibly damage lung tissues.

The airway obstruction occurs when the bronchioles constrict (bronchospasm) and mucous secretions increase causing the patient to experience difficulty breathing (dyspnea).

PNEUMONIA

Pneumonia is an infection in the lungs that can be caused by a variety of microorganisms including viruses, bacteria, or fungus. It often starts after an upper respiratory infection. Symptoms can occur 2 to 3 days after a cold or sore throat. Symptoms include fever, chills, cough, rapid breathing, wheezing and/or grunting respirations, labored breathing, vomiting, chest pain, abdominal pain, loss of appetite, decreased activity, and, in extreme cases, signs of hypoxia (low oxygen levels) or cyanosis such as a bluish tint around the mouth or fingernails. There are vaccines to prevent certain types of pneumonia. Pneumonia is treated based on the underlying cause. Viral pneumonia is usually treated symptomatically. That is, bronchodilators, antipyretics (fever reducing), analgesics such as ibuprofen, cough medications that include expectorants, mucolytics, as well as suppressants to help the patient sleep. Bacterial and fungal pneumonia are treated with antimicrobials as well as the above treatment for viral pneumonia. The antimicrobial is chosen based on the specific microorganism causing the pneumonia. Antimicrobials are discussed in Chapter 13. Antipyretics such as ibuprofen are discussed in Chapter 12. Pneumonia is contagious and is spread from person to person via droplets in the air from coughing and sneezing.

TUBERCULOSIS

Tuberculosis (TB) is caused by the acid-fast bacillus *Mycobacterium tuberculosis*. The pathogen is frequently referred to as the tubercle bacillus. It is a major health problem in the world and kills more persons than any other infectious disease. More than 1½ billion people in the world may have TB and many do not know it. Each year there are more than 8 million new bases of TB. Many of the new cases of TB can be attributed, in part, to the increased number of persons with acquired immunodeficiency syndrome (AIDS). Active TB develops in these people because of their compromised immune system. It can also be attributed to the increasingly crowded living conditions in urban areas. Individuals susceptible to TB are those with alcohol addiction, AIDS, and those in a debilitative condition.

Tuberculosis is transmitted from one person to another by droplets dispersed in the air through coughing and sneezing. The organisms are inhaled into the alveoli (air sacs) of the lung. The tubercle bacilli can spread from the lungs to other organs of the body via the blood and lymphatic system. If the body's immune system is strong or intact, the phagocytes stop the multiplication of the tubercle bacilli. When the immune system is compromised, the tubercle bacilli spread in the lungs and to other organs. Dissemination of tuberculosis bacilli can be found in the liver, kidneys, spleen, and other organs. Symptoms of TB include anorexia, cough, sputum production, increased fever, night sweats, weight loss, and positive acid-fast bacilli (AFB) in the sputum. Medication to treat and prevent TB is discussed in Chapter 13.

CHRONIC BRONCHITIS

Chronic bronchitis is an inflammation of the bronchi that persists for a long period of time or repeatedly occurs. It is a form of COPD. Smoking is the main cause for bronchitis. Second-hand smoke may also cause chronic bronchitis. Air pollution, infection, and allergies make it worse. Patients who develop chronic bronchitis have excess mucous production that irritates the bronchial causing the patient to have a persistent productive cough.

Patients exhibit a gurgling lung sound (rhonchi) both on inspiration and expiration. The excess mucus blocks the airway causing a build up of carbon dioxide in the blood (hypercapnia) and a decrease in oxygen (hypoxemia) which leads to respiratory acidosis.

BRONCHIECTASIS

Brochiecstasis is the enlargement and distension of the airways so that pockets are formed where infection can develop. This condition alters the lining of the airways and damages the lung's ability to filter air. Dust, mucus, and bacteria accumulate in the lungs, causing infection.

EMPHYSEMA

Emphysema is a progressive COPD. The alveoli become enlarged and damaged, trapping air in the over expanded alveoli preventing an adequate exchange of oxygen and carbon dioxide.

Emphysema is caused by smoking cigarettes, by inhaling contaminants from the environment, or by the lack of the $alpha_1$-antitrypsin protein. The lung contains bacteria that release proteolytic enzymes that destroy alveoli. The $alpha_1$-antitrypsin protein inhibits proteolytic enzymes and protects the alveoli.

Excess mucus as well as the residue from cigarette smoking and airborne pollutants find their way down the airways and plug the terminal bronchioles. The network of alveoli then loses their fiber and become inelastic and unable to spring back to size after expanding during inspiration. Alveoli enlarge as many of the alveolar walls are destroyed. Air becomes trapped in the overexpanded alveoli leading to inadequate gas exchange (O_2 and CO_2).

ASTHMA

Acute asthma is a reactive airway disease (RAD) that occurs when lung tissue is exposed to extrinsic (environmental) or intrinsic (internal) factors that stimulate the bronchoconstrictive response. This causes bronchospasms that result in the patient wheezing and having difficulty breathing. More than 500,000 patients are hospitalized and 5000 die from asthma each year making acute asthma the third leading cause of preventable hospitalizations in the United States.

There are a variety of allergens (something that causes an allergic reaction) that can trigger an asthma attack. These include humidity, air pressure changes, temperature changes, smoke, fumes (exhaust, perfume), stress, emotional upset, and allergies to animal dander, dust mites, and drugs such as aspirin, indomethacin, and ibuprofen.

Allergens attach to mast cells and basophils in connective tissues causing an antigen-antibody reaction to occur. Mast cells stimulate release of chemical mediators. These chemicals constrict the bronchi, increase mucous secretions, stimulate the inflammatory response, and cause pulmonary congestion.

Chemical mediators include histamines (proteins that are potent vasodilators), cytokines (small proteins that mediate and regulate the immune system, inflammatory response and hematopoiesis [red cell production]), serotonin (CNS neurotransmitter), ECF-A (eosinophil chemotatic factor of anaphylaxis) and leukotrines. Histamine and ECF-A are strong bronchoconstrictors that stimulate the contraction of bronchial smooth muscles. Cyclic adenosine monophosphate (cyclic AMP or cAMP) maintains bronchodilation. Histamines, ECF-A, and

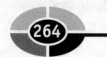

leukotrienes inhibit the action of cAMP resulting in bronchoconstriction. An increase in the serum level of eosinophils indicates that the inflammatory response has occurred.

The first line of treatment for an acute asthma attack is administering sympathomimetics (beta-adrenergic agonists), which promote the production of cAMP and thereby cause bronchodilation.

Long-term management includes controlling extrinsic factors that caused the attack, educating the patient and the patient's family, school officials, and employers about how to reduce exposure to those factors, and using various combinations of medications depending on the severity of the disease.

Medications to treat COPD

There are four types of medications used to treat this disease.

Bronchodilator

Bronchodilators relax smooth muscles around the bronchioles restoring airflow to the lungs. Sympathomimetics are bronchodilators that increase the production of cyclic AMP, causing dilation of the bronchioles by acting as adrenergic agonistic.

Some sympathomimetics are selective to particular adrenergic receptors, which are referred to as alpha$_1$, beta$_2$ and beta$_2$-adrenergic. Other sympathomimetics are non-selective sympathomimetic that affect all types of adrenergic receptor sites.

Epinephrine (adrenalin) is a non-selective sympathomimetic that is given subcutaneously, IV, or via an endotracheal tube in emergency situations to restore circulation and increase airway patency.

Selective beta$_2$-adrenergic agonists have fewer side effects then epinephrine and are given by aerosol or as a tablet. These include albuterol (Proventil, Ventolin), isoetharine HCl (Bronkosol), metaproterenol sulfate (Alupent), samleterol (Serevent), and Terbulaline SO$_4$ (Brethine).

Ipratropium bromide (Atrovent) is an anticholinergic drug that inhibits vagal-mediated response by reversing the action of acetylcholine, producing smooth muscle relaxation. It is a newer medication that dilates bronchioles with few systemic effects. Ipratropium bromide (Atrovent) is used five minutes before glucocorticoid (steroid) or cromolyn are inhaled so the bronchioles dilate enabling the steroids to be deposited in the bronchioles. Sometimes ipratropium bromide is combined with albuterol sulfate (Combivent) to treat chronic bronchitis for more effective and longer duration than if each is used alone.

Methylxanthine (xanthine) derivatives are a second group of bronchodilators used to treat asthma. They include aminophylline, theophylline, and caffeine, which stimulate the central nervous system (CNS) to increase respirations, dilate coronary and pulmonary vessels, and increase urination (diuresis).

Leukotriene Modifiers

Bronchoconstrictors cause the contraction of smooth muscle around the bronchi restricting airflow to the lungs. Leukotriene (LK) is the primary bronchoconstrictor that increases migration of eosinophils, increases mucous production, and increases edema in the bronchi resulting in bronchoconstriction.

There are two types of Leukotriene (LK) modifers: LT receptor antagonists and LT synthesis inhibitors. These are effective in reducing the inflammatory symptoms of asthma triggered by allergic and environmental stimuli.

Leukotriene (LK) modifiers include Zafirlukast (Accolate), zileuton (Zyflo) and nontelukast sodium (Singulair).

Anti-inflammatory

Chronic obstructive pulmonary disease causes inflammation in the respiratory tract that results in respiratory distress for the patient. Glucocorticoids (steroids) are the primary medication given to reduce the inflammation. You'll learn more about glucocorticoids (steroids) in Chapter 12.

Glucocorticoids (steroids) can be administered orally, via aerosol inhalation, intramuscularly, and intravenously. Glucocorticoids used for aerosol inhalation use beclomethasone (Beconase, Vanceril), dexamethasone (decadron), flunisolide (Aerobid, Nasalid), or triamcinolone (Azmacort, Kenalog, Nasacort).

Glucocorticoids used for other routes include betamethasones (Celestone), cortisone acetate (Cortone acetate, Cortistan), dexamethasone (Decadron), hydrocortisone (Cortef, Hydrocortone), methylprednisolone (Medrol, Solu-Medtol, Depo-Medrol); and prednisolone, prednisone, and triamcinolone (Aristocort, Kenacort, Azmacort).

Expectorant

As you learned previously in this chapter, an expectorant—referred to as mucolytics—liquefies and loosens thick mucous secretions so they can be removed through coughing. A commonly prescribed expectorant for chronic obstructive pulmonary disease is acetylcysteine (Mucomyst), which is administered by nebulizor five minutes after the patient receives a bronchodilator.

Acetylcysteine should not be mixed with other medications and can cause nausea, vomiting, oral ulcers (stomatitis), and a runny nose. Acetylcysteine is also an antidote for acetaminophen overdose if given within 12 to 24 hours after the overdose.

Mast Stabilizer Drugs

Mast cells release histamines, leukotrienes and other mediators of the inflammatory process. Mast cell stabilizer drugs inhibit the early asthmatic response and the late asthmatic response. They have no bronchodilator effect nor do they have any effect on any inflammatory mediators already released in the body. They are indicated for the prevention of bronchospasms and bronchial asthma attacks. They are administered by aerosol inhalation. The exact action of the drugs have not been determined. However, they are believed to have a modest effect in lowering the required dose of corticosteroids. The most common mast stabilizer drugs are cromolyn (Intal) and nedocromil (Tilade).

A list of drugs utilized in the treatment of lower respiratory tract disorders is provided in the Appendix. Detailed tables show doses, recommendations, expectations, side effects, contraindications, and more; available on the book's Web site (see URL in Appendix).

Summary

Respiratory diseases interfere with air passages or gas exchanges of the respiratory system. They are grouped together according to the portion of the respiratory tract they affect. These are the upper respiratory tract and the lower respiratory tract.

Diseases that affect the upper respiratory tract are called upper respiratory infections (URIs). These include the common cold, acute rhinitis (not the same as allergic rhinitis), sinusitis, acute tonsillitis, and acute laryngitis.

Diseases that affect the lower respiratory tract are called lower respiratory infections (LRIs). Lower respiratory infections include pneumonia and tuberculosis.

Some conditions obstruct or restrict tracheobronchial tubes and prevent the exchange of gas within the lungs. These conditions are referred to as chronic obstructive pulmonary disease. These include bronchitis, bronchiectasis, emphysema and asthma.

Some patients treat URIs with home remedies to treat the infection, however these don't kill the bacteria or virus that causes the infection. Home remedies at times do help to ease the symptoms of the disease.

When home remedies don't work, patients often use over-the-counter drugs or prescription drugs. The most commonly used are antihistamines (blocks histamines produced by the body), decongestants (reduces swollen nasal mucous membranes), antitussives (suppress the coughing reflex), and expectorants (loosens mucus).

Patients suffering from chronic obstructive pulmonary disease take prescription medication to ease the symptoms of COPD. These include bronchodilators (dilates bronchial tubes), steroids (reduces inflammation), leukotriene-modifiers (reduce inflammation and decrease bronchoconstriction).

Quiz

1. Compliance is
   (a) the ability of the lungs to be contracted.
   (b) the ability of the lungs to be distended.
   (c) the ability of the lungs to exchange gases.
   (d) none of the above.

2. All cases of pharyngitis are caused by bacteria.
   (a) True
   (b) False

3. The common cold is referred to as
   (a) rhinovirusites.
   (b) nasoitis.
   (c) rhinitis.
   (d) all of the above.

4. A runny nose is caused by nasal congestion
   (a) True
   (b) False

5. Acute laryngitis is an infection that causes swelling (edema) of the vocal cords
   (a) True
   (b) False

6. Bronchiectasis is a form of
   (a) URI.
   (b) acute pulmonary disease.
   (c) chronic obstructive pulmonary disease.
   (d) none of the above.

7. Constriction of the bronchioles is called bronchospasm.
   (a) True
   (b) False

8. The lack of the alpha$_1$-antitrypsin protein causes
   (a) bronchiectasis.
   (b) bronchitis.
   (c) emphysema.
   (d) asthma.

9. The lung contains bacteria that release proteolytic enzymes that destroy alveoli.
   (a) True
   (b) False

10. The vagus nerve releases acetylcholine when stimulated, which causes the tracheobronchial tube to contract.
    (a) True
    (b) False

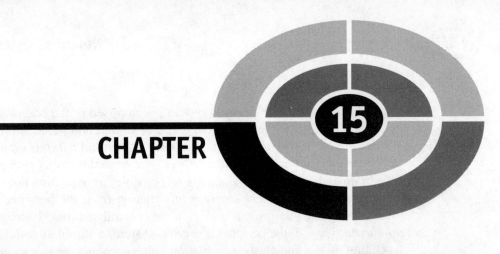

CHAPTER 15

Nervous System Drugs

The nervous system is our Internet over which sensory impulses travel the neural pathways to the brain. There they are interpreted and analyzed for an appropriate response. Another impulse is then generated by the brain and transmitted along the same pathway to tell appropriate parts of the body to respond.

Sometimes those responses are voluntary, such as using your hand to swat a bug from your nose. Involuntary responses include your heartbeat. Some responses can be a combination, such as breathing. You can hold your breath and you can make yourself breathe faster but your involuntary nervous system will take over and slow down your breathing or make you take a breath. Medication is available to interrupt impulses that flow along the neural pathway and prevent the body from responding normally to a stimulant. Likewise, there are medications that cause an impulse to stimulate parts of the body. These include drugs that increase the heart rate.

In this chapter, you'll learn about medications that affect the central nervous system and the peripheral nervous system.

A Brief Look at the Nervous System

In order to understand the therapeutic effects of medication used to treat the nervous system, you'll need to have an understanding of the anatomy and physiology of the system. The nervous system is comprised of the brain, spinal cord, nerves, and ganglia. Collectively, they receive stimuli and transmit information.

There are two nervous systems. These are the central nervous system (CNS) and the peripheral nervous system (PNS). The central nervous system consists of the brain and spinal cord, which are responsible for regulating body function. The central nervous system receives information from the peripheral nervous system, which is interpreted, and then the central nervous system sends an appropriate signal to the peripheral nervous system to stimulate cellular activity. Depending on the signal, the stimulation either increases or blocks nerve cells, which are called neurons.

The peripheral nervous system is organized into two divisions. These are the somatic nervous system (SNS) and the autonomic nervous system (ANS). The somatic nervous system acts on skeletal muscles to produce voluntary movement. The autonomic nervous system, known as the visceral system, is responsible for involuntary movement and controls the heart, respiratory system, gastrointestinal system, and the endocrine system (glands).

The autonomic nervous system is further divided into the sympathetic and parasympathetic nervous systems (see Autonomic Nervous System).

The sympathetic nervous system is called the adrenergic system and uses the norephinephrine neurotransmitter to send information. The parasympathetic system, called the cholinergic system, uses the acetylcholine neurotransmitter to transmit information.

Both the sympathetic and parasympathetic nervous systems innervate organs within the body. The sympathetic system excites the organ while the parasympathetic system inhibits the organ. For example, the sympathetic system increases the heart rate while the parasympathetic system decreases the heart rate.

NEUROLOGICAL PATHWAYS

Neurological pathways extend from locations in the spinal cord to various areas of the body. These pathways contain two types of nerve fibers. These preganglionic and postganglionic fibers are connected together by a ganglion. The preganglionic nerve fiber carries messages from the central nervous system to the ganglion. The postganglionic nerve fiber transmits that message to specific tissues and organs from the ganglion.

Neurological pathways in the sympathetic nervous system originate from the thoracic (T1 to T12) and the upper lumbar segments (L1 and L2) of the spinal cord. This is why the sympathetic nervous system is also referred to as the thoracolumbar division of the autonomic nervous system.

The preganglionic fibers of the sympathetic nervous system extend from the spinal cord to the ganglionic fiber. These are relatively short. However, sympathetic postganglionic fibers are long from the ganglion to the body cells.

Neurological pathways in the parasympathetic nervous system originate from cranial nerves III, VII, IX, and X from the brain stem and the sacral segments S2, S3, and S4 from the spinal cord. This is why the parasympathetic nervous system is also known as the craniosacral division of the autonomic nervous system.

Preganglionic fibers are long from the spinal cord to the ganglion and the postganglionic fibers are short from the ganglion to the body cells.

Central Nervous System Stimulants

Medication is given to stimulate the central nervous system in order to induce a therapeutic response. These include medications that treat narcolepsy, attention deficit disorder (ADD), obesity, and reversal of respiratory distress.

There are four major groups of medications that stimulate the central nervous system. These are amphetamines, caffeine, analeptics, and anorexiants. Amphetamines stimulate the cerebral cortex of the brain. Caffeine also stimulates the cerebral cortex and stimulates respiration by acting on the brain stem and medulla. Analeptics have an effect on the brain stem and medulla as caffeine does. Anorexiants inhibit appetite by stimulating the cerebral cortex and the hypothalamus.

Amphetamines, analeptics, and anorexiants are commonly referred to as "uppers" when used to prevent sleep. Anorexiants and amphetamines can produce psychological dependence and the body can become tolerant to its effect if abused. Abruptly discontinuing these medications may result in withdrawal symptoms including depression. Amphetamines are also taken to decrease weight and increase energy enabling the patient to perform work quickly without rest.

Analeptics are substances which stimulate breathing and heart activity. Methylphenidate (Ritalin) is an analeptic often prescribed for children with Attention Deficit Hyperactivity Disorder (ADDHD).

Amphetamines, analeptics, and anorexiants stimulate the release of the neurotransmitters norepinephrine and dopamine from the brain and from the peripheral nerve terminals of the sympathetic nervous system. The result is euphoria and increased alertness. The patient can also experience sleeplessness, restlessness, tremors, and irritability; cardiovascular problems (increased heart rate, palpitations, dysrhythmias and hypertension). Some examples of anorexiants and

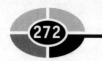

analeptics are benzphetamine (Didrex), deithylpropion (Tenuate), felfluramine (Pondimin), and phentermine (Phentride). Caffeine is also a stimulant found in many beverages, foods, OTC drugs, and prescription drugs. Caffeine is found in many drugs including Anacin, Excedrin, Cafergot, Fiorinal, and Midol.

See amphetamine-like drugs provided in the Appendix. Detailed tables show doses, recommendations, expectations, side effects, contraindications, and more; available on the book's Web site (see URL in Appendix).

MIGRAINE HEADACHES

Migraines are a debilitating neurovascular disorder that affects 28 million people over the age of 11. The cause of migraines is not clearly understood although research indicates the expansion of blood vessels and the release of certain chemicals—such as dopamine and serotonin—causes inflammation and pain. Dopamine and serotonin are found normally in the brain. A migraine can occur if an abnormal amount of these chemicals are present or if the blood vessels are unusually sensitive to them.

Patients who have migraines experience intense, throbbing, headache pain which is often accompanied by nausea, photophobia (sensitivity to light), phonophobia (sensitivity to sound), and temporary disability. Migraines are sometimes preceded by an aura such as a breeze, odor, a beam of light, or a spectrum of colors. Migraines can occur on one side of the head (unilateral) and the pain is frequently reported as pulsating or throbbing.

Treatment of migraine is divided into prevention and symptomatic relief. There are six categories of medication used to prevent migraines. These are blood-vessel constrictors and dilators (see Chapter 26), antiseizure drugs (discussed later in this chapter), antidepressants (discussed later in this chapter), beta-blockers (see Chapter 26), and analgesics (see Chapter 16). Patients are given a selected combination of these medications to prevent migraines. The prescriber determines the most effective combination for each patient based on the patient's response to these medications.

Commonly prescribed medications to prevent migraines are amitriptyline, divaproex sodium, propranol, timolol, topiramate, bupropion, cyproheptadine, diltiazem, doxepin, fluvoxamine, ibuprofen, imipramine, and methysergide. Methysergide is particularly effective. However, there are side effects that might make this drug less tolerable.

Bringing about symptomatic relief from the pain associated with migraines and other migraine symptoms is achieved by prescribing antiemetics (anti-nausea, see Chapter 18), ergot alkaloids and related compounds, NSAIDS (see Chapter 12), and other analgesic (nonopioids); opioids, and triptans (see chart).

Other Triptans	
Almotriptan	6.25–12.5 mg and repeat one dose if necessary; use with greater caution in patients with liver and kidney impairment; less side effects reported
Eletriptan	20–40 mg tablets repeated in 2 hours; high drug-drug interaction
Frovatriptan	2.5 mg at onset and may repeat after 2 hours; has longest half life with a slow onset of action
Naratriptan	1–2.5 mg tablets and repeat after 4 hours; onset of action is slower but has the second longest half life; has less side effects
Rizatriptan	5–10 mg repeated in two hours; fast acting
Zolmitriptan	2.5–5 mg dose with 2 hour repeats available PO and nasal spray; increased risk of drug-drug interaction.

A list of drugs utilized in the treatment of migrane headaches is provided in the Appendix. Detailed tables show doses, recommendations, expectations, side effects, contraindications, and more; available on the book's Web site (see URL in Appendix).

CNS Depressants

Central nervous system depressants are medications that suppress the transmission of information throughout the central nervous system. There are seven broad classifications of central nervous system depressants. These are sedative-hypnotics, general and local anesthetics (discussed later in this chapter), analgesics, narcotic analgesics (Chapter 16), anticonvulsants, antipsychotics, and antidepressants (discussed later in this chapter)

SEDATIVE-HYPNOTICS

Sedative-hypnotics are commonly referred to as sedatives and are the mildest form of central nervous system depressant. Sedative-hypnotics are given in low doses to diminish the patient's physical and mental responses without affecting the patient's consciousness.

With increased doses, the patient experiences a hypnotic effect causing the patient to fall asleep. Even higher doses of sedative-hypnotics anesthetize the patient. Such is the case of the ultra-short-acting barbiturate thiopental sodium (Pentothal) that produces anesthesia.

Sedative-hypnotics and barbituates were first used to reduce tension and anxiety. However, other medications have been developed for this use. Chronic use of any sedative-hypnotic should be avoided.

It is important to understand that sedative-hypnotics are not the same as sleep medications purchased over-the-counter such as Nytol, Sominex, Sleep-eze, and Tylenol PM. Over-the-counter sleep medications such as diphenhydramine contain an antihistamine not barbiturates to achieve sedation.

Short-acting sedative-hypnotics are ideal for patients who need assistance falling asleep but who must awaken early without experiencing a lingering aftereffect from the medication. Intermediate-acting sedative-hypnotics are useful to sustain sleep. Patients may experience residual drowsiness (hangover) after awakening.

The use of sedative-hypnotics for sleep (hypnotic) should be short term or there is a chance that the patient could become dependent on the medication or develop a tolerance. Patients who take high doses of sedative-hypnotics over long periods must gradually discontinue the medication rather than abruptly stopping the drug which can cause withdrawal symptoms. Sedative-hypnotics should not be administered to patients who have severe respiratory disorders or who are pregnant.

Before a patient is prescribed a sedative-hypnotic to aid with sleep, the patient should try non-pharmacological methods that promote sleep such as:

- Arise at a specific hour in the morning.
- Take few or no daytime naps.
- Avoid heavy meals or strenuous exercise before bedtime.
- Take a warm bath, read, or listen to music before bedtime.
- Decrease exposure to loud noises.
- Avoid watching disturbing television before sleep.
- Avoid drinking a lot of fluids before sleep.
- Drink warm milk before sleep.

See sedative-hypnotic–benzodiazepine provided in the Appendix. Detailed tables show doses, recommendations, expectations, side effects, contraindications, and more; available on the book's Web site (see URL in Appendix).

BARBITURATES

Barbiturates are a type of sedative-hypnotic that is used to induce sleep, as an anesthetic, and in high doses to control epileptic seizures. Barbiturates are classified by duration of action referred to as ultrashort-acting, short-acting, intermediate acting, and long-acting.

Ultrashort-acting barbiturates such as thiopental sodium (Pentothal) is a commonly used anesthetic. Secobarbital (Seconal) and pentobarbital (Nembutal) are short-acting barbiturates that induce sleep. For longer periods of sleep, patients are prescribed intermediate acting such as amobarbital (Amytal), aprobarbital (Alurate) and bubatabarbital (Butisol). Phenobarbital and mephobarbital are long-acting barbiturates used for controlling epileptic seizures.

Barbiturates are Class II Controlled Substances and should be prescribed for no more than two weeks because of the adverse side effect. Barbiturates increase CNS depression in the elderly and should not be used for sleep.

See sedative-hypnotic: barbituates and others provided in the Appendix. Detailed tables show doses, recommendations, expectations, side effects, contraindications, and more; available on the book's Web site (see URL in Appendix).

Other Barbiturates			
Short-acting:	Secobarbital sodium (Seconal Sodium) Class II	Preoperative sedation Used to induce sleep	PO 100–200 mg before surgery; hypnotic PO/IM 100–200 mg h.s.; Status epilepticus: IV; 5.5 mg/kg; repeat in 3–4 hours; with spinal anesthesia IV; 50–100 mg.; infused over 30 seconds; maximum dose of 250/mg
Intermediate-acting	Amobarbital sodium (Amytal Sodium)	Sleep sustainers	PB 50–60%; half life 20–40 hours; Sedative: PO 30–50 mg bid-tid; Hypnotic PO/IM 65–200 mg h.s., IV: 65–200 mg

Other Barbiturates	(continued)		
Other	Chloral hydrate Class IV	No hangover and less respiratory depression; give with meals or fluids to prevent gastric irritation	Pregnancy category C; PB 70%–80%; half life 8–10 hours; PO 250 mg tid before meals; Hypnotic: PO 500 mg–1g h.s.
Other	Paraldehyde Class IV	Exhaled via the lungs; strong odor and disagreeable taste; seldom used; has been used to control delirium tremens (DTS) in alcoholics; can be used for drug poisoning	Status epilepticus and tetanus to control convulsions; Pregnancy category C, PB UK; half life 7.5 hours; Sedative PO 5–10 mL q4–6h PRN in water or juice; maximum dose of 30 mL; Hypnotic: PO 10–30 mL h.s.

ANESTHETIC AGENTS

Anesthetic agents depress the central nervous system causing a loss of consciousness. They are classified as general and local.

Anesthetic agents were introduced in surgery in the early 1800s in the form of nitrous oxide (laughing gas), which continues to be used today for dental procedures. Other anesthetic agents became widely used by the mid-1800s. These included ether and chloroform. Ether is a highly flammable liquid with a pungent odor that causes nausea and vomiting and is seldom used today. Chloroform is toxic to the liver and is no longer used.

General anesthetics are used for general surgery, cardiac surgery, neurosurgery, and pediatric surgery. They are administered by an anesthesiologist or a nurse anesthetist. They are inhaled through a mask or breathing tube.

A general anesthetic can consist of one medication or a combination of medications—called balanced anesthesia—depending on the patient's age, weight, medical history, general health, and allergies.

This balanced approach is used when administering general anesthetics to patients in phases to minimize cardiovascular problems, decrease the amount of general anesthetic needed, reduce possible post-anesthetic nausea and vomiting, minimize the disturbance of organ function, and increase recovery from anesthesia with fewer adverse reactions.

The night before the surgery, the patient is given a hypnotic to assist with a good night's sleep. On the day of the surgery, premedication may be given to the patient about one hour before surgery. Premedication typically consists of two medications. One is a benzodiazepine such as lorazepan (Ativan). This medication sedates and decreases anxiety. The other is an anticholinergic such as atropine to decrease secretions. A short-acting barbiturate such as thiopental sodium (Pentothal) is then administered in the operating room to induce anesthesia. The patient is then given inhaled gas and oxygen to maintain anesthesia. Sometimes the anesthetic is administered IV. Depending on the nature of the operation, the patient may also receive a muscle relaxant.

The patient experiences four stages of anesthesia, some of which are not observable because they occur rapidly. These stages are:

Stage one: analgesia

The patient experiences analgesia (a loss of pain sensation) but remains conscious and can carry on a conversation.

Stage two: excitement

The patient may experience delirium or become violent. Blood pressure rises and becomes irregular, and breathing rate increases. This stage is typically bypassed by administering a barbiturate such as sodium pentothal before the anesthesia.

Stage three: surgical anesthesia

Skeletal muscles relax. Breathing becomes regular. Eye movement slows then stops. It is at this point when surgery begins.

Stage four: medullary paralysis

Breathing and other vital functions cease to function because the respiratory center (medulla oblongata) is paralyzed. Death results if the patient is not revived quickly. Careful administration of the anesthesia prevents reaching this stage.

A list of Anesthetic Drugs is provided in the Appendix. Detailed tables show doses, recommendations, expectations, side effects, contraindications, and more; available on the book's Web site (see URL in Appendix).

Commonly administered intravenous anesthetic agents	
Ketamine (Ketalar)	Affects the senses, and produces a dissociative anesthesia (catatonia, amnesia, analgesia) in which the patient may appear awake and reactive, but cannot respond to sensory stimuli. These properties make it especially useful in developing countries and during warfare medical treatment. Ketamine is frequently used in pediatric patients because anesthesia and analgesia can be achieved with an intramuscular injection. It is also used in high-risk geriatric patients and in shock cases, because it also provides cardiac stimulation.
Thiopental (Pentothal)	A barbiturate that induces a rapid hypnotic state of short duration. Because thiopental is slowly metabolized by the liver, toxic accumulation can occur; therefore, it should not be continuously infused. Side effects include nausea and vomiting upon awakening.
Opioids	Fentanyl, sufentanil, and alfentanil are frequently used prior to anesthesia and surgery as a sedative and analgesic, as well as a continuous infusion for primary anesthesia. Because opioids rarely affect the cardiovascular system, they are particularly useful for cardiac surgery and other high-risk cases. Opioids act directly on spinal cord receptors, and are frequently used in epidurals for spinal anesthesia. Side effects may include nausea and vomiting, itching, and respiratory depression.
Propofol (Diprivan)	Nonbarbiturate hypnotic agent and the most recently developed intravenous anesthetic. Its rapid induction and short duration of action are identical to thiopental, but recovery occurs more quickly and with much less nausea and vomiting. Also, propofol is rapidly metabolized in the liver and excreted in the urine, so it can be used for long durations of anesthesia, unlike thiopental. Hence, propofol is rapidly replacing thiopental as an anesthetic agent.

TOPICAL ANESTHETIC AGENTS

Topical anesthetic agents (see chart) are solutions, liquid sprays, ointments, creams, and gels that are applied to mucous membranes, broken or unbroken skin surfaces, and burns to decrease the sensitivity of nerve endings in the affected area.

The first topical anesthetic agent was TAC, which is a combination of tetracaine, adrenaline (epinephrine), and cocaine, and was used for face and scalp lacerations. A version of TAC called LET is used today. LET is a combination of lidocaine, epinephrine, and tetracaine. Lidocaine replaced cocaine. LET gel is

generally preferred over TAC as analgesia for skin that is not intact because LET has a superior safety record and is more cost-effective than TAC.

Perhaps the most well known topical anesthetic for intact skin is EMLA. EMLA is commonly used to anesthetize skin before IM injections, venipuncture, and simple skin procedures such as curettage or biopsy. EMLA is most effective if administered 90 minutes before the procedure.

ELA-Max (4% Liposomal Lidocaine) is another topical anesthetic for intact skin that works faster than EMLA. EL-Max is an over-the-counter medication that uses the liposomal delivery system. Liposomes are tiny lipid (fat) balls that deliver moisture to the skin. Because of their small molecular size, they are able to penetrate the cell wall reasonably well and can be used to deliver medications.

Other topical anesthetics can be delivered using iontophoresis—a therapy that uses a local electric current to introduce the ions of a medicine into the tissues—and anesthetic patch.

Topical Anesthetic Agents	
TAC (0.5% tetracaine, 1:2,000 epinephrine, and 11.8% cocaine)	2 to 5 mL (1 mL per cm of laceration) applied to wound with cotton or gauze for 10 to 30 minutes; Onset: effective 10 to 30 minutes after application; Duration: not established; May be as effective as lidocaine for lacerations on face and scalp; Rare severe toxicity, including seizures and sudden cardiac death.
LET (4% lidocaine, 1:2,000 epinephrine, and 0.5% tetracaine)	1 to 3 mL directly applied to wound for 15 to 30 minutes; Onset: 20 to 30 minutes Duration: not established; Similar to TAC for face and scalp lacerations; less effective on extremities; No severe adverse effects reported
EMLA (2.5% lidocaine and 2.5% prilocaine)	Thick layer (1 to 2 g per 10 cm^2) applied to intact skin with covering patch of Tegaderm; Onset: must be left on for 1 to 2 hours Duration: 0.5 to 2 hours; Variable, depending on duration of application; Contact dermatitis, methemoglobinemia (very rare)
Iontophoresis	Small current applied to lidocaine-soaked sponges on intact skin; Onset: 10 minutes; Duration: 10 to 20 minutes; Good for small procedures, depth of anesthesia greater than EMLA; Stinging sensation; may burn skin if high current

Other Local Anesthetic Agents	
Procaine (Novocaine)	Short-acting ($1/2$ to 1 hour)—ester, first synthetic local anesthetic, relatively safe due to rapid metabolism in the plasma, fast onset-short duration, not good for topical anesthesia
Cocaine	Ester, only local anesthetic that is a vasoconstrictor, only local anesthetic that produces euphoria, used by ENTs for surgical procedures because it reduces pain and controls bleeding.
Tetracaine (Pontocaine)	Long-acting—ester—used for spinal anesthesia and topical
Bupivicaine	Long-acting—amide—can be cardiotoxic at high concentrations, used for infiltration, epidural and nerve blocks.

LOCAL ANESTHESIA

A local anesthetic (see chart) blocks pain at the site where the medication is administered without affecting the patient's consciousness. It is commonly used for dental procedures, suturing of skin lacerations, short-term surgery at a localized area, spinal anesthesia by blocking nerve impulses (nerve block) below the insertion of the anesthetic, and diagnostic procedures such as lumbar punctures.

Local anesthetics are divided into two groups according to their basic chemical structure. These are esters and amides. An ester is a chemical compound formed from the reaction between an acid and an alcohol. Amides are an organic chemical compound formed by reaction of an acid chloride, acid anhydride, or ester with an amine. Amides have a lower incidence of causing an allergic reaction than esters.

See local anesthetics listing provided in the Appendix. Detailed tables show doses, recommendations, expectations, side effects, contraindications, and more; available on the book's Web site (see URL in Appendix).

SPINAL ANESTHESIA

Spinal anesthesia is a local anesthetic injected into the spinal column in the third or fourth lumbar space to produce a regional neural block. If it is given too high, the respiratory muscles could be affected and respiratory distress or failure could result. There are 4 types of spinal anesthesia: subarachnoid block, epidural block, the saddle block, and a caudal block.

A subarachnoid block is the injection into the subarachnoid space in the third or fourth lumbar space to produce anesthesia.

The epidural block occurs when the anesthetic is injected into the outer covering (dura mater) of the spinal cord near the sacrum.

The saddle block is given at the lower end of the spinal column to block the perineal area for procedures such as childbirth.

The caudal block is placed near the sacrum.

The patient may experience headaches and hypotension as a result of these procedures because of a change in cerebrospinal fluid pressure when the needle is inserted into the spine. The patient should remain in the supine position following the procedure and increase fluid intake.

Autonomic Nervous System

The autonomic nervous system—also known as the visceral system—involuntarily regulates smooth muscles and glands including the heart, respiratory system, GI tract, peristalsis (digestion), bladder, and eyes.

The autonomic nervous system has two sets of nerves. These are the sensory neurons (afferent) and the motor neurons (efferent). Sensory neurons send impulses to the central nervous system, which are transmitted to the brain where they are interpreted. The brain then sends a response to the motor neuron's brain through the spinal cord that directs specific organ cells to respond to the sensory neuron's impulse.

Previously in this chapter you learned that the autonomic nervous system has two branches. These are the sympathetic branch and parasympathetic branch. Both branches act on the same organ cells but in an opposite way. The sympathetic branch stimulates a response and the parasympathetic branch depresses a response by the organ cell. Together, they keep the organ in balance (homeostasis).

The sympathetic branch stimulates a response using norepinephrine, a neurotransmitter. Medications that mimic the effect of norepinephrine are called adrenergic drugs or sympathomimetics (mimic sympathetic nervous system actions) (see chart). These drugs are also known as adrenergic agonists because they start a response at the adrenergic receptor sites. There are four types of adrenergic receptors. These are alpha$_1$, alpha$_2$, beta$_1$, and beta$_2$. (see chart)

The parasympathetic branch depresses a response using adrenergic blockers—also known as sympatholytics. Lytic means to stop effect. Adrenergic blockers prevent the norepinephrine response at the adrenergic receptor sites.

The parasympathetic branch is sometimes referred to as the cholinergic system because an acetylcholine neurotransmitter is used to innervate muscle cells at the end of the neuron. Acetylcholine stimulates receptor cells to produce a

Receptor	Physiologic responses
Alpha$_1$	Increases force of contraction of heart. Vasoconstriction: increases blood pressure. Mydriasis: dilates pupils of the eyes. Glandular (salivary): decreases secretions. Bladder & prostate: capsule increases contraction and ejaculation.
Alpha$_2$	Inhibits the release of norepinephrine, dilates blood vessels, and produces hypotension; decreases gastrointestinal motility and tone.
Beta$_1$	Increases heart rate and force of contraction; increases rennin secretion, which increases blood pressure
Beta$_2$	Dilates bronchioles; promotes GI and uterine relaxation; promotes increase in blood sugar through glycogenolysis in the liver; increases blood flow in the skeletal muscles.

response. However, the enzyme acetylcholinesterase can inactivate the acetylcholine before it reaches the receptor cell.

Drugs that mimic acetylcholine are cholinergic agonists because they initiate a response. These are also known as cholinergic drugs or parasympathomimetics (see chart).

Drugs that block the effect of acetylcholine are called anticholinergic, or parasympatholytics. They are also known as cholinergic antagonists because they inhibit the effect of acetylcholine on the organ.

There are two types of cholinergic receptors. These are nicotinic or muscarinic. Nicotinic receptors are stimulated by alkaloids nicotine. Muscarinic receptors are stimulated by muscarine.

Sympathetic Stimulants	Parasympathetic Stimulants
Sympathomimetics (adrenergics, adrenomimetics, or adrenergic agonists)	**Direct-acting**
Increase blood pressure	*Parasympathomimetics (cholinergics, or cholinergic agonists)*
Increase pulse rate	Decrease blood pressure
Relax bronchioles	Decrease pulse rate
Dilate pupils of eyes	Constrict bronchioles
Uterine relaxation	Constrict pupils of eyes
Increase blood sugar	Increase urinary contraction
	Increase peristalsis
	Indirect-acting
	Cholinesterase Inhibitors (anticholinesterase)
	Increase muscle tone

Sympathetic Depressants	Parasympathetic Depressants
Sympatholytics (adrenergic blockers, adrenolytics, or adrenergic antagonists)	*Parasympatholytics (anticholinergics, cholinergic antagonists, or antispasmodics)*
Decrease blood pressure	Increase pulse rate
Decrease pulse rate	Decrease mucus secretions
Constrict bronchioles	Decrease gastrointestinal motility
	Increase urinary retention
	Dilate pupils of eyes

THE FIGHT OR FLIGHT RESPONSE

Norepinephrine and acetylcholine neurotransmitters produce a fight or flight response (see chart). In a fight response, eyes dilate so you can see better and lungs inspire more oxygen while increasing your heart rate. Blood vessels constrict increasing blood pressure. Smooth muscles along the bladder and the GI tract relax so that energy is not expended on digestion. Salivary glands reduce the secretion of saliva giving the person the dry mouth feeling in an emergency.

The flight response is really a misnomer because it doesn't help you run away. Instead, the flight response is really the opposite of fight and allows the individual to relax and function normally. In the flight response or the non-fight mode, pupils constrict, the heart rate slows, the GI tract reduces function, and breathing slows down.

Body Tissue/Organ	Sympathetic (Fight) Response	Parasympathetic (Flight) Response
Eye	Dilates pupil	Constricts pupil
Lungs	Dilates bronchioles	Constricts bronchioles and increases secretions
Heart	Increases heart rate	Decreases heart rate
Blood vessels	Constricts	Dilate
Gastrointestinal	Relaxes smooth muscles	Increases peristalsis
Bladder	Relaxes bladder muscle	Constricts bladder
Uterus	Relaxes uterine muscle	
Salivary gland		Increases salivation

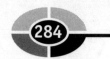

ADRENERGICS AND ADRENERGIC BLOCKERS

Andrenergics are medications that stimulate alpha$_1$-receptors and beta$_2$-adrenergic receptors. Alpha$_1$-receptors are located in the smooth muscle of vascular (vessels) tissues. Beta$_2$-adrenergic receptors are in the smooth muscle of the lungs, arterioles of skeletal muscles, and the uterine muscles. Adrenergics also stimulate the dopaminergic receptor located in the renal, mesenteric, coronary, and cerebral arteries to dilate and increase blood flow. Dopamine is the only adrenergic that can activate this receptor.

Adrenergic blockers inactivate these receptors in three ways:

1. They promote reuptake of the transmitter back into the neuron (nerve cell terminal).
2. Transmitters are transformed or degraded by enzymes making them unable to attach to a receptor. Two enzymes that inactive norepinephrine are monoamine oxidase (MAO) and catechol-o-methyl-transferase (COMIT). MAO is inside the neuron and COMIT is outside the neuron.
3. Transmitters are diffused away from receptors.

Sympathomimetic drugs stimulate andrenergic receptors and are classified into three categories according to its effect on organ cells. These categories are:

1. Direct-acting sympathomimetics—directly stimulate receptors.
2. Indirect-acting sympathomimetics—stimulate the release of norepinephrine from terminal nerve endings.
3. Mixed-acting sympathomimetics—have the effect of both direct-acting sympathomimetics and indirect-acting sympathomimetics. They simulate the adrenergic receptor sites and stimulate the release of norepinephrine from terminal nerve endings. Ephedrine is an example of a mixed-acting sympathomimetic and is used to treat idiopathic orthostatic hypotension and hypotension resulting from spinal anesthesia. Ephedrine also stimulates beta$_2$-receptors to dilate bronchial tubes and is used treat mild forms of bronchial asthma.

Many adrenergic medications stimulate more that one adrenergic receptor site. For example, epinephrine (Adrenalin) acts on alpha$_1$-, beta$_1$-, beta$_2$-receptor sites. These receptor sites include an increase in blood pressure, pupil dilation, increase in heart rate (tachycardia), and bronchodilation.

Epinephrine (Adrenalin) is used to treat cardiogenic and anaphylactic shock because it increases blood pressure, heart rate, and airflow through the lungs through bronchodilation. Because it affects three different receptors, it lacks selectivity.

Alpha-adrenergic blockers inhibit the response at the alpha-adrenergic receptor sites. There are two types of alpha-adrenergic blockers: selective and nonselective blockers. Both types decrease symptoms of benign prostatic hypertrophy (BPH) (enlarged prostate) and promote vasodilation and treat peripheral vascular disease such as Raynaud's disease.

Doxazosin (Cardura) is a selective $alpha_1$-blocker and phentolamine (Regitine) is a nonselective alpha adrenergic blocker. Both can be used to treat hypertension.

However, alpha-adrenergic blockers can cause orthostatic hypotension (drop in blood pressure when an individual stands up), dizziness, and reflex tachycardia. They are not as frequently prescribed as beta-blockers.

Beta-adrenergic blockers (see chart)—also known beta blockers—decrease heart rate and decrease blood pressure resulting in bronchoconstriction. Therefore, beta-adrenergic blockers should be used with caution for patient's who have COPD or asthma.

Other Adrenergics	
Ephedrine HCl ($alpha_1$, $beta_1$, $beta_2$)	PO 25–50 mg tid/qid; SC/IM: 25–50 mg; IV: 10–25 mg PRN; maximum dose 150 mg/24 hr; effective for relief of hay fever, sinusitis, and allergic rhinitis; may be used for treating mild cases of asthma; Pregnancy category C: PB UK; half life 3–6 hours.
Norepinephrine bitartrate (Levophed) ($alpha_1$, $beta_1$):	Potent vasoconstrictor; IV: 4 mg in 250–500 mL of D_5W or NSS infused initially 8–12 μg/min; then 4 μg/min; titrated according to blood pressure; Pregnancy category CD PB: UK; half life: UK.
Metaraminol bitartrate (Aramine) ($alpha_1$, $beta_1$)	V/Inf: 15–100 mg in 500 mg D_5W at a rate adjusted according to blood pressure; Pregnancy category C; PB UK; half life UK.
Dobutamine HCl (Dobutrex) ($beta_1$)	To treat cardiac decompensation due to depressed myocardial contractility which may result from organic heart disease, cardiac surgery. IV: 2.5–20 μg/kg/min initially; increase dose gradually; maximum dose of 40 μg/kg/min. Pregnancy category: C; PBUK; half life 2 min.
Dopamine HCl (Intropin) ($alpha_1$, $beta_1$) IV/Inf	1–5 μg/kg/min initially; gradually increase 5–10 μg/kg/min to a maximum of 50 μg/kg/min; it does not decrease renal function in doses <5 μg/kg/min. Pregnancy category C; PB: UK; half life 2 min.

There are also two types of beta-adrenergic blockers: selective and non-selective. For example, metoprolol tartrate (Lopressor) is a selective beta-adrenergic blocker that blocks beta$_1$ receptors to decrease pulse rate and decrease blood pressure. Propranolol NCl (Inderal) is a non-selective beta-adrenergic blocker that blocks both beta$_1$ and beta$_2$ receptors resulting in a slower heart rate, decreased cardiac output, and lower blood pressure.

Other Beta Blockers	
Doxazosin mesylate (Cardura) alpha$_1$	Mild to moderate hypertension; PO: 1 mg/d; titrate dose up to maximum of 16 mg/d; maintenance 4–8 mg/day. Pregnancy category C; PB 95%; half life 3 h.
Carvedilol (Coreg) alpha$_1$, beta$_1$, beta$_2$	Use for hypertension and mild to moderate heart failure; can be used with a thiazide diuretic; PO: 6.25 mg bid; may increase to 12.5 mg bid to maximum 50 mg/d; Pregnancy category: C; PB UK; half life 7–10 h.
Labetalol (Normodyne) alpha$_1$, beta$_1$, beta$_2$	Mild to severe hypertension; angina pectoris; PO: 100 mg bid; dose may be increased to a maximum of 2.4 g/day. IV: 20 mg OR 102 mg/kg; repeat 20–80 mg at 10-min interval to maximum dose of 300 mg/day. Pregnancy category C; PB 50%; half life 6–8 hours.
Nadolol (Corgard) beta$_1$, beta$_2$	Management of hypotension and angina pectoris. Contraindicated in bronchial asthma and severe COPD. PO: 40–80 mg/d; maximum 320 mg/day. Pregnancy category: C; PB 30%; half life 10–24 h.

Selective Beta Adrenergics	
Metoprolol tartrate (Lopressor)—beta$_1$	Management of hypertension, angina pectoris, postmyocardial infarction. Hypertension: PO: 50–100 mg/d in 102 divided doses; maintenance 100–450 mg/d in divided doses to maximum of 450 mg/d in divided doses. Myocardial infarction: IV: 5 mg q2 min x 3 doses, then PO: 100 mg bid. Pregnancy category C; PB 12%; half life 3–4 h.
Atenolol (Tenormin)—beta$_1$	Mild to moderate hypertension and angina pectoris. May be used in combination with antihypertensive drugs. PO: 25–100 mg/d. Pregnancy category: C; PB 6–16%; half life 6–7h Esmolol HCl (Brevibloc)—beta$_1$. Supraventricular tachycardia, atrial fibrillation/flutter, and hypertension. Contraindications: heart block, bradycardia, cardiogenic shock, uncompensated CHF; IV: Loading dose 500 μ/kg/min for 1 min; then 50 μg/kg/min for 4 min. Pregnancy category C; PB UK; half life 9 min.

Cholinergics

Cholinergics mimic the parasympathetic neurotransmitter acetylcholine. Acetylcholine (Ach) is a neurotransmitter located in the ganglions and terminal nerve endings of parasympathetic nerves that connect to receptors in organs, tissues, and glands.

There are two types of cholinergic receptors. These are muscarinic receptors and nicotinic receptors. Muscarinic receptors stimulate smooth muscles and slow the heart rate. Nicotinic receptors affect skeletal muscles. Some cholinergic medications are selective and affect either muscarinic receptor or nicotinic receptors while other cholinergic medications are non-specific and affect both receptors.

Direct-acting cholinergics act on the receptors to activate a tissue response. Indirect-acting cholinergic drugs inhibit the action of cholineresterase (acetylcholinesterase) by forming a chemical complex that permits acetylcholine to persist and attach to the receptor. These drugs are called cholinesterase inhibitors or anticholinesterase drugs.

Pilocarpine is a commonly used direct-acting cholinergic that is used to treat glaucoma. Pilocarpine reduces intraocular pressure by constricting pupils and opening the Canal of Schlemm enabling aqueous humor (fluid) to drain.

There are two types of cholinesterase inhibitors. These are reversible inhibitors and irreversible inhibitors. A reversible inhibitor binds to the cholinesterase enzyme for a period of time and then unbinds enabling the cholinesterase enzyme to properly function. An irreversible inhibitor permanently binds to the cholinesterase enzyme.

Cholinergics stimulate (see chart) the bladder, constrict pupils (miosis), increase neuromuscular transmission, and provide muscle tone to the GI tract. Other effects include a decreased heart rate and blood pressures while increasing secretion of the salivary glands.

See direct-acting cholinergic list is provided in the Appendix. Detailed tables show doses, recommendations, expectations, side effects, contraindications, and more; available on the book's Web site (see URL in Appendix).

Anticholinergics

Anticholinergics drugs (see chart) inhibit acetylcholine by occupying the acetylcholine receptors. Anticholinergics are also called parasympatholytics, cholinergic blocking agents, cholinergic or muscarinic antagonists, antiparasympathetic agents, antimuscarinic agents, or antispasmodics.

Anticholinergics drugs block parasympathetic nerves thereby enabling impulses from sympathetic nerves to take control. Anticholinergic and adrenergic drugs produce many of the same responses.

A list of anticholinergic drugs are provided in the Appendix. Detailed tables show doses, recommendations, expectations, side effects, contraindications, and more; available on the book's Web site (see URL in Appendix).

Antiparkinsonism-Anticholinergic Drugs

Antiparkinsonism-anticholinergic drugs are used to treat the early stages of Parkinson's disease. These are typically combined with levodopa to control parkinsonism or alone to treat pseudoparkinsonism. These are the parkinsonism-like side effects of phenothiazines, which is an antipsychotic medication.

Drugs for Parkinsonism

Parkinsonism, better known as Parkinson's disease, is a chronic neurological disorder that affects balance and locomotion at the extrapyramidal motor tract. It is considered a syndrome because it has a combination of symptoms. Parkinsonism has three major features. These are rigidity, bradykinesia (slow movements), and tremors.

Rigidity is the abnormal increase in muscle tone that causes the patient to make postural changes such a shuffling gate, the chest and head is thrust forward, and knees and hips are flexed. The patient walks without swinging his arms. These movements are slow (bradykinesia) and the patient exhibits involuntary tremors of the head and neck which may be more prevalent at rest and pill-rolling movements of the hands. Another characteristic symptoms is the masked facies (no facial expression) common in patients with Parkinson's disease.

There are four types of drugs used to treat Parkinson's disease: dopaminergics, dopamine agonists, MAO-B inhibitors, and anticholinergics which have been discussed previously in this chapter.

Dopaminergics decrease the symptoms of Parkinson's disease by permitting more levodopa to reach the nerve terminal where levodopa is transformed into dopamine and the tremors are reduced.

Dopamine agonists stimulate the dopamine receptors and reduce the symptoms of Parkinson's disease. MAO-B inhibitors inhibit the catabolic enzymes that break down dopamine thereby extending the effects of dopamine. However they can cause a hypertensive crisis if taken with certain foods (see Table 15-1).

Table 15-1. MAO inhibitors can cause a hypertensive crisis if taken with these foods.

Foods	Effects
Cheese (cheddar, Swiss, bleu)	Sweating, tremors
Bananas, raisins	Bounding heart rate
Pickled foods	Increased blood pressure
Red wine, beer	Increased temperature
Cream, yogurts	
Chocolate, coffee	
Italian green beans	
Liver	
Yeast	
Soy sauce	

Avoid taking barbiturates, tricyclic antidepressants, antihistamines, central nervous system depressants, and over-the-counter cold medications with MAO inhibitors.

A list of drugs utilized in the treatment of Parkinson's Disease is provided in the Appendix. Detailed tables show doses, recommendations, expectations, side effects, contraindications, and more; available on the book's Web site (see URL in Appendix).

MUSCLE SPASMS AND PAIN

Muscle spasms and pain are associated with traumatic injuries and many chronic debilitating disorders such as multiple sclerosis. Spasms are caused by hyperexcitable neurons stimulated by cerebral neurons or from lack of inhibition of the stimulus in the spinal cord or at the skeletal muscles.

Muscle relaxants are used to treats muscle spasms. There are two groups of muscle relaxants: centrally acting and peripherally acting. Centrally acting muscle relaxants depress neuron activity in the spinal cord or in the brain. They are used to treat acute spasms from muscle trauma, but are less effective for treating spasms caused by chronic neurological disorders.

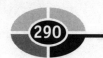

Centrally acting muscle relaxants

Carisoprodol (Soma), Cyclobenzaprine (Flexeril) and Methocarbamol (Robaxin).

These drugs decrease pain, increase range of motion and have a sedative effect on the patient. Centrally acting muscle relaxants should not be taken concurrently with central nervous system depressants such as barbiturates, narcotics, and alcohol.

Diazepam (Valium) and Baclofen (Lioresal)

These are used to treat acute spasms from muscle trauma and for treating spasms caused by chronic neurologic disorders.

Dantrolene sodium (Dantrium)

This is a peripherally acting muscle relaxant. Peripherally acting muscle relaxants depress neuron activity at the skeletal muscles and have a minimal effect on the central nervous system. These are most effective for spasticity or muscle contractions caused by chronic neurologic disorders. This is also used to treat malignant hypertension which is an allergic reaction to anesthesia.

MYASTHENIA GRAVIS

Myasthenia gravis is a disease where nerve impulses don't reach the nerves in muscle endings (myoneural junction) because of an inadequate secretion of or loss of acetylcholine due to action of acetylcholinesterase, an enzyme that destroys acetylcholine at the myoneural junction.

Patients experience fatigue and muscle weakness—particularly in respiratory muscles, facial muscles, and muscles in the extremities. They have drooping eyelids (ptosis) and difficulty in chewing and swallowing and their respiratory muscles become paralyzed which leads to respiratory arrest. Acetylcholinesterase (ACE inhibitors) are used to treat the symptoms of this disease. They include ambenonium (Mytelase), edrophonium Cl (Tensilon), Neostigmine bromide (Prostigmin), and Pyridostigmine bromide (Mestinon).

MULTIPLE SCLEROSIS

Multiple sclerosis (MS) is an autoimmune disease affecting the central nervous system. Multiple lesions of the myelin sheath that surround the nerve fibers occur that are called plaque. Myelin enables nerves to conduct impulses.

Because some axons are spared, symptoms are different in each patient. The absence of the myelin causes impulses to jump or not transmit at all. MS patients can live a normal life span. At times patients don't experience symptoms and other times symptoms can become severe and debilitating. These patients are said to have relapsing-remitting multiple sclerosis. Other patients have no periods of remission.

There is no cure for MS. However, the disease is treated symptomatically using several medications.

Corticosteroids

These are used for treating periods when the patient experiences symptoms of MS (exacerbations). These are also known as attacks, relapses and flare-ups.

Interferonß-1B (betaseron) and interferonß-1a (avonex)

These are used to reduce the frequency and severity of relapses.

Copolymer 1

This drug is in clinical trials and appears to decrease the disease's activity.

Copaxone (glatiramer acetate injection)

This drug reduces new brain lesions and the frequency of relapses in people with relapsing-remitting multiple sclerosis.

ALZHEIMER'S DISEASE

Alzheimer's disease is a form of dementia common in older people that affects the patient's ability to carry out daily activities. Part of the patient's brain that controls thought, memory, and language becomes impaired.

Four and a half million Americans are afflicted with Alzheimer's disease. Alzheimer's disease affects 5% of people between 65 and 74 years of age and half of those older than 85 years. Alzheimer's disease is not part of the aging process.

Although the cause of Alzheimer's disease remains unknown, investigators have discovered Alzheimer's patients have abnormal clumps of amyloid plaques and tangled bundles of fibers called neurofibrillary tangles in parts of their brain.

There are also low levels of chemicals that carry messages between nerve cells in the brain. Amyloid plaques, neurofibrillary tangles, and decreased chemical levels impair thinking and memory by disrupting these messages and causing nerve cells to die. The course of the disease varies from person to person. Eventually, the patient loses mental capacity and the ability to carry out daily activities. This can range from mild memory problems to severe brain damage.

Although there isn't a treatment that stops Alzheimer's disease, there are medications that provide some relief to patients who are in the early and middle stages of the disease.

Tacrine (Cognex), donepezil (Aricept), rivastigmine (Exelon), and galantamine (Reminyl)

These drugs prevent some symptoms from becoming worse for a limited time.

Memantine (Namenda)

This medication is used to treat moderate to severe cases.

Tranquilizers, mood elevators, and sedatives

These can help control behavioral symptoms such as sleeplessness, agitation, wandering, anxiety, and depression.

A list of anticholinergic drugs is provided in the Appendix. Detailed tables show doses, recommendations, expectations, side effects, contraindications, and more; available on the book's Web site (see URL in Appendix).

Effects of Cholinergic and Anticholinergic Drugs		
Body Tissue	Cholinergic Response	Anticholinergic Response
Cardiovascular*	Decreases heart rate, lowers blood pressure due to vasodilation, and slows conduction of atrioventricular node.	Increases heart rate with large doses. Small doses can decrease heart rate.
Gastrointestinal+	Increases the tone and motility of the smooth muscles of the stomach and intestine. Peristalsis is increased and the sphincter muscles are relaxed.	Relaxes smooth muscle tone of GI tract, decreasing GI motility and peristalsis. Decreases gastric and intestinal secretions.

*Tissue responses to large doses of cholinergic drugs
+ Major tissue responses to normal doses of cholinergic drugs

Effects of Cholinergic and Anticholinergic Drugs *(continued)*		
Body Tissue	**Cholinergic Response**	**Anticholinergic Response**
Genitourinary	Contracts the muscles of the urinary bladder, increases tone of the ureters, and relaxes the bladder's sphincter muscles. Stimulates urination.	Relaxes the bladder detrusor muscle and increases constriction of the internal sphincter. Urinary retention can result.
Eye+	Increases papillary constriction, or miosis (pupil becomes smaller), and increases accommodation (flattening or thickening of eye lens for distant or near vision).	Dilates pupils of the eye (mydriasis) and paralyzes ciliary muscle (cycloplegia), causing a decrease in accommodation.
Glandular*	Increases salivation, perspiration, and tears	Decreases salivation, sweating, and bronchial secretions.
Bronchi (lung)*	Stimulates bronchial smooth muscle contraction and increases bronchial secretions.	Dilates the bronchi and decreases bronchial secretions.
Striated muscle+	Increases neuromuscular transmission and maintains muscle strength and tone.	Decreases tremors and rigidity of muscles.
Central nervous system		Drowsiness, disorientation, and hallucination can result from large doses.

*Tissue responses to large doses of cholinergic drugs
+ Major tissue responses to normal doses of cholinergic drugs

EPILEPSY

Epilepsy is a seizure disorder where there is an abnormal electric discharge from the cerebral neurons that result in loss or disturbance of consciousness and convulsion (abnormal motor reaction). Epilepsy affects 1% of people in the United States.

Half the epilepsy cases are secondary to trauma, brain anoxia, infection, lesions, or cerebrovascular disorder (CVA) [commonly referred to as a stroke]. Cause of the other half is unknown (idiophatic). Seventy-five percent of persons with seizures had their first seizure before 18 years of age. There are various types of seizures defined by the international classification of seizures. These include grand mal (tonic-clonic), petit mal (absence), and psychomotor seizures.

Epilepsy is treated by using anticonvulsant medication.

Hydantoins (phenytoin, mephenytoin, ethotoin)

These treat grand mal (tonic-clonic) seizures and psychomotor seizures.

Barbiturates (Phenobarbital, mephobarbital, primidone)

These are used for treating grand mal and acute episodes or status epilepticus; meningitis, toxic reactions, and eclampsia

Succinimides (ethosuximide)

These are used to treat absence seizures and may be used in combination with other anticonvulsants.

Oxazolidones (trimethadione)

This is used to treat petit mal seizures and may be used in combination with other drugs or singly for treating refractory petit mal seizures.

Benzodiazepines (diazepam, clonazepam)

These are effective in controlling petit mal seizures.

Carbamazepine

This is effective in treating refractory seizure disorders that have not responded to other anticonvulsant therapies. It is also used to control grand mal and partial seizures and a combination of these seizures.

Valproate (valproic acid)

This is used to treat petit mal, grand mal, and mixed types of seizures.

Anticonvulsant medication works one of three ways:

1. It can suppress the sodium influx by binding to the sodium channel prolonging the channel's inactivation and preventing neurons from firing.
2. It suppresses the calcium influx preventing stimulation of the T calcium channel.
3. It increases the action of the gamma-aminobutyric acid (GABA) inhibiting neurotransmitters throughout the brain and thereby suppressing seizure activity.

A list of drugs utilized in the treatment of epilepsy is provided in the Appendix. Detailed tables show doses, recommendations, expectations, side effects, contraindications, and more; available on the book's Web site (see URL in Appendix).

Antipsychotics

Psychosis is a disorder that is characterized by a number of symptoms. These include difficulty processing information and reaching a conclusion; experiencing delusions or hallucinations; being incoherent or in a catatonic state; or demonstrating aggressive violent behavior.

Psychosis is divided into major categories, once of which is schizophrenia. Schizophrenia is a chronic psychotic disorder where patients exhibit either positive or negative symptoms. Positive symptoms are exaggeration of normal function such as agitation, incoherent speech, hallucination, delusion, and paranoia. Negative symptoms are characterized by a decrease or loss of motivation or function such as social withdrawal, poor selfcare, and a decrease in the content of speech. Negative symptoms are more chronic and persistent than positive symptoms.

Psychosis is caused by an imbalance in the neurotransmitter dopamine in the brain. Antipsychotic medication, also known as dopamine antagonists, block the D_2 dopamine receptors in the brain thereby reducing the psychotic symptoms.

A number of antipsychotic medications block the chemoreceptor trigger zone and vomiting (emetic) center of the brain. In doing so, it produces an antiemetic effect. Although blocking dopamine improves the patient's thought processes and behavior, it can cause side effects.

These include symptoms of Parkinsonism (see Parkinsonism previously discussed in this chapter). Patients who undergo long-term treatment for psychosis using antipsychotic medications also might be prescribed drugs to treat the symptoms of Parkinsonism.

Antipsychotic medications are divided into two categories. These are sometimes called traditional and atypical. The typical category of antipsychotic medication is further subdivided into phenothiazines and nonphenothiazines.

Phenothiazines block norepinephrine causing sedative and hypotensive effects early in treatment.

Nonphenothiazines include butyrophenone haloperidol (Haldol) whose pharmacologics are similar to phenothiazines as it alters the effects of dopamine by blocking the dopamine receptor sites.

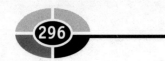

Atypical antipsychotic drugs are used to treat schizophrenia and other psychotic disorders for patients who do not respond to the typical antipsychotic medication.

A list of antipsychotic drugs is provided in the Appendix. Detailed tables show doses, recommendations, expectations, side effects, contraindications, and more; available on the book's Web site (see URL in Appendix).

Phenothiazines

Phenothiazines are divided into three groups. These are aliphatic, piperazine, and piperidine. Each category has different side effects (see Table 15-2). The aliphatic group produces a strong sedative effect, decreases blood pressure, and may moderate extrapyramidal symptoms (EPS). Chlorpromazine is a member of this group.

The piperzine group produces a low sedative effect and a strong antiemetic effect, more EPS, and little effect on blood pressure. Included in this group are prochlorperazine (Compazine), fluphenazine (Prolixin), perphenazine (Trilafon), and trifluoperazine (Stelazine).

The piperidine group includes mesoridazine besylate (Serentil) and thioridazine HCl (Mellaril). These produce few EPS or anti-emetic effects and can cause hypotension.

Anxiolytics

Anxiolytics are medications used to treat anxiety and insomnia. These have replaced sedatives that were traditionally used because they have fewer and less potent side effects, especially if an overdose of the medication is given to the patient. Benzodizepine is the major group of anxiolytics.

Anxiolytics are prescribed when the patient's anxiety reaches a level where the patient becomes disabled and is unable to perform normal activities. Anxiolytics have a sedative-hypnotic effect on the patient, but not an antipsychotic effect.

There are two types of anxiety: primary anxiety and secondary anxiety. Primary anxiety is not caused by a medical condition or drug use but may be situational. Secondary anxiety is caused by a medical condition or by drug use. Anxiolytics are usually not administered for secondary anxiety unless the secondary cause is severe or untreatable. Instead, the secondary cause is treated.

Benzodizepines are prescribed to treat severe or prolonged anxiety, but are also used to treat convulsions, hypertension, and as a sedative-hypnotic and

Table 15-2.   The effects of categories of antipsychotics.

Group	Sedation	Hypotension	EPS	Antiemetic
Aliphatic	+++	+++	++	++
(Chlorpromazine and triflupromazine)				+++
Piperazine	++	+	+++	+++
Piperidine	+++	+++	+	–
Nonphenothiazines				
Haloperidol	+	+	+++	++
Loxapine	++	++	+++	–
Molindone	+/++	+	+++	–
Thiothixene	+	+	+++	–
Atypical antipsychotics				
Risperidone	+	+	+/0	–

Key: ---no effect; + mild effect; ++ moderate effect; +++severe effect

pre-operative medication. Benzodizepines include chlordiazepoxide (Librium), diazepam (Valium), chlorazepatge dipotassium (Tranxene), oxazepam (Serax), lorazepam (Ativan), and alprazolam (Xanax).

Depression

About 20% of Americans are depressed; however, one-third receives medical or psychiatric help for their depression. Depression is characterized by mood changes and loss of interest in normal activities. Patients who are depressed might have insomnia, fatigue, a feeling of despair, and an inability to concentrate. Some may have suicidal thoughts. Depression is associated with two-third of all suicides.

   Depression is caused by a number of factors including genetic predisposition, social and environmental factors, and biologic conditions such as insufficient monoamine neurotransmitter (norepinephrine and serotonin).

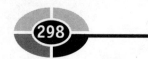

There are three types of depression:

REACTIVE (EXOGENOUS)

Reactive depression has a sudden onset and lasts for months and is usually caused by an event such as the loss of a loved one. Benzodiazepine is used to treat reactive depression.

MAJOR (UNIPOLAR)

Major depression is characterized by losing interest in work and home. The patient is unable to complete tasks and falls into a deep depression. Causes of major depression can include genetic predisposition, social and environmental factors, and biologic conditions. Benzodiazepines are the drugs of choice to treat major depressions.

BIPOLAR AFFECTIVE (MANIC-DEPRESSIVE)

Bipolar affective is when the patient undergoes moods swings from manic (euphoric) to depressive (dysphoric). Lithium is prescribed for bipolar affective disorders.

Antidepressants are used to treat depressions, however they also can mask suicidal tendencies (Table 15-3). There are four groups of antidepressants. These are tricyclics, second-generation antidepressants (Serontonin Reuptake Inhibitors or SSRIs), atypical antidepressants, and Monoamine oxidase (MAO) inhibitors.

Tricyclics are the most commonly prescribed drug to treat major depression. Tricyclics include clomipramine HCl (Anafranil), desipramine HCl (Norpramin, Pertofrane), doxepin HCl (Sinequan), imipramine HCl (Tofranil), Nortriptyline HCl (Aventyl), Protriptyline HCl (Vivactil), and trimipramine maleate (Surmontil).

Second-generation antidepressants have fewer side effects than tricyclics. They do not cause hypotension, sedation, anticholinergic effects, or cardiotoxicity. Second-generation antidepressants include

- SSRI: fluoxetine HCl (Prozac), paroxetine HCl (Paxil), sertraline HCl (Zoloft), fluvoxamine (Luvox)
- Atypical: amoxapine (Asendin), bupropion HCl (Wellbutrin), maprotiline HCl (Ludiomil), nefazodone HCl (Serzone), trazodone HCl (Desyrel)

Table 15-3. Side effects of antidepressants.

Category	Anticholinergic effect	Sedation	Hypotension	GI distress	Cardiotoxicity	Seizures	Insomnia/Agitation
Tricyclic Antidepressants							
Amitriptyline (Elavil)	++++	++++	+++	−	++++	+++	−
Clomipramine (Anafranil)	++++	++++	++	−	++++	++	−
Desipramine (Norpramin)	+	++	++	−	++	++	+
Doxepin (Sinequan)	+++	++++	++	−	++	++	−
Imipramine (Tofranil)	+++	+++	+++	+	++++	++	+
Nortriptyline (Aventyl)	+	+++	+	−	+++	++	−
Protriptyline (Vivactil)	+++	+	++	−	+++	+	+
Trimipramine (Surmontil)	+++	++++	+++	−	++++	++	−
Selective Serotonin Reuptake Inhibitors							
Fluoxetine (Prozac)	−	+	−	+++	−	0/+	++
Fluvoxamine (Luvox)	−	++	−	+++	−	−	++
Paroxetine (Paxil)	−	+	−	+++	−	−	++
Sertraline (Zoloft)	−	+	−	+++	−	−	++

Table 15-3. Side effects of antidepressants. *(continued)*

Category	Anticholinergic effect	Sedation	Hypotension	GI distress	Cardiotoxicity	Seizures	Insomnia/ Agitation
Atypical (Heterocyclic) Antidepressants							
Amoxapine (Asendin)	+++	++	+	–	+	+++	++
Bupropion (Wellbutrin)	++	–	0/+	+	+	++++	++
Nefazodone (Serzone)	+	++	+	+	0/+	–	–
Trazodone (Desyrel)	–	+++	++	+	+	+	–
Maprotiline (Ludiomil)	+++	+++	+	–	++	++	–
Monoamine Oxidase Inhibitors	+	+	++	+	–	–	++

Monamine Oxidase Inhibitors (MAOI). The enzyme monoamine oxidase inactivates norepinephrine, dopamine, epinephrine, and serotonin. By inhibiting monoamine oxidase, the levels of these neurotransmitters rise. Examples of these drugs includes isocarboxazid (Marplan), phenelzine sulfate (Nardil), and tranycypromine sulfate (Parnate).

A list of drugs utilized in the treatment of depression is provided in the Appendix. Detailed tables show doses, recommendations, expectations, side effects, contraindications, and more; available on the book's Web site (see URL in Appendix).

Summary

There are many medications that either interfere with impulses transmitted over the neural pathways or stimulate those impulses. Medications that interfere with impulses are called inhibitors and usually compete with neurotransmitters for receptor sites. That is, the medication gets to the receptor site before the neurotransmitters blocking the neurotransmitters from delivering the impulse to the receptor site. Medications that cause an impulse to be generated are called stimulants.

There are four major groups of medications that stimulate the central nervous system. These are amphetamines, caffeine, analeptics, and anorexiants. Amphetamines stimulate the cerebral cortex of the brain. Caffeine also stimulates the cerebral cortex and stimulates respiration by acting on the brain stem and medulla. Analeptics have a similar effect on the brain stem and medulla as caffeine. Anorexiants inhibit appetite by stimulating the cerebral cortex and the hypothalamus.

There are seven broad classifications of medications that depress the central nervous system. These are sedative-hypnotics, general and local anesthetics, analgesics, narcotic analgesics, anticonvulsants, antipsychotics, and antidepressants.

Sedative-hypnotics diminish the patient's physical and mental responses without affecting the patient's consciousness. General anesthetics cause a loss of consciousness and relieve pain. Local anesthetics block pain at the site where the medication is administered without affecting the patient's consciousness.

Analgesics are drugs that reduce pain such aspirin, acetaminophen, and ibuprofen. Narcotic analgesics are drugs that reduce pain and produce a state of stupor or drowsiness by blocking the transmission of pain signals in the brain.

Anticonvulsants are medications that prevent or lessen the likelihood that a patient will experience convulsions, which are abnormal motor reactions such as those found in epilepsy. Antipsychotics are drugs used to minimize symptoms of psychosis. Psychosis is a disorder that is characterized by one of a number of symptoms such as difficulty processing information and reaching a conclusion. Antidepressants are medications used to treat depressions.

The next chapter continues our exploration of drugs that affect the central nervous system by examining narcotic agonists. A narcotic agonist is a medication that relieves pain—called an analgesic.

Quiz

1. Amphetamines
   (a) inhibit the release of neurotransmitters.
   (b) stimulate the release of neurotransmitters.
   (c) lower the heart rate.
   (d) None of the above.

2. Patients who experience migraines
   (a) can be treated with a combination of migraine medications.
   (b) should not be treated with a combination of migraine medications.
   (c) should be treated with amphetamines.
   (d) should be treated with Prozac.

3. Muscarinic receptors
   (a) stimulate smooth muscles.
   (b) stimulate skeletal muscles.
   (c) increase the heart rate.
   (d) All of the above.

4. Tricyclic medications are used to treat depression.
   (a) True
   (b) False

5. Anticholinergics drugs inhibit acetylcholine.
   (a) True
   (b) False

6. Beta-adrenergic blockers
   (a) decrease blood pressure.
   (b) decrease the heart rate.
   (c) cause bronchoconstriction.
   (d) All of the above.

7. Selective blockers affect specific receptors while non-selective blockers affect multiple receptors.
   (a) True
   (b) False

8. Indirect-acting sympathomimetics
   (a) stimulate receptors.
   (b) stimulate the release of norepinephrine from terminal nerve endings.
   (c) stimulate both receptors and the release of norepinephrine from terminal nerve endings.
   (d) None of the above.

9. The saddle block can be used during childbirth
   (a) True
   (b) False

10. A local anesthetic blocks pain at the site where the medication is administered without affecting the patient's consciousness.
    (a) True
    (b) False

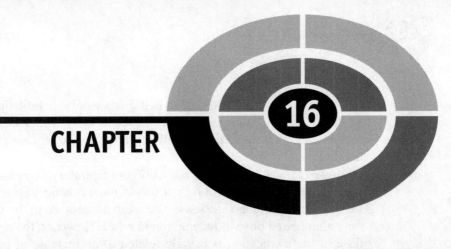

CHAPTER 16

Narcotic Agonists

Pain is something all of us feel; yet it is difficult for healthcare providers to accurately assess because pain is whatever you say it is. You know it hurts when you twist an ankle or have a pounding headache. All you want is fast relief. You want a magic pill to make the pain go away. The pill may be a narcotic agonist that blocks transmission of impulses from the site of the injury to the area of the brain that interprets pain.

This chapter explores pain and how healthcare providers assess pain and manage pain. You'll also learn about narcotic and non-narcotic analgesics and how they are used to treat pain.

A Close Look at Pain

Narcotic agonists are medications that relieve pain. These are safe and effective when properly administered. These medications are opioid based and are used to treat acute or chronic pain from trauma, tumor growth, and from surgical procedures. They are also used to treat pain caused by the progression of diseases or complications from other conditions.

For example, pain from sickle cell crisis can be debilitating and require the patient to receive a narcotic analgesic such as morphine. This medication blocks the pain and creates a euphoric effect giving the patient relief from the pain of the disease.

However, fear of inducing addiction or respiratory depression interferes with pain management. Addiction is rare in clinical practice. Some patients who are treated with opioid analgesics can develop a tolerance to the medication requiring an increased dose to maintain pain relief. However, the need to increase the dose of the medication is usually related to an increase in pain due to disease progression or complications. Physical dependence on a medication occurs when the physiological condition of the patient is altered.

Increased doses of opioid analgesics also expose the patient to adverse side effects such as respiratory depression. Opioid analgesics can cause some respiratory depression. However, this effect usually does not occur with long-term use such as with cancer patients. Prescribers avoid this side effect by titrating doses over time to deliver pain relief without adversely affecting the respiratory system.

Influences on Administrating Pain Medication

The concerns about addiction and the potential for adverse side effects of opioid analgesics influence how the medication is administered. Patients may avoid or postpone taking pain medication until the pain is unbearable for fear of becoming addicted or developing a tolerance for the medication. This is especially true with patients who suffer chronic debilitating diseases. They realize pain increases as the disease progresses and they are fearful that the medication will lose its effectiveness.

Some healthcare providers are also hesitant about administering pain medication for some of the same reasons patients refuse to take the drug. Furthermore, healthcare providers might be skeptical that the patient is actually in pain since pain is subjective and difficult to measure in the clinical setting.

Many studies have demonstrated that women, the elderly, children, and those addicted to illegal drugs are at greater risk for being undertreated for acute pain. These studies indicate that some healthcare providers believe females react emotionally and pain is not as severe as reported. Others believe the elderly and children do not feel pain as acutely as other patients. And many healthcare providers believe addicts are simply seeking drugs to forego withdrawal symptoms even when it is clear that the addict is suffering pain from an acute injury or illness.

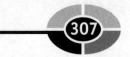

Components of Pain

There are two components of pain. These are the physical sensation of pain and the psychological component. The physical sensation of pain occurs when nerve endings are stimulated causing it to send an impulse along the nerve pathways to the brain, which transmits a pain response.

The psychological component is a person's emotional response to pain based on a person's pain threshold. The pain threshold is the level of nerve-ending stimulation that causes the person to have the feeling of unbearable pain.

For example, applying heat to the skin will cause the sensation of pain. However, the point beyond which pain becomes unbearable (pain tolerance) varies widely among individuals. Pain tolerance is also different for the same person depending on the circumstance in which sensation is detected. For example, a toothache might hurt more when you're home than at work where you have a lot of distractions from the pain.

The Gate Control Theory

The gate control theory is an attempt to describe the mechanism of pain transmission. The dorsal horn of the spinal cord contains a gate mechanism that alters the transmission of painful sensations from peripheral nerve fiber to the thalamus and cortex of the brain. The thalamus and the cortex is where painful sensations are recognized as pain.

The transmission flows through the gate mechanism. The gate is closed by large diameter, low-threshold afferent fibers and is opened by small diameter, high-threshold afferent fibers. In addition to these two sets of fibers, the gate is also influenced by descending control inhibition from the brain to close the gate.

When the patient experiences slower-acting painful stimuli, the large-diameter fibers are stimulated. This causes the gate to close, stopping transmission of the painful stimuli.

Nonpharmacological pain relief treatments, such as a massage, are based on the gate control theory to ease the patient's pain.

Defining Pain

Pain is whatever the patient who is experiencing pain says it is. Healthcare providers describe pain in terms of intensity, duration, frequency, and type of pain. However, these terms are subjective and characterized by the patient.

Pain is classified in six ways.

1. Acute pain is the presence of severe discomfort or an uncomfortable sensation that has a sudden onset and subsides with treatment. For example, a fractured bone causes acute pain since the uncomfortable sensation occurs suddenly when the bone is broken and subsides when the bone is immobilized in a cast. Pain associated with myocardial infarction (heart attack), appendicitis, and kidney stones are also examples of acute pain. Acute pain can be treated with NSAIDs or opioid analgesics.

2. Chronic pain is a persistent or recurring pain that continues for six months or more. This is the pain from cancer and rheumatoid arthritis and other chronic conditions. Chronic pain is treated with combinations of NSAIDs and opioid analgesics as well as medications to reduce swelling and anxiety.

3. Visceral pain is the dull and aching pain caused by stimulating nerve endings in smooth muscle or sympathetically innervated organs. Visceral pain is referred pain. This makes it difficult to localize the source of the pain. Pain of a myocardial infarction (MI) is an example of visceral pain. MI can be described as crushing chest pain and also described as pain in the left arm or hand and even the shoulder, left back, or the left ear. Visceral pain is best treated with opioid analgesics.

4. Somatic pain is pain occurring from skeletal muscles, fascia, ligaments, vessels and joint. Somatic pain is an aching, throbbing pain over the affected area. Somatic pain is best treated with nonsteroidal anti-inflammatory agents.

5. Neuropathic pain is a burning, shooting, and sometimes tingling pain that is caused by peripheral nerve injury. This is caused by the invasion of a cancerous tumor or nerve damage. Neuropathic pain is treated with a combination of medications such as anticonvulsants, tricyclic antidepressants, and opioid analgesics.

6. Psychogenic pain is pain caused by psychiatric illness or psychosocial stimuli such as anxiety, depression, and fear. Drug therapy alone may bring brief relief. Psychotherapy may bring long-lasting relief from psychogenic pain.

Pain Assessment

The most common method used to assess pain is the pain scale. One of the pain scales ranges from zero to 10. Zero is freedom from pain; 10 is the most severe pain. There are a number of variations of this pain scale including the Face Rating Scale and the Color Scale. The face rating scale uses expressions of cartoon faces to assess pain while the color scale uses colors ranging from blue to red where blue is freedom from pain and red is the most severe pain.

In addition to rating the intensity of the patient's pain, you also must assess other characteristics of pain. These are onset, duration, frequency, what started the pain (precipitating cause), and what relieves the pain.

Patients who are in chronic pain should keep a pain diary. A pain diary helps the healthcare professional develop a pain management plan. The patient is asked to keep a timed record of the pain experience to include when the pain starts, what starts it, how bad it is, what relieves the pain, and any other factors that may explain how the patient is responding to the pain. This record can help the healthcare provider and the patient plan effective pain management.

The pain management plan contains both pharmacological and nonpharmacological strategies for managing the patient's pain. Pharmacological strategies involve using pain medication. Nonpharmacological strategies involve treatments other than medication. These include massage, imagery, music, distraction, humor, acupuncture, chiropractic interventions, hypnosis, herbal therapies, therapeutic touch, and transcutaneous electronerve stimulation. Surgical interventions are also sometimes performed to relieve pain.

Pharmacologic Management of Pain

Pharmacologic management of pain involves administering pain medication to relieve the patient's pain. These include non-narcotic analgesics, nonsterioidal anti-inflammatory drugs (NSAIDs), narcotic analgesics, and salicylates.

Non-narcotic analgesics (see chart) are used to treat mild to moderate pain. Many of these medications are not addictive and available over-the-counter. Non-narcotic analgesics are used to treat headaches, menstrual pain (dysmenorrheal), pain from inflammation, minor abrasions, muscular aches and pain, and mild-to-moderate arthritis. Non-narcotic analgesics also lower elevated body temperature (antipyretic). Non-narcotic analgesics include acetaminophen and NSAIDs (aspirin, ibuprofen, and COX-2 inhibitors), which were discussed in Chapter 12.

See non-narcotic analgesics in the Appendix. Detailed tables show doses, recommendations, expectations, side effects, contraindications, and more; available on the book's Web site (see URL in Appendix).

NARCOTIC ANALGESICS

Narcotic analgesics are known as narcotic agonists, and act on the central nervous system to provide relief from moderate and severe pain. Narcotic analgesics are also used to suppress coughing by acting on the respiratory and cough centers in the medulla of the brain stem.

Opioids are a category of narcotic analgesics. All relieve pain and all, except meperidine (Demerol), have an antitussive (cough suppression) and antidiarrheal effect.

See Narcotic agonist-opiate analgesic and Opioid agonist listed in the Appendix. Detailed tables show doses, recommendations, expectations, side effects, contraindications, and more; available on the book's Web site (see URL in Appendix).

NARCOTIC AGONIST-ANTAGONISTS

A narcotic agonist-antagonist (agonist) is an opioid narcotic mixed with naloxione (antagonist) to try to curb a form of drug misuse. Although the exact mechanism of action is unknown, these agents have both agonist and antagonist effects on the opioid receptors. Generally, these drugs are less potent and have a

Other Narcotic Analgesics of the Opium and Synthetic Group	
Drug	Purpose
Codeine (sulfate, phosphate), CSS II	For mild to moderate pain
Hydromorphone HCl (Dilaudid) CSS II	For severe pain
Levorphanol tartrate (Levo-Dromoran) CSS II	For moderate to severe pain
Meperidine (Demerol) Synthetic narcotic CSS II	For moderate pain
Fentanyl (Duragesic, Sublimaze) CSS II	Short-acting potent—used with short-term surgery; patches for controlling chronic pain
Sufentanil (Duragesic, Sublimaze) CSS II	Short-acting potent—used as part of balanced anesthesia
Methadone (Dolophine)	Similar to morphine but longer duration of action; used in drug abuse programs

lower dependency potential than opioids and withdrawal symptoms are not as severe. Commonly used narcotic agonist-antagonists are Pentazocine (Talwin), Butorphanol tartrate (Stadol), duprenorphine (Buprenex), and nalbuphine hydrochloride (Nubain). Their pharmacokinetics, adverse, and side effects are similar to morphine.

See Narcotic Agonist-Antagonists listed in the Appendix. Detailed tables show doses, recommendations, expectations, side effects, contraindications, and more; available on the book's Web site (see URL in Appendix).

NARCOTIC ANTAGONISTS

Narcotic antagonists (see chart) are antidotes for overdoses of narcotic analgesics. They have a higher affinity to the opiate receptor site than the narcotic analgesic and block the narcotic analgesic from binding to the opiate receptor site. They also reverse the respiratory and CNS depression caused by the narcotics.

Naloxone (Narcan) is a narcotic antagonist and can be used to determine if an unconscious patient has used an opioid narcotic drug. If the patient wakes up after Narcan is administered intravenously, the patient is likely to have ingested or injected an opioid narcotic.

Summary

Pain is sensed when a nerve ending is stimulated sending an impulse along the neural pathway to the brain that interprets the impulse as pain. Pain is assessed in a patient by asking the patient to describe the intensity of the pain on a pain scale—the higher the value, the more severe the pain. Besides intensity, pain is assessed according to onset, duration, frequency, what started the pain (precipitating cause), and what relieves the pain.

There are six classifications of pain: acute pain, chronic pain, visceral pain, somatic pain, neuropathic pain, and psychogenic pain. Pain can be treated nonpharmacologically or pharmacologically.

Nonpharmacological pain treatment includes massage, imagery, music, distraction, humor, acupuncture, chiropractic interventions, hypnosis, herbal therapies, therapeutic touch, and transcutaneous electronerve stimulation. Surgical interventions are also sometimes performed to relieve pain.

Pharmacological pain treatment involves administering medication that relieves the patient of pain. There are four categories of pain medication: non-narcotic analgesics, nonsterioidal anti-inflammatory drugs (NSAIDs), narcotic analgesics, and salicylates (discussed in Chapter 12).

Narcotic analgesics are opioid narcotics that can induce respiratory depression. The effects of a narcotic analgesic can be reversed by administering a narcotic antagonist.

Many patients and healthcare providers are concerned that a patient will become addicted to narcotic analgesics or develop a tolerance for these drugs. Both can occur. However, proper pain management can alleviate these potential problems.

This chapter concludes the look at pain medications. In the next chapter, we'll take a look at medications that are used to control the immune system.

Quiz

1. Physical sensation of pain
   (a) occurs when nerve endings are stimulated causing it to send an impulse along the nerve pathways to the brain.
   (b) is a person's emotional response to pain based on a person's pain threshold.
   (c) occurs when the brain stimulates nerve endings at the site of the injury.
   (d) none of the above.

2. Nonpharmacological pain relief treatments use the
   (a) Pain Oppression theory.
   (b) Pain Suppression theory.
   (c) Brain Suppression theory.
   (d) Gate Control theory.

3. The presence of severe discomfort or an uncomfortable sensation that has a sudden onset and subsides with treatment is
   (a) neuropathic pain.
   (b) visceral pain.
   (c) chronic pain.
   (d) acute pain.

4. The color scale uses colors ranging from blue to red where blue is freedom from pain and red is the most severe pain.
   (a) True
   (b) False

5. Naloxone (Narcan) is the antidote to an opioid narcotic.
   (a) True
   (b) False

6. Pain occurring from skeletal muscles, fascia, ligaments, vessels, and joints is called
   (a) neuropathic pain.
   (b) visceral pain.
   (c) chronic pain.
   (d) none of the above.

7. Surgical interventions are sometimes performed to relieve pain.
   (a) True
   (b) False

8. Patients who are in chronic pain should
   (a) stay in bed.
   (b) keep a pain diary.
   (c) avoid vacations.
   (d) none of the above.

9. Most opioids suppress coughs.
   (a) True
   (b) False

10. Music can help relieve pain.
   (a) True
   (b) False

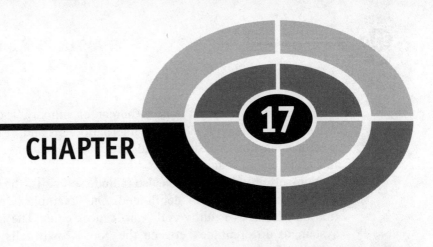

Immunologic Agents

The body's immune system is its natural defense against microorganisms that cause diseases (pathogens) and against cells that are not the body's own cells, such as transplanted organs. The immune system also treats its own abnormal cells, such as cancer cells, as foreign and attacks it with the same energy as it attacks microorganisms.

However, when the immune system is compromised through diseases including HIV, the body loses its ability to fight off microorganisms and destroy its own abnormal cells. The patient encounters more episodes of infection that can ultimately lead to death.

In this chapter, you'll learn about the therapies used to assist the immune system combat preventable diseases and you'll also learn about medications that inhibit the growth of HIV.

A Brief Look at Immunity

The immune system is the body's way of combating the invasion of microscopic organisms such as bacteria, viruses, molds, spores, pollens, protozoa, and cells from transplant donors (human or animal). The immune system prevents an invasion from attacking internal organs and, if that fails, the immune system neutralizes, destroys, and eliminates any non-self proteins and cells, including microorganisms.

Non-self proteins and cells also include self cells (the body's own cells) that have become infected or debilitated. One example is malignant transformation that changes healthy cells into cancer cells. The ability of the immune system to differentiate between the body's own cells and non-self cells is called self-tolerance.

The immune system is able to recognize self-cells by using unique proteins that are on the surface of all self-cells. Think of these proteins as an identification code. Foreign cells have a different identification code. These are called antigens and stimulate the immune response of a host.

When bacteria invade your body, your immune system detects the bacteria's surface protein as not being a self-cell. This triggers your immune system to launch an attack against the bacteria.

The immune system originates in the bone marrow. Mature immune system cells are released from the bone marrow into the bloodstream where they circulate throughout the body looking for invaders.

There are three processes necessary for immunity: inflammation, antibody-mediated immunity (humoral immunity), and cell-mediated immunity (CMI).

INFLAMMATION

This is discussed in detail in Chapter 12.

ANTIBODY-MEDIATED IMMUNITY

Antibody-mediated immunity occurs when the immune system produces antibodies that neutralize, eliminate, or destroy an antigen (foreign protein). Antibodies are produced by B lymphocytes. The body must be exposed to sufficient amounts of an antigen before the immune system produces an antibody to combat the antigen. Patients can be given vaccinations that stimulate the immune system to generate antibodies before the microorganism actually invades the body. In this way, the antibodies already exist and can attack at the first sign of the microorganism.

CELL-MEDIATED IMMUNITY

Cell-mediated immunity, also known as cellular immunity, uses T-leukocytes (referred to as natural killer cells or NK cells) to attack non-self cells. Cell-mediated immunity also causes the body to release cytokines, which regulate the activities of antibody-mediated immunity and inflammation.

Cell-mediated immunity is especially useful in identifying and ridding the body of self-cells that are infected by organisms that live within host cells and self-cells that mutate at the DNA level transforming them into abnormal and potentially harmful cells. Cell-mediated immunity is critically important in preventing development of cancer and metastasis after exposure to carcinogens.

HIV and the immune system

Human immunodeficiency virus (HIV) is a retrovirus that gradually destroys the immune system's function. When the retrovirus becomes active, the patient develops acquired immunodeficiency syndrome (AIDS), which is characterized by profound immunological deficits, opportunistic infection, secondary infections, and malignant neoplasms.

HIV disables and kills CD4+ T cells, which lowers the immune system's capability to fight infection. The number of CD4+ T cells triggers other cells in the immune system to attack invading organisms. HIV lowers the CD4+ T cell count and thereby inhibits other immune system cells to go on the attack.

A healthy person who is not HIV positive, has between 800 and 1200 CD4+ T cells per cubic millimeter (mm^3) of blood. HIV reduces this count to 200 mm^3. This is equal to or less than 14%. Infected patients are particularly vulnerable to opportunistic infections and cancers.

In addition to the T-cell count, the viral load (VL) is a test used to evaluate the status of the patient's immune system. The higher the number, the higher the viral load.

HIV is transmitted in three ways: injection of infected blood or blood products, sexual contact, and maternal–fetal transmission. Occupational exposure to HIV accounts for a small number of transmissions usually from a needle-stick.

HIV uses three enzymes to genetically encode, replicate, and assemble a new HI virus within a host cell. HIV can replicate only inside cells. These enzymes are reverse transcriptase, integrase, and protease.

The HI virus enters the cell through the CD4 molecule on the cell surface. Once inside the cell, the virus is uncoated with the help of the reverse transcriptase enzyme enabling the virus' single stranded RNA to be converted into DNA.

The viral DNA migrates to the nucleus of the cell where it is spliced into the host DNA with the help of the integrase enzyme. Once combined, the HIV DNA is called the provirus and is duplicated each time the cell divides. The protease enzyme assists in the assembly of a new form of the viral particles.

Patients with HIV undergo Highly Active Antiretroviral Therapy (HAART) that uses antiretroviral medications designed to slow or inhibit reverse transcriptase and protease enzymes. The Food and Drug Administration approved the first reverse transcriptase (RT) inhibitor in 1987. The first protease inhibitor was approved in 1995. No integrase inhibitors have been approved as yet.

HAART decreases the viral load to undetectable levels, thereby preserving and increasing the number of CD4+ T cells. HAART also prevents resistance to disease and keeps the patient in good clinical condition and prevents secondary infections and cancer.

The patient must adhere to HAART therapy as the virus becomes resistant and the antiretroviral agents lose their therapeutic effect. In addition, patients must avoid opportunistic infections and aggressive prophylaxis and treatment of opportunistic infections that do occur is recommended. Nutritional therapy, complementary therapy, and supportive care are also necessary.

Antiretroviral therapy is offered to patients who have less than 500 CD4+ T cells mm³ or whose plasma HIV RNA levels are greater than 10,000 copies/mL (B-DNA assay) or 20,000 copies/mL (R-PCR assay). Therapy should be considered for all HIV-infected patients who have detectable HIV RNA in plasma. There are risks and benefits to early initiation of antiretroviral therapy in the asymptomatic HIV-infected patient.

Potential Benefits

- Control of viral replication and mutation
- Reduction of viral burden
- Prevention of progressive immunodeficiency
- Maintenance of the normal immune system
- Reconstruction of the normal immune system
- Delay in the progression to acquired immunodeficiency syndrome and prolongation of life
- Decreased risk of selection of resistant virus
- Decreased risk of drug toxicity
- Possible decreased risk of viral transmission

Potential Risks

- Reduction in quality of life from adverse drug effects
- Inconvenience of taking the regimen of medications

- Earlier development of drug resistance
- Transmission of drug-resistant virus
- Limitation in future choices of antiretroviral agents as a result of development of resistance
- Unknown longterm toxicity of antiretroviral drugs
- Unknown duration of effectiveness of current antiretroviral therapies

HIV medication

There are four classes of medication approved by the FDA for treatment of HIV (see Charts). These are:

Nonnucleoside Reverse Transcriptase Inhibitors (NNRTIs)

NNRTIs bind to reverse transcriptase, a protein HIV needs to make more copies of itself. In doing so, reverse transcriptase becomes disabled. Drugs within this category include Delavirdine (Rescriptor, DLV), Efavirenz (Sustiva, EFV), and Neviapine (Viramune, NVP).

Nucleoside Reverse Transcriptase Inhibitors (NRTIs)

NRTIs are faulty version reverse transcriptase. Reproduction of HIV is stalled when HIV uses NRTI instead of the normal reverse transcriptase. Drugs within this category include Abacavir (Ziagen, ABC), Abacavir, Lamivudine (Epzicom), Abacavir, Lamivudine, Zidovudine (Trizivir), Didanosine (Videx, ddI, Videx EC), Emtricitabine (Emtriva, FTC, Coviracil), Emtricitabine, Tenofovir DF (Truvada), Lamivudine (Epivir, 3TC), Lamivudine, Zidovudine (Combivir), Stavudine (Zerit, d4T), Tenofovir DF (Viread, TDF), Zalcitabine (Hivid, ddC), and Zidovudine (Retrovir, AZT, AZV).

Protease Inhibitors (PIs)

PI disables protease, a protein that HIV needs to make more copies of itself. Drugs within this category include Amprenavir (Agenerase, APV), Atazanavir (Reyataz, ATV), Fosamprenavir (Lexiva, FPV), Indinavir (Crixivan, IDV), Lopinavir, Ritonavir (Kaletra, LPV/r), Nelvinavir (Viracept, NFV), Ritonavir, (Norvir, RTV), and Saquinavir (Fortovase, SQV; Invirase).

Fusion Inhibitors

Fusion Inhibitors prevent HIV from entry into cells. They include Enfuviritide (Fuzeon, T-20).

A list of drugs utilized in the treatment of HIV is provided in the Appendix. Detailed tables show doses, recommendations, expectations, side effects, contraindications, and more; available on the book's Web site (see URL in Appendix).

HIV therapy and pregnancy

Special care must be taken when an HIV patient is pregnant. The objective is to reduce the risk of transmission of HIV to the fetus. Before the onset of labor, the patient is given 100 mg of ZDV five times daily, initiated at 14 to 34 weeks of gestation and continued throughout the pregnancy.

The patient is given ZDV intravenously in a 10-hour loading dose of 2 mg per kg of body weight, followed by a continuous infusion of 1 mg per kg of body weight per hour at beginning of labor and until delivery.

The newborn is then given PO ZDV at 2 mg/kg/per dose every 6 hours for the first 6 weeks of life, beginning 8 to 12 hours after birth.

Postexposure prophylaxis

Postexposure prophylaxis is administered to all healthcare workers according to the Public Health Service Statement on the Management of Occupational Exposures to HIV and Recommendations. The policy for postexposure prophylaxis is institution specific and should be available to all employees.

Basic and Expanded Postexposure Prophylaxis Regimens

Regimen Category	Application	Drug Regimen
Basic	Occupational HIV exposures for which there is a recognized transmission risk.	4 week (28 d) of both zidovudine 600 mg every day in divided doses (i.e., 300 mg twice a day, 200 mg three times a day, or 100 mg every 4 h) and lamivudine 150 mg twice a day
Expanded	Occupational HIV exposures that pose an increased risk for transmission (e.g., larger volume of blood and/or higher virus titer in blood)	Basic regimen plus either indinavir 800 mg every 8 hr or nelfinavir 750 mg three times a day

Vaccines

The immune system develops antibodies to attack a pathogen using one of two methods: active immunity and passive immunity.

Active immunity occurs when the immune system generates antibodies on the first exposure to the pathogen. This immune response is relatively slow, resulting in the patient showing the signs and symptoms of the disease.

However, the immune system remembers the pathogen and is quick to dispatch antibodies should the pathogen attack a subsequent time. This happens faster than the initial response and can generally eliminate the pathogen before the patient experiences the signs and symptoms of the disease. The patient may have a life-long immunity to the pathogen thanks to the body's active natural immunity.

Active natural immunity can also occur through immunization when the patient receives a vaccination against the pathogen. The vaccination contains a small amount of the pathogen to stimulate the production of antibodies, but insufficient in strength to develop the signs and symptoms of the disease.

There are five ways in which the pathogen in vaccines is produced.

1. Whole or components of an inactivated (dead) microorganism
2. Live, but weakened microorganisms
3. Toxoids, which are inactivated toxins produced by some microorganisms
4. Conjugates, which are vaccines that link a protein (toxoid) from an unrelated organism to the outer coat of the disease-causing microorganism. The result is a substance that is recognized by the immature immune system of young infants. *Haemophilus influenzae* type b is an example.
5. Recombinant subunit vaccine is where DNA of a pathogen is inserted into a cell or organism. The cell or organism then produces massive quantities of the pathogen that are used in place of the whole pathogen. Examples are hepatitis B and LYMErix for Lyme disease.

A booster dose of a vaccine is sometimes required to maintain sufficient immunity. The immune system has a memory and when the vaccinated individual is later exposed to the actual pathogen, the body can mount a rapid immune response and prevent the disease. This is called artificially acquired immunity.

Passive immunity occurs when the patient receives antibodies from another source rather than generating his or her own antibodies. Newborns have natural passive immunity to protect them from pathogens. The newborn receives natural passive immunity from antibodies that cross the placenta. Antibodies may

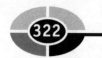
also be acquired from a pool of antibodies from human or animal sources. This is acquired passive immunity.

Passive immunity is transient—lasting no more than several weeks to a few months. The individual does not mount his or her own immune response to antigens. Acquired passive immunity is important when time does not permit active vaccination alone, when the exposed individual is at high risk for complications of the disease, or when the person suffers from an immune system deficiency that renders that person unable to produce an effective immune response.

Preventing Diseases

More than 20 infectious diseases in the United States can be prevented by vaccination. Some vaccines are routinely administered to both children and adults. Other vaccines are given under special circumstances to military personnel, travellers whose destination are certain foreign countries, and the chronically ill.

These preventable diseases include adenovirus, cholera, diphtheria, *Haemophilus influenzae* type b (Hib), hepatitis A, hepatitis B, influenza, Japanese encephalitis, Lyme disease, measles, meningococcal disease, poliomyelitis, rabies, rotavirus, rubella, tetanus, tuberculosis, typhoid, varicella, and yellow fever.

The Center for Disease Control (CDC) recommends a schedule for vaccination for children Web site (http://www.cdc.gov/mmwr/preview/mmwrhtml/mm5351-Immunizationa1.htm).

ADULT IMMUNIZATIONS

Adults are frequently overlooked when it comes to vaccination because emphasis is placed on preventing children from developing preventable diseases. However, the CDC suggests adults review their immunizations on decade birthdays (20, 30, 40, 50, and 60).

Adults should also review their immunizations every time they travel to a foreign country regardless of their age. The CDC provides information regarding appropriate immunizations on their Web site (http://www.cdc.gov/).

ADVERSE EVENTS OF VACCINE

Biologic products such as vaccines do not undergo the pharmacokinetic process that is associated with other drug therapies. Vaccines are generally safe. Some common mild reactions include swelling at the injection site and fever. Absolute contraindications for the use of vaccines include anaphylactic reaction to a specific vaccine or component of another vaccine or moderate or severe illness.

Healthcare providers are expected to report vaccine adverse events to public health officials who report these to the CDC every week using the Vaccine Adverse Events Reporting System (VAERS), which is used to provide compensation for injury and death caused by vaccination.

ARE YOU VACCINATED?

Patients may not know if they've been vaccinated. Therefore, healthcare professionals perform a blood test to determine detectable levels of antibodies in the bloodstream for preventable diseases such as Rubella.

If antibodies are detected in sufficient quantity, then the patient is immune to the disease. If the antibodies are not detected, then the patient needs to be revaccinated. Healthcare professionals are required to be vaccinated for many common communicable diseases in order to prevent acquiring the disease and passing the disease along to patients.

NURSING ACTIONS FOR VACCINATIONS

Here are the steps that should be followed when vaccinating a patient:

- Obtain immunization history.
- Obtain medical history of immune deficiency diseases such as malignancy (cancer) or HIV.
- Obtain pregnancy history and pregnancy test.
- Obtain drug history including high-dose immunosuppressants, blood transfusions, and immune globulin.
- Obtain a complete allergy history include drugs, foods, and environmental allergies.
- Do not administer vaccines to a pregnant patient.
- Determine if anyone in the patient's household is not vaccinated or is immunodeficient.
- Assess for symptoms of moderate to severe acute illness with or without fever.
- Adhere to storage requirements for the vaccine to ensure its potency.
- Administer vaccine within stated time limit after preparation.

- If more than one vaccine is being administered at the same time, use different injection sites.
- Do not mix vaccines in the same syringe.
- Observe patient for signs and symptoms of adverse reactions to vaccines.
- Keep epinephrine available in the case of anaphylactic reaction.
- Document that a Vaccine Information Statement (VIS) is available from the CDC for each vaccine administered and is provided to the patient/family. Be sure to include the date of vaccination, route and site, vaccine type, manufacturer, lot number, and expiration date, name, address, and title of individual administering vaccine.
- Provide patient with a record of immunizations.

PATIENT EDUCATION FOR VACCINATIONS

Here are facts that patients should know about vaccinations:

- Explain risk of contracting vaccine-preventable diseases.
- Female patients of childbearing age must avoid becoming pregnant within a month of receiving the vaccine.
- Provide the patient or family with current Vaccine Information Statements (VISs) available from CDC for each vaccine administered. Be sure to include the date of vaccination, route and site, vaccine type, manufacturer, lot number, and expiration date, name, address, and title of individual administering vaccine.
- Remind patient or family to bring the VIS record to all visits.
- Provide patient or family with date for return for next vaccination.
- Discuss common side effects of receiving the vaccine.
- Tell patient or family to contact healthcare provider if they see signs of a serious reaction to the vaccine.

IMMUNOSUPPRESSANTS

The development of organ transplants—which include kidneys, liver, heart, lungs, and pancreas—has led to the development of immunosuppressant drugs. These drugs are meant to suppress the body's natural reaction to reject the foreign protein so the person doesn't reject the transplanted organ. Some of these drugs include azathioprine (Imuran), cyclosporine (Sandimmune), muromonab-DC3 (Orthoclone OKT3), mycophenolate mofetil (Cell Cept), and tacrolimus (FK506 Prograf).

Some of the side effects of these drugs include nausea and vomiting and an increased risk of tumor growth. Significant leukopenia and thrombocytopenia may occur. These drugs are expensive and must be continued for the life of the patient.

Summary

The immune system provides a natural defense against pathogens and against abnormal cells that might lead to cancer. This system differentiates between self-cells and non-self cells by protein on the surface of the cell. Abnormal self-cells are considered non-self cells. Microorganisms are antigens and considered non-self cells and cause the immune system to generate antibodies that neutralize and destroy the antigen.

There are three processes to produce immunity: inflammation, antibody-mediated immunity (humoral immunity), and cell-mediated immunity (CMI).

Human immunodeficiency (HIV) is a retrovirus that destroys the immune system. When the retrovirus becomes active, the patient exhibits acquired immunodeficiency syndrome (AIDS).

Highly Active Antiretroviral Therapy (HAART) is the use of antiretroviral medications designed to slow or inhibit reverse transcriptase and protease enzymes which replicate HIV. The patient must adhere to HAART therapy or the virus becomes resistant and the antiretroviral agents lose their therapeutic effect. There are four classes of medication approved by the FDA for treatment of HIV: NNRTI, NRTI, PI, and Fusion Inhibitors.

A vaccine contains a small amount of a pathogen that is enough to stimulate the production of antibodies, but not sufficient for the patient to acquire the disease. Once antibodies for a specific pathogen are generated, the immune system can quickly regenerate the antibodies when the pathogen invades the body again.

In the next chapter we look at medications that are used to treat gastrointestinal and digestive diseases.

Quiz

1. The immune system is able to recognize self-cells by
   (a) using unique RNA that are on the surface of all self-cells.
   (b) using unique lipids that are on the surface of all self-cells.
   (c) using unique proteins that are on the surface of all self-cells.
   (d) none of the above.

2. Antibody-mediate immunity occurs when the immune system produces
   (a) antibodies that neutralize, eliminate or destroy an antigen (foreign protein).
   (b) antigens that neutralize, eliminate or destroy an antibody (foreign protein).
   (c) antibodies that generate an antigen (foreign protein).
   (d) antigens that generate antibodies (foreign protein).

3. HIV is transmitted via
   (a) injection of infected blood or blood products.
   (b) sexual contact.
   (c) maternal–fetal transmission.
   (d) all of the above.

4. Cell-mediated immunity, also known as Cellular Immunity, uses T-leukocytes referred to as natural killer cells (NK cells) to attack non-self cells.
   (a) True
   (b) False

5. Cell-mediated immunity is especially useful in identifying and ridding the body of self-cells that are infected by organisms that live within host cells.
   (a) True
   (b) False

6. NNRTI inhibits HIV by
   (a) binding to HAART.
   (b) binding to protease.
   (c) binding to reverse transcriptase.
   (d) none of the above.

7. A newborn whose mother is HIV positive should not be treated for HIV unless the newborn shows signs and symptoms of HIV.
    (a) True
    (b) False

8. When administering a vaccination, which of the following would you have on hand?
    (a) immune globulin
    (b) whole blood
    (c) plasma
    (d) epinephrine

9. Passive immunity can also occur through immunization by giving the patient a vaccination against the pathogen.
    (a) True
    (b) False

10. The HIV virus enters the cell through the CD4 molecule on the cell surface.
    (a) True
    (b) False

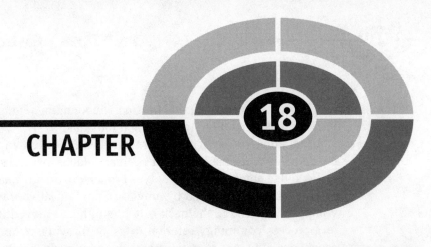

CHAPTER

18

Gastrointestinal System

At some point, all of us have had a bellyache—especially right before an exam—that suddenly disappeared once the exam was over. However, a stomach ache and other ailments of the gastrointestinal system are not as easily cured by removing stress. Some require more sophisticated treatment with medication.

Problems with the gastrointestinal system can include vomiting, ingesting toxins, diarrhea, constipation, peptic ulcers, and gastroesophageal reflux disease. Each is treatable with the proper medication.

In this chapter, you'll learn about common gastrointestinal disorders and about the medications that are frequently prescribed to treat these conditions.

A Brief Look at the Gastrointestinal System

The gastrointestinal (GI) system consists of the alimentary canal and the digestive tract that begins with the oral cavity and extends to the anus. The major structures of the GI system are the oral cavity (mouth, tongue, and pharynx), esophagus, stomach, small intestine (duodenum, jejunum, and ileum), large intestine (cecum, colon, rectum), and the anus.

In addition to these major structures, the GI system has several accessory organs and glands that include the salivary glands, pancreas, gallbladder, and liver.

Food that enters the oral cavity is broken down into small pieces in the mouth. Starches are then digested by amylase found in saliva. Small pieces of food are voluntarily moved to the back of the mouth and moved down to the esophagus in a process commonly referred to as swallowing. When the food reaches the esophagus, it is moved to the stomach and intestines with an involuntary movement called peristalsis.

The esophagus is a tube connecting the oral cavity to the stomach and is lined with mucous membranes that secrete mucus. The esophagus has two sphincters. These are the superior (hyperpharyngeal) sphincter and the lower sphincter that prevents gastric juices from entering the esophagus (gastric reflux).

The stomach is a hollow organ that holds between 1000 to 2000 mL of contents that takes about 2–3 hours to empty. It, too, has two sphincters. These are the cardiac sphincter (located at the opening of the esophagus), and the pyloric sphincter (that connects the stomach to the head of the duodenum).

The stomach has mucosal folds containing glands that secrete gastric juices used to break down food (digest) into its chemical elements. Lipid-soluble drugs and alcohol are absorbed in the stomach. There are four types of cells in the stomach. These are:

Chief Cells

Chief cells secrete proenzyme pepsinogen (pepsin).

Parietal Cells

Parietal cells secrete hydrochloric acid (HCl)

Gastrin-Producing Cells

Gastrin-producing cells secrete gastrin, which is a hormone that regulates the release of enzymes during digestion.

Mucus-Producing Cells

Mucus-producing cells release mucus that protect the stomach lining from the gastric juices.

The small intestine extends from the ileocecal valve at the stomach to the duodenum. The cecum is attached to the duodenum, which is the site where most medication is absorbed. Most foods are also absorbed in the small intestine.

The duodenum releases secretin, which is a hormone that suppresses gastric acid secretion. This results in the intestinal juices having a higher pH than the gastric juices in the stomach. The hormone cholecystokinin is also released. It simulates the flow of bile into the duodenum. Hormones, bile, and pancreatic enzymes trypsin, chymotrypsin, lipase, and amylase digest carbohydrates, protein, and fat in preparation for absorption in the small intestine.

The small intestine lead into the large intestine where undigested material from the small intestine is collected. The large intestine also absorbs water and secretes mucus while moving the undigested material—using peristaltic contractions—to the rectum where it is eliminated through defecation.

VOMITING

Vomiting (emesis) is the expulsion of gastric contents of the stomach through the esophagus and out the oral cavity. Vomiting is sometimes preceded by nausea, which is a queasy sensation, although vomiting can occur without nausea. Vomiting can occur for a number of reasons. These include motion sickness, viral and bacterial infections, food intolerance, surgery, pregnancy, pain, shock, effects of selected drugs, radiation, and disturbances of the middle ear affecting equilibrium.

Vomiting occurs when two major centers in the cerebrum are stimulated. These are the chemoreceptor trigger zone (CTZ) that lies near the medulla and the vomiting center in the medulla. The CTZ receives impulses from drugs, toxins, and the vestibular center in the ear. These impulses are transmitted by the neurotransmitter dopamine to the vomiting center. The neurotransmitter acetylcholine is also a vomiting stimulant. Sensory impulses such as odor, smell, taste, and gastric mucosal irritation are transmitted directly to the vomiting center.

When the vomiting center is stimulated, motor neurons respond causing contraction of the diaphragm, the anterior abdominal muscles, and the stomach. The glottis closes, the abdominal wall moves upward, and the stomach contents are forced up the esophagus.

When vomiting occurs, try to identify the cause before treating the patient. Begin treatment with nonpharmacological measures such as drinking weak tea, flattened carbonated beverages, gelatin, Gatorade, and for children, Pedialyte. Crackers and dry toast may also be helpful.

Nausea and vomiting that occur during the first trimester of pregnancy should be treated with nonpharmacologic remedies since amtimetics can cause possible harm to the fetus.

If dehydration occurs because vomiting is severe, intravenous fluids may be needed to restore body fluid balance.

If nonpharmacological measures fail, then administer antiemetic medication. There are two groups of antiemetics: nonprescription and prescription. Nonprescription antiemetics are purchased over-the-counter and used to prevent motion sickness. They have little effect controlling severe vomiting. They must be taken 30 minutes before traveling and are not effective once vomiting occurs.

Antihistamine antiemetics such as diphenhydrinate (Dramamine), meclizine hydrochloride (Antivert), and diphenhydramine hydrochloride (Benadryl) are over-the-counter medications that prevent nausea, vomiting, and dizziness (vertigo) caused by motion by inhibiting stimulation in the middle ear. They also cause drowsiness, dryness of the mouth, and constipation.

Several over-the-counter drugs—such as bismuth subsalicylate (Pepto-Bismol)—act directly on the gastric mucosa to suppress vomiting. Such drugs can be taken for gastric discomfort or diarrhea. Do not give Pepto-Bismol to children who are vomiting who might be at risk for Reyes syndrome as it contains salicylates.

Phosphorated carbodydrate solution (Emetrol), a hyperosmolar carbohydrate is also available over-the-counter. It decreases nausea and vomiting by changing the gastric pH or by decreasing smooth muscle contractions of the stomach. This drug has a high sugar content and should not be used by diabetics.

Prescription antiemetics act as antagonists to dopamine, histamine, serotonin, and acetylcholine. Antihistamines and anticholinergics act on the vomiting center and decrease stimulation of the CTZ and vestibular pathways.

There are eight classifications of prescription antiemetics.

ANTIEMETICS

Antihistamines

Antihistamines are used to decrease nausea and vomiting that occur after surgery. They are also used for the management of motion sickness and to treat allergic symptoms. Examples are Vistaril, Atarax, and Phenergan.

See antihistamines in the Appendix. Detailed tables show doses, recommendations, expectations, side effects, contraindications, and more; available on the book's Web site (see URL in Appendix).

Anticholinergics

Anticholinergics are used to prevent and treat nausea, vomiting and motion sickness. They are also used to treat vertigo that is associated with vestibular system disease. Scopolamine is an example of an anticholinergic agent.

See anticholinergics in the Appendix. Detailed tables show doses, recommendations, expectations, side effects, contraindications, and more; available on the book's Web site (see URL in Appendix).

Dopamine antagonists

Dopamine antagonists suppress emesis by blocking dopamine receptors in the CTZ. These include phenothiazines, butyrophenones, and metoclopramide. Common side effects are extrapyramidal symptoms (EPS)—caused by blocking the dopamine receptors—and hypotention. Phenothiazines are the largest group of antiemetics. They are also used for anxiety (see Chapter 15). Dopamine antagonists suppress emesis by blocking dopamine receptors. They act by inhibiting the CTZ. Not all phenothiazines are effective antiemetics. The dose is generally smaller when phenothiainerase is used as an antiemetic. Promethazine (Phenergan) is a phenothiazine. It was introduced as an antihistamine with sedative side effects and can be used for motion sickness.

Phenothiazines and the miscellaneous antiemetics such as benzquinamide, diphenidol, metclopramide, and trimethobenzamide act on the CTZ center.

Chlorpromazine (Thorazine) and prochlorperazine edisylate (Compazine) are tranquilizers used for both psychosis and vomiting.

Butyrophenones include haloperidol (Haldol) and droperidol (Inapsine). They block dopamine$_2$ receptors in the CTZ. Extrapyramidal side effects (EPS) are likely to occur if these drugs are used over an extended period of time. Hypotension can also occur.

Metoclopramide (Reglan) suppresses emesis by blocking the dopamine and serotonin receptors in the CTZ. High doses can cause sedation and diarrhea. The occurrence of EPS is more prevalent in children than adults.

Benzodiazepines

Benzodiazepines indirectly control nausea and vomiting. Lorazepam (Ativan) is the choice drug in this category and may be given with metoclopramide.

Serotonin antagonists

Serotonin antagonists suppress nausea and vomiting by blocking the serotonin receptors in the CTZ and the afferent vagal nerve terminals in the upper GI tract. Two serotonin antagonists—ondanestron (Zofran) and granisetron (Kytril)—are effective in suppressing chemotherapy-induced emesis. They do not block the dopamine receptors. Therefore, they do not cause EPS. Zofran is commonly used to prevent and treat post-operative nausea and vomiting.

Glucocorticoids

Glucocorticoids (corticosteroids) include Dexamethasone (Decadron) and methylprednisolone (Solu-Medrol). They are administered intravenously for short-term use. This reduces the side effects caused by using glucocorticoids. (See Chapter 12 for a discussion on the use of steroids.)

Cannabinoids (for cancer patients)

The cannabinoids act on the cerebral cortex and have the same side effects and adverse reactions as antihistamines and anticholinergic. These include drowsiness, dry mouth, blurred vision, tachycardia, and constipation. Cannabinoids include dronabinol and nabilone. These drugs should not be administered to glaucoma patients because they dilate the pupils (mydriasis). They are contraindicated for use in patients with psychiatric disorders and also used as an appetite stimulant for patients with AIDS. Side effects include mood changes, euphoria, drowsiness, dizziness, headaches, depersonalization, nightmares, confusion, incoordination, memory lapse, dry mouth, orthostatic hypotension, hypertension, and tachycardia. Less common symptoms include depression, anxiety, and manic psychosis.

MISCELLANEOUS

Miscellaneous antiemetics include benzquinamide hydrochloride (Emete-Con), diphenidol (Vontrol), and trimethobenzamide (Tigan). They do not act strictly as antihistamines, anticholinergics, or phenothiazides. They suppress the impulses to the CTZ. Diphenidol also prevents vertigo by inhibiting impulses to the vestibular area. Benzquinamide appears to have antiemetic, antihistaminic, and anticholinergic effects. It inhibits stimulation to the CTZ center and decreases activity in the vomiting center. It can also increase cardiac output and elevate blood pressure. Side effects and adverse reactions of the miscellaneous antiemetics include drowsiness and anticholinergic symptoms such as dry mouth, increased heart rate, urine retention, constipation, and blurred vision. Benzquinamide should be used cautiously in clients with cardiac problems such as dysrhythmias. It can cause CNS stimulation, including nervousness, excitement, and insomnia. Trimethobenzamide can cause hypotension, diarrhea, and EPS.

A list of antiemetic drugs are in the Appendix. Detailed tables show doses, recommendations, expectations, side effects, contraindications, and more; available on the book's Web site (see URL in Appendix).

EMETICS—INDUCING VOMITING

When a patient ingests a toxic substance, it is critical that the toxin be expelled or neutralized before the body can absorb it. However, vomiting should not be induced if the toxin is a caustic substance such as ammonia, chlorine bleach, lye, toilet cleaners, or battery acid. Regurgitating these substances can cause additional injury to the esophagus. Vomiting should also be avoided if petroleum distillates are ingested. These include gasoline, kerosene, paint thinners, and lighter fluid.

In cases where vomiting is contraindicated, the patient should be administered activated charcoal, which is available in tablets, capsules, or suspension. Charcoal absorbs (detoxifies) ingested toxic substances, irritants, and intestinal gas. Activated charcoal can be given as a slurry (30 grams in at least 8 oz. of water) or 12.5–50 grams in aqueous or sorbitol suspension. It is usually given as a single dose.

In cases where vomiting is desired, use one of two ways to expel a toxin:

The nonpharmacological treatment is to induce vomiting by stimulating the gag reflex by placing a finger or a toothbrush in the back of the patient's throat.

Pharmacological treatment involves administering an emetic to induce vomiting. Ipecac is the most commonly used emetic. Ipecac, available over the counter, should be purchased as a syrup—not a fluid extract. The syrup induces vomiting by stimulating the CTZ in the medulla and acts directly on the gastric mucosa.

Ipecac should be taken with at least eight or more ounces of water or juice (do not use milk or carbonated beverages). If vomiting does not occur within 20 minutes, then the dose should be repeated. If vomiting cannot be induced, then administer activated charcoal. The absorption of ipecac is minimal. Protein-binding is unknown and the half life is short. Duration of action is only 20–25 minutes. Do not attempt to induce vomiting if the patient is not fully awake and alert.

ANTI-DIARRHEA

Diarrhea is defined as frequent liquid stools that can be caused by foods, fecal impaction, bacteria (*Escherichia coli, Salmonella*), virus (*parvovirus, rotavirus*), toxins, drug reaction, laxative abuse, malabsorption syndrome caused by lack of digestive enzymes, stress and anxiety, bowel tumor, and inflammatory bowel disease such as ulcerative colitis or Crohn's disease.

Diarrhea can be mild (lasting one bowel movement) or severe (lasting several bowel movements). Intestinal fluids are rich in water, sodium, potassium, and bicarbonate, and diarrhea can cause minor or severe dehydration and electrolyte imbalances. The loss of bicarbonate places the patient at risk for developing metabolic acidosis. Severe diarrhea can be life threatening in young, elderly, and debilitated patients.

Diarrhea is a symptom of an underlying cause. Therefore, you must treat the underlying cause while treating the diarrhea. Diarrhea can be treated with a combination of medications and nonpharmacological measures such as clear liquids and oral solutions—Gatorade, Pedialyte, or Ricolyte—and intravenous electrolyte solutions.

For example, traveler's diarrhea also known as Montezuma's Revenge is an acute condition usually caused by *E. coli* that last less than 2 days but it can become severe. A patient experiencing traveler's diarrhea may be given fluoro-quinolone antibiotics and loperamide (Immodium) to slow peristalsis and decrease the frequency of the stools. Fluoroquinolone treats the underlying cause of diar-rhea and loperamide treats the diarrhea itself.

Anti-diarrhea medications decrease the hypermotility (increased peristalsis) that stimulates frequent bowel movements. Antidiarrheals should not be used for longer than 2 days and should not be used if a fever is present. Anti-diarrhea medication is available in four classifications.

See antidiarrheals listed in the Appendix. Detailed tables show doses, recom-mendations, expectations, side effects, contraindications, and more; available on the book's Web site (see URL in Appendix).

Opiates

Opiates decrease intestinal motility thereby decreasing persistalsis. Constipation is a common side effect. Examples are tincture of opium, paregoric (camphorated opium tincture), and codeine. Opiates are frequently combined with other antidiar-rheal agents and can cause central nervous system (CNS) depression when taken with alcohol, sedatives, or tranquillizers. Duration of action is about 2 hours.

Opiate-Related Agents

Opiate-related agents are drugs that are synthetic compounds similar to opiates. These drugs include diphenoxylate (Lomotil) (50% atropine to discourage abuse; amount of atropine is subtherapeutic) and loperamide. Both are synthetic drugs that are chemically related to meperidine (Demerol). Loperamide causes less CNS depression than diphenoxylate and can be purchased over-the-counter. It protects against diarrhea longer than a similar dose of Lomotil, reduces fecal volume, and decreases intestinal fluid and electrolyte losses. These drugs can cause nausea, vomiting, drowsiness, and abdominal distention. Tachycardia, para-lytic ileus, urinary retention, decreased secretions, and physical dependence can occur with prolonged use.

Absorbents

Adsorbents coat the wall of the GI tract and adsorb bacteria or toxins that are causing the diarrhea. Adsorbents include kaolin and pectin, which are combined in the over-the-counter drug Kaopectate, and other antidiarrheals. Pepto-Bismol is considered an adsorbent because it adsorbs bacterial toxins. Bismuth salts can also be used for gastric discomfort. Colestipol and cholestyramine (Questran) are prescription drugs that have been used to treat diarrhea.

Anti-Diarrhea Combinations

Anti-diarrhea combinations are miscellaneous antidiarrheals that include colistin sulfate, furazolidone, loperamide, lactobacillus, and octreotide acetate. You may know these brand names drugs to alleviate diarrhea: Lomotil (diphenoxylate HCl with atropine sulfate) and parepectolin (paregoric, kaolin, pectin, alcohol). Most contain a synthetic narcotic ingredient.

CONSTIPATION

Constipation is the accumulation of hard fecal material in the large intestine. It is a common occurrence for the elderly due to insufficient water intake and poor dietary habits. Other factors that cause constipation are fecal impaction, bowel obstruction, chronic laxative use, neurologic disorders such as paraplegia, a lack of exercise, and ignoring the urge to have a bowel movement. Drugs such as anticholinergics, narcotics, and certain antacids can also cause constipation.

Constipation can be treated nonpharmacologically and pharmacologically. The nonpharmacological approach is to include bulk (fiber) and water in the patient's diet and have the patient exercise and develop routine bowel habits. The normal number of bowel movements is between 1–3 per day to 1 to 3 per week. Normal bowel movements vary from person to person.

The pharmacological approach is to administer laxatives and cathartics to eliminate fecal matter. Laxatives promote a soft stool and cathartics promote a soft-to-watery stool with some cramping. Harsh cathartics that cause a watery stool with abdominal cramping are called purgatives. Frequency of the dose determines whether the drug acts as a laxative or a cathartic.

Laxatives should be avoided if there is any question that the patient has an intestinal obstruction, severe abdominal pain, or symptoms of appendicitis, ulcerative colitis, or diverticulitis. Most laxatives stimulate peristalsis. Laxative abuse from chronic use of laxatives is a common problem, especially with the elderly. Dependence can become a problem.

There are four types of laxatives.

Osmotics (saline)

Osmotic laxatives (hyperosmolar) are salts or saline products, lactulose, and glycerin. The saline products are composed of sodium or magnesium, and a small amount is systemically absorbed. They pull water into the colon and increase water in the feces to increase bulk, which stimulates peristalsis. Saline cathartics cause a semiformed-to-watery stool depending on dose. However, they are contraindicated for patients who have congestive heart failure.

Osmotic laxatives contain three types of electrolyte salts: sodium salts (sodium phosphate or phospho-soda, sodium biphosphate), magnesium salts (magnesium hydroxide (milk of magnesia), magnesium citrate, magnesium sulfate (Epsom salts), and potassium salts (potassium bitartrate, potassium phosphate). Serum electrolytes should be monitored to avoid electrolyte imbalance. Good renal function is needed to excrete any excess salts.

High doses of salt laxatives are used for bowel preparation for diagnostic and surgical procedures. Also used for bowel preparation is polyethylene glycol (PEG) with electrolytes, commonly referred to as Colyte or GoLYTELY. PEG is administered in amounts of 3 to 4 liters over 3 hours. Patients may be advised to keep GoLYTELY refrigerated to make it more palatable. PEG is an isotonic, nonabsorbable osmotic substance that contains sodium salts. Therefore, patients with renal impairment or cardiac disorder can use potassium chloride.

Lactulose, another saline laxative, is not absorbed and draws water into the intestines and promotes water and electrolyte retention. Lactulose decreases the serum ammonia level and is useful in liver diseases such as cirrhosis. Glycerin acts like lactulose by increasing water in the feces in the large intestine. The bulk that results from the increased water in the feces stimulates peristalsis and defecation. Patients who have diabetes mellitus should avoid lactulose because it contains glucose and fructose.

Adequate renal function is needed to excrete excess magnesium. Patients who have renal insufficiency should avoid magnesium salts. Hypermagnesemia can result from continuous use of magnesium salts, causing symptoms such as drowsiness, weakness, paralysis, complete heart block, hypotension, flushing, and respiratory depression. Side effects from excess use are flatulence, diarrhea, abdominal cramps, nausea, and vomiting.

Stimulants (contact or irritants)

Stimulant laxatives increase peristalsis by irritating sensory nerve endings in the intestinal mucosa. Stimulant laxatives include those containing phenolphthalein

(Ex-Lax, Feen-A-Mint, Correctol), bisacodyl (Dulcolax), cascara sagrada, senna (Senokot), and castor oil (purgative). Bisacodyl and phenolphthalein are two of the most frequently used and abused laxatives because they can be purchased over-the-counter.

Results occur in 6 to 12 hours. Stimulant laxatives such as bisacodyl are used to empty the bowel before diagnostic tests (for example, barium enema) because they are minimally absorbed from the GI tract. Most are excreted in feces. However, a small amount of bisacodyl absorption excreted in the urine changes the color to reddish-brown. With excessive use, fluid and electrolyte imbalances can occur (especially potassium and calcium). Mild cramping and diarrhea are side effects.

Caster oil is a harsh laxative (purgative) that acts on the small bowel and produces a watery stool within 2 to 6 hours. Therefore, this shouldn't be taken at bedtime. Caster oil is used mainly for bowel preparation and seldom used to correct constipation. Caster oil should not be used in early pregnancy because it stimulates uterine contractions and spontaneous abortion can occur. Prolonged use of Caster oil can damage nerves resulting in loss of intestinal muscular tone.

Bulk-forming

Bulk-forming laxatives are natural fibrous substances that promote large, soft stools by absorbing water into the intestines and increasing fecal bulk and peristalsis. Bulk-forming laxatives are non-absorbable. Defecation usually occurs within 8 to 24 hours but can take up to 3 days after the start of therapy for the stool to become soft and formed.

Powdered bulk-forming laxatives come in flavored and sugar-free preparations and should be mixed in a glass of water or juice, stirred. The patient should drink it immediately, followed by a half to a full glass of water. Insufficient fluid intake can cause the drug to solidify in the GI tract, resulting in intestinal obstruction. Bulk-forming laxatives do not cause dependence and may be used by patients with diverticulosis, irritable bowel syndrome, ileostomy and colostomy.

Calcium polycarbophil (FiberCon), methylcellulose (Citrucel), fiber granules (Perdiem), and psyllium hydrophilic mucilloid (Metamucil) are examples of bulk-forming laxatives. Patients with hypercalcemia should avoid calcium polycarbophil because of the calcium in the drug. Metamucil is a nondigestible and nonabsorbent substance that when mixed with water, becomes a viscous solution. There is no protein-binding or half-life for the drug. It is excreted in the feces. There are no systemic effects. Nausea can occur with excessive use. The dry form can cause abdominal cramps.

Emollients

Emollients (surfactants) are stool softeners (surface-acting drugs) and lubricants used to prevent constipation and decrease straining during defecation by lowering surface tension and promoting water accumulation in the intestine and stool.

Emollients are frequently prescribed for patients after a myocardial infarction (heart attack) or surgery and are also given prior to administration of other laxatives in treating fecal impaction. Docusate calcium (Surfak), docusate potassium (Dialose), docusate sodium (Colace), and docusate sodium with casanthranol (Peri-Colace) are examples of stool softeners.

Lubricants such as mineral oil increase water retention in the stool. Mineral oil absorbs essential fat-soluble vitamins A, D, E, and K. Some of the minerals can be absorbed into the lymphatic system. Side effects include nausea, vomiting, diarrhea, and abdominal cramping. They are not indicated for children, the elderly, or patients with debilitating conditions because they can aspirate the mineral oil, resulting in lipid pneumonia.

Emollients are contraindicated in patients with inflammatory disorders of the GI tract, such as appendicitis, ulcerative colitis, undiagnosed severe pain that could be due to an inflammation of the intestines (diverticulitis, appendicitis), pregnancy, spastic colon, or bowel obstruction.

A list of stimulant drugs is provided in the Appendix. Detailed tables show doses, recommendations, expectations, side effects, contraindications, and more; available on the book's Web site (see URL in Appendix).

PEPTIC ULCER

A peptic ulcer is a sore or hole in the lining of the stomach or duodenum and is a term used to describe a lesion in the esophagus, stomach, or duodenum. More specific names are used to describe an ulcer located at a specific site. Duodenal ulcers (the first part of the small intestine) are more common than other types of peptic ulcers. Peptic ulcers are caused by hypersecretion of hydrochloric acid and pepsin that erode the GI mucosal lining.

Anyone can get an ulcer. Most ulcers are caused by an infection with the bacterium *Helicobacter pylori*—not spicy food, acid, or stress—and can be cured with antibiotics in about two weeks. The most common ulcer symptom is burning pain in the stomach: $1/2$–$1 1/2$ hours after eating with gastric ulcers; 2–3 hours for a duodenal ulcer.

Gastric secretions in the stomach maintain a pH between 2 and 5. Pepsin, a digestive enzyme, activates at pH 2 and the acid-pepsin complex of gastric secretions cause mucosal damage. If gastric secretions increase to pH 5, pepsin declines. The gastric mucosal barrier (GMB) is a thick, viscous, mucous lining and is a defense against corrosive substances. The two sphincter muscles—cardiac and pyloric—act as barriers to prevent reflux of acid into the esophagus and the duodenum. Esophageal ulcers result from reflux of acidic gastric secretion into the esophagus as a result of a defective or incompetent cardiac sphincter.

Gastric ulcers frequently occur because of a breakdown of the GMB.

Duodenal ulcers are caused by hypersecretion of acid from the stomach that passes to the duodenum because of

- insufficient buffers to neutralize the gastric acid in the stomach.
- a defective or incompetent pyloric sphincter.
- hypermotility of the stomach.

Treatment of peptic ulcers is given in two-drug, three-drug, and four-drug regimens, or a combination medication consisting of multiple drugs combined into one package.

However, the American College of Gastroenterology no longer recommends two-drug regimens since they are not as effective as other treatment regimens. The different classes of medication that may be combined are listed below.

GASTROESOPHAGEAL REFLUX DISEASE (GERD)

Gastroesophageal reflux disease is an inflammation of the esophageal mucosa caused by reflux of stomach contents into the esophagus. GERD is caused by a malfunction of the esophageal sphincter brought about by smoking and obesity.

GERD is treated using common anti-ulcer drugs that neutralize the gastric contents and reduce gastric acid secretion. Once the content is neutralized, the esophageal mucosa has time to heal—freeing the patient of symptoms of GERD.

There are eight groups of anti-ulcer drugs used to treat GERD. These are:

Tranquilizers

Tranquilizers have minimal effect preventing and treating ulcers. However, they reduce vagal stimulation and decrease anxiety. Librax is a commonly prescribed tranquilizer to treat GERD. Librax is a combination of the anxiolytic chlordiazepoxide (Librium) and the anticholineratic clidinium (Quarzan) and is used in the treatment of ulcers.

Anticholinergic

Anticholinergics (antimuscarinics, parasympatholytics) relieve pain by decreasing GI motility and secretion and by inhibiting acetylcholine and blocking histamine and hydrochloric acid. Anticholinergics delay gastric emptying time and are used frequently to treat duodenal ulcers.

Anticholinergics should be taken before meals to decrease the acid secretion that occurs with eating. They should not be taken with antacids because antacids can slow the absorption of antichloinergic administration. Side effects include dry mouth, decreased secretions, tachycardia, urinary retention, and constipation. However, because gastric emptying time is delayed, gastric secretions can be stimulated and actually aggravate the ulceration.

Antacids

Antacids promote ulcer healing by neutralizing hydrochloric acid and reducing pepsin activity. Antacids don't coat the ulcer. There are two types of antacids: Those that have a systemic effect and antacids without a systemic effect. A systemic effect occurs when the antacid is absorbed.

Sodium bicarbonate is a systemic antacid that has many side effects including sodium excess that causes hypernatremia and water retention. Sodium bicarbonate also causes metabolic alkalosis related to the excess bicarbonate. Therefore, sodium bicarbonate is seldom used to treat peptic ulcers.

Calcium carbonate is most effective in neutralizing acid, however one third to one half of the drug can be systemically absorbed resulting in acid rebound. Hypercalcemia and "milk-alkali syndrome" can result from excessive use of calcium carbonate. Calcium carbonate is intensified if taken with milk products.

Nonsystemic antacids are composed of alkaline salts such as aluminum (aluminum hydroxide, aluminum carbonate) and magnesium (magnesium hydroxide, magnesium carbonate, magnesium trisilicate, and magnesium phosphate). A small degree of systemic absorption occurs with these drugs—mainly with aluminum.

Magnesium hydroxide has greater neutralizing power than aluminum hydroxide, however magnesium compounds can be constipating in long-term use. A combination of magnesium and aluminum salts neutralizes gastric acid without causing constipation or severe diarrhea. Simethicone (an anti-gas agent) is found in many antacids.

Histamine2 (H2 blockers)

Histamine2 blockers prevent acid reflux in the esophagus by blocking the H2 receptors of the parietal cells in the stomach. This results in a reduction of gastric acid secretion and concentration. Histamine2 blockers also cause head-aches, dizziness, constipation, pruritus, skin rash, gynecomastia, decreased libido, and impotence. Examples include Cimetidene (Tagamet) Famotidene (Pepsid) Ranitidine (Zantac).

Proton pump inhibitors

Proton pump inhibitors (gastric acid secretion inhibitors, gastric acid pump inhibitors) inhibit gastric acid secretion 90% greater than the H2 blockers because they block the final step of acid production. Both omeprazole (Prilosec) and lansoprazole (Prevacid) are proton pump inhibitors used for the treatment of peptic ulcers and GERD. Those with hepatic impairment should take these drugs with caution and have liver enzymes monitored regularly.

Pepsin inhibitor

Pepsin inhibitors such as sucralfate (Carafate) are mucosal protective drugs that are non-absorbable and combine with protein to form a viscous substance that covers the ulcer. This protects it from acid and pepsin. Pepsin inhibitors do not neutralize acid or decrease acid secretions.

Prostaglandin E1 analogue

Prostaglandin analogue antiulcer drugs such as misoprostol (Cytotec), prevents and treats peptic ulcers by suppressing gastric acid secretion and increasing cytoprotective mucus in the GI tract. Prostaglandin analogue also moderately decreases pepsin secretion. Prostaglandin analogue is ideal for patients who have gastric distress from taking NSAIDS such as aspirin or indomethacin. Prostaglandin analogue should not be taken during pregnancy and by any women of childbearing age.

Gastrointestinal stimulants

Gastrointestinal stimulants are used to treat nocturnal heartburn caused by GERD and primarily prescribed for patients who do not respond to other drugs or non-drug therapy. Gastrointestinal stimulants increase gastric emptying time prevent-ing acid reflux into the esophagus. Gastrointestinal stimulants also enhance the release of acetylcholine at the mysenteric plexus. Cisapride (Propulsid) is an example of a gastrointestinal stimulant.

Gastrointestinal stimulants should not be used for patients who have cardiac dysrhythmias especially ventricular tachycardia, ventricular flutter, or fibrillation.

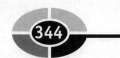

Nor should it be used for patients with ischemic heart disease, congestive heart failure, uncorrected electrolyte disorders (hypokalemia, hypomagnesemia), and renal or respiratory failure. An EKG should be done before and during therapy.

See the list inhibitor drugs listed are in the Appendix. Detailed tables show doses, recommendations, expectations, side effects, contraindications, and more; available on the book's Web site (see URL in Appendix).

Summary

The gastrointestinal (GI) system consists of the alimentary canal and the digestive tract that begins with the oral cavity and extends to the anus. When the GI system malfunctions or is invaded by a microorganism, the patient might experience vomiting, diarrhea, constipation, peptic ulcers, and gastroesophageal reflux disease.

Vomiting (emesis) is the expulsion of gastric contents of the stomach through the esophagus and out the oral cavity. It is caused by motion sickness, viral and bacterial infections, food intolerance, surgery, pregnancy, pain, shock, and the effects of selected drugs, radiation, and disturbances of the middle ear affecting equilibrium. Antiemetic medication is administered to prevent or stop vomiting.

A patient can be induced to vomit to regurgitate ingested toxins by administering an emetic. Activated charcoal should be administered if the patient ingested caustic material.

Diarrhea is a frequent liquid stool that can be caused by foods, fecal impaction, bacteria, a virus, or a number of other conditions. Diarrhea can be stopped by administering anti-diarrhea medication and treating the underlying cause.

Constipation is the accumulation of hard fecal material in the large intestine. Constipation can be relieved by administering laxatives to promote a soft stool and cathartics to promote a soft-to-watery stool with some cramping.

A peptic ulcer is a sore or hole in the lining of the stomach or duodenum or a lesion in the esophagus, stomach, or duodenum. Most ulcers are caused by a bacterial infection. Treatment of peptic ulcers is to give a two-drug, three-drug, and four-drug regimen, or combination medication consisting of multiple drugs combined into one package.

Gastroesophageal reflux disease (GERD) is an inflammation of the esophageal mucosa caused by reflux of stomach content into the esophagus. One of eight groups of anti-ulcer drugs is used to treat GERD.

Quiz

1. What cells produce hydrochloric acid in the stomach?
   (a) Gastrin-producing cells
   (b) Parietal cells
   (c) Mucus-producing cells
   (d) None of the above

2. Vomiting is caused by
   (a) viral and bacterial infections.
   (b) motion sickness.
   (c) surgery.
   (d) all of the above.

3. Ipecac should not be taken with
   (a) eight or more ounces of water.
   (b) eight or more ounces of juice.
   (c) milk.
   (d) none of the above.

4. Laxatives should be avoided if there is any question that the patient has an intestinal obstruction or severe abdominal pain.
   (a) True
   (b) False

5. Stimulant laxatives increase peristalsis by irritating sensory nerve endings in the intestinal mucosa.
   (a) True
   (b) False

6. GERD is caused by
   (a) a malfunctioning of the stomach mucosa.
   (b) a malfunctioning of the pepsin pump.
   (c) a malfunctioning of the esophageal sphincter.
   (d) none of the above.

7. Dopamine antagonists suppress emesis by blocking dopamine receptors in the CTZ.
   (a) True
   (b) False

8. Serotonin antagonists suppress nausea and vomiting by
   (a) blocking the glucocorticoids.
   (b) blocking the serotonin receptors in the CTZ and the afferent vagal nerve terminals in the upper GI tract.
   (c) blocking the dexamethasone.
   (d) blocking the dopamine receptors.

9. An emetic is administered to a patient who ingests toilet cleaner
   (a) True
   (b) False

10. Emollients are frequently prescribed for patients after a myocardial infarction.
    (a) True
    (b) False

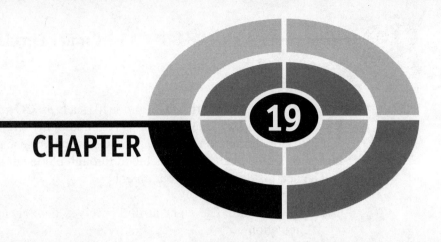

CHAPTER 19

Cardiac Circulatory Medications

The cardiovascular system is the highway within the body that distributes oxygen, nutrients and hormones and transports waste products, such as carbon dioxide, so they can be removed from the body.

When this highway falters the flow of traffic slows down, sometimes coming to a complete stop, backing up other systems of the body, and ultimately causing death to tissues and organs.

Fortunately, there are medications that can be taken to treat and prevent cardiovascular disorders. In this chapter, you'll learn about drugs that affect the heart and drugs that keep the vascular system humming.

A Brief Look at the Cardiovascular System

The cardiovascular system includes the heart, blood vessels (arteries and veins), and blood. Blood rich in oxygen, nutrients, and hormones moves through vessels called arteries that narrow to arterioles. Capillaries transport oxygenated blood to cells and absorb waste products such as CO_2, urea, creatinine, and ammonia. The deoxygenated blood is returned to the circulation by the venules and veins for elimination of waste products by the lungs and kidneys. The pumping action of the heart circulates blood through blood vessels.

The heart is divided into four chambers.

1. Right atrium. The right atrium receives deoxygenated blood from the circulation.
2. Right ventricle. The right ventricle pumps unoxygenated blood to the pulmonary artery to the lungs for gas exchange (CO_2 for O_2).
3. Left atrium. The left atrium receives oxygenated blood via the pulmonary vein.
4. Left ventricle. The left ventricle pumps the blood into the aorta for systemic circulation.

THE HEART

The heart muscle, called the myocardium, has a fibrous covering called the pericardium. The endocardium is a three-layered membrane that lines the interior of the heart chambers.

The heart has four valves—two atrioventricular (tricuspid and mitral) and two semilunar (pulmonic and aortic). Atrioventricular valves control bloodflow between the atria and ventricles. Semilunar valves control the bloodflow between the ventricles and the pulmonary artery and the aorta.

There are three major coronary arteries: the right, left, and circumflex. Each provides nutrients to the myocardium. Blockage in one or more of these arteries can result in a myocardial infarction ("heart attack.")

The myocardium is capable of generating and conducting its own electrical impulses. The impulse begins in the sinoatrial (SA) node and moves to the atrioventricular (AV) node. The heart beats about 60 to 80 beats a minute. The ventricle can beat independently at a rate of about 30 to 40 beats per minute.

Drugs can affect cardiac contraction by stimulating or inhibiting the heart. Contractions are also influenced by the autonomic nervous system (ANS). The sympathetic nervous system increases heart rate and the parasympathetic nervous system decreases heart rate. (See Chapter 15.)

BLOOD PRESSURE AND CARDIAC PERFORMANCE

Resistance develops as the blood travels through the circulatory system. This resistance is known as blood pressure. The average systemic arterial pressure (blood pressure) is 120/80 mmHg. The higher the resistance, the higher the blood pressure.

The total volume of blood expelled by the heart in a minute is referred to as cardiac output. The average cardiac output is 4 to 8 L/min. The amount of blood ejected from the left ventricle during each heartbeat is called the stroke volume. The average stroke volume is 70 mL/beat.

As blood flows into the ventricles the ventricles fill and stretch. The force in which blood flows into the ventricle is called preload. The force used to contract the ventricle is called the heart's contractility. The resistance to blood ejected by the ventricle is called the afterload. Afterload is the opposing pressure in the aorta and systemic circulation to the contraction of the ventricle.

Drugs can be used to ease the workload of the heart by increasing or decreasing the preload and afterload resulting in adjusting the stroke volume and cardiac output. Vasodilators decrease the preload and afterload decreasing arterial pressure and cardiac output. Vasopressors increase the preload and afterload increasing the arterial pressure and cardiac output.

CIRCULATION

There are two types of circulation.

1. Pulmonary circulation. The pulmonary circulation is when the heart pumps deoxygenated blood that contains CO_2 from the right ventricle through the pulmonary artery to the lungs. Oxygenated blood returns to the left atrium by the pulmonary vein.
2. Systemic (peripheral) circulation. In systemic circulation, the heart pumps blood from the left ventricle to the aorta into the general circulation. Blood is carried by the arteries to the arterioles down to the capillary beds where nutrients in the blood are exchanged with waste products at the cellular level. Blood then returns through the venules to the veins back to the heart.

BLOOD

Blood is composed of plasma, red blood cells (erythrocytes), white blood cells, (leukocytes) and platelets. Plasma is the fluid component of blood that is comprised of 90% water and 10% solutes, and constitutes 55% of the total blood volume.

Plasma contains glucose, protein, lipids, amino acids, electrolytes, minerals, lactic and pyruvic acids, hormones, enzymes, oxygen, and carbon dioxide.

Blood provides nutrients including oxygen to body cells. Oxygen is carried in the hemoglobin of red blood cells (RBCs). The white blood cells are the major defense mechanism of the body and act by engulfing microorganisms. Platelets are present in the blood. They gather at the site of a wound and aggregate (stitch together) to form a clot to stop the bleeding.

Cardiac drugs

Cardiac drugs regulate heart contraction, heart rate, and heart rhythm. Cardiac drugs also regulate blood flow to the heart muscle. There are three groups of cardiac drugs: glycosides, antianginals, and antidysthythmics.

Glycosides, known as digitalis glycosides, inhibit the sodium-potassium pump and increase intracellular calcium. This causes the cardiac muscle fibers to contract better. Glycosides have three effects on the heart:

1. A positive inotropic action that increases cardiac muscle contraction.
2. Negative chronotropic action that decrease the heart rate.
3. A negative dromotropic action that decreases conduction of the electrical stimulus.

The effects of glycosides improve heart, peripheral, and kidney function because

- Cardiac output is increased.
- Preload is decreased, improving blood flow to the periphery and kidneys.
- Edema decreases.
- Fluid excretion increases.
- Fluid retention in the lung and extremities is decreased.

Glycoside preparations are also used to correct atrial fibrillation and atrial flutter (cardiac dysrhythmia).

Glycosides include digoxin (Lanoxin), inamrinone lactate (Inocor) and milrinone lactate (Primacor), and positive inotropic bipyridines. The antidote for glycoside toxicity is digoxin immune Fab (Ovine, Digibind).

A list of drugs utilized in the treatment of the heart is provided in the Appendix. Detailed tables show doses, recommendations, expectations, side effects, contraindications, and more; available on the book's Web site (see URL in Appendix).

Heart Failure Medication

Heart failure is treated by using vasodilators to decrease venous blood return to the heart. This results in a decrease in cardiac filling, decreased ventricular stretching, and decreased oxygen demand on the heart.

Vasodilators work in three ways. They

- Reduce cardiac afterload, which increases cardiac output.
- Dilate the arterioles of the kidneys to improve renal perfusion and increase fluid loss.
- Improve circulation to the skeletal muscles.

Examples of vasodilators include: hydralozine (apresoline), and Minoxidil (Lonitin).

Heart failure is also treated with angiotensin-converting enzyme (ACE) inhibitors. Angiotensin-converting enzyme (ACE) inhibitors dilate venules and arterioles to improve renal blood flow and decreases blood fluid volume. Angiotensin-converting enzyme (ACE) inhibitors moderately decrease the release of aldosterone; sodium retention is reduced as is fluid retention.

Diuretics are also prescribed to treat heart failure. Diuretics, which will be discussed in detail later in this chapter, are the first line of treatment for reducing fluid volume and are frequently prescribed with digoxin. Spironalactone (Aldactone) is a potassium-sparing diuretic and is effective in treating moderate to severe heart failure. It is more effective than ACE inhibitors. Beta-blockers have been contraindicated for patients in heart failure.

Antianginal Drugs

Antianginal drugs (see Table 19-1) are used to treat angina pectoris by increasing blood flow either by increasing oxygen supply or by decreasing oxygen demand of the heart. Angina pectoris is acute cardiac pain caused by inadequate blood flow as a result of plaque occlusion in the coronary arteries of the myocardium or spasms of the coronary arteries. The decreased blood flow causes a decrease in oxygen to the myocardium, which is the cause of the pain. Anginal attacks may last for a few minutes and can lead to myocaradial infarction (heart attack).

There are three types of angina.

1. Classic (stable). Classic angina occurs with stress and exertion and is caused by the narrowing or partial occlusion of coronary arteries.

2. Unstable (preinfarction). Unstable angina occurs over the course of a day with progressive severity and is caused by the narrowing or partial occlusion of coronary arteries. This often indicates an impending heart attack—a medical emergency.

3. Variant (Prinzmetal, vasospastic). Variant angina occurs at rest and is due to a vessel spasm (vasospasm).

Stress tests, cardiac profile laboratory tests, and cardiac catherization may be needed to determine the degree or blockage in the coronary arteries. A combination of pharmacologic and nonpharmacologic measures (avoiding heavy meals, smoking, extremes in weather changes, strenuous exercise, and emotional stress) is necessary to control and prevent anginal attacks. Proper nutrition, moderate exercise, adequate rest, and relaxation techniques may be used to prevent attacks.

Antianginals

Nitrates

Nitrates reduce venous tone resulting in decreased workload of the heart and increased vasodilation. These are used to treat variant angina pectoris. The most commonly prescribed nitrate is nitroglycerin. There are various types of organic nitrates. Isosorbide dinitrate (Isordil, Sorbitrate) can be administered sublingually (SL) by tablets and orally by chewable tablets, immediate release tablets, sustained-release tablets, and capsules. Isosorbide mononitrate (Monoket, Imdur) can be given orally by immediate-release or sustained-release tablets.

Beta-Blockers

Beta-blockers (see Chapter 15) decrease the workload of the heart and decrease the heart's oxygen demands. Beta-blockers include atenolol (Tenormin), metoprolol tartrate (Lopressor), nadolol (Corgard), and propranolol HCl (Inderal)

Calcium Channel Blockers

Calcium channel blockers decrease the workload of the heart and decrease the heart's oxygen demands and are used to treat variant angina pectoris. Calcium channel blockers include amlodipine (Norvasc), bepridil HCl (Vascor), and diltiazem HCl (Cardizem), Felodipine (Plendil), and verapamil HCl (Calan, Isoptin).

See nitrates and calcium channel blockers in the Appendix. Detailed tables show doses, recommendations, expectations, side effects, contraindications, and more; available on the book's Web site (see URL in Appendix).

Table 19-1.   Effects of antianginal drugs on angina.

Drug Group	Variant (Vasospastic) Angina	Classic (Stable) Angina
Nitrates	Relaxation of coronary arteries, which decreases vasospasms and increases oxygen supply	Dilation of veins, which decreases preload and decreases oxygen demands
Beta blockers	Not effective	Decreases heart rate and contractility, which decreases oxygen demand
Calcium channel blockers	Relaxation of coronary arteries, which decreases vasospasms and increases oxygen supply	Dilation of arterioles, which decreases after load and decreases oxygen demand. Verapamil and diltiazem decrease heart rate and contractility.

Antidysrhythmics

Antidysrhythmics are drugs that restore normal cardiac rhythm and are used to treat cardiac dysrhythmias. A cardiac dysrhythmia is a disturbed heart rhythm. It is also known as arrhythmia—absence of heart rhythm. A disturbed heart rhythm is any deviation from the normal heart rate or heart pattern including slow rates (bradycardia) and fast rates (tachycardia). The electrocardiogram (ECG) is used to identify the type of dysrhythmia.

Table 19-2 lists the actions of antidysrhythmics and Table 19-3 describes classes of antidysrhythmic drugs.

Table 19-2.   Antidysrhythmic actions.

Mechanisms of Action
Block adrenergic stimulation of the heart
Depress myocardial excitability and contractility
Decrease conduction velocity in cardiac tissue
Increase recovery time (repolarization) of the myocardium
Suppress automaticity (spontaneous depolarization to initiate beats)

Table 19-3. Classes and actions of antidysthythmic drugs.

Classes	Actions	Examples/Side Effects
Class I Sodium channel blockers IA IB IC	 Slows conduction; prolongs repolarization Slows conduction and shortens repolarization Prolongs conduction with little to no effect on repolarization	Procainamide (Pronestyl, Procan) (*less cardiac depression than quinidine, abdominal pain/cramping, nausea, diarrhea, vomiting, flushing, rash, pruritus, lupus-like syndrome with rash*). Quinidine sulfate, polygalactorate, gluconate (Quinidex, Cadioquin) (*nausea, vomiting, diarrhea, confusion, and hypotension*). Lidocaine (Xylocaine) (*cardiovascular depression, bradycardia, and hypotension; dizziness, lightheadedness, and confusion*) Flecainide (Tambocor) (*nausea, vomiting, diarrhea, confusion*)
Class II Beta blockers	Reduces calcium entry; decreases conduction velocity, automaticity, and recovery time (refractory period)	Esmolol (Brevibloc) (*Generally well tolerated, with transient and mild side effects*) Propranolol HCl (Inderal) (*Decreased sexual ability, drowsiness, difficulty sleeping, unusual tiredness/weakness*)
Class III Prolong repolarization	Prolongs repolarization during ventricular dysrhythmias. Prolongs action potential duration.	Adenosine (Adenocard) (*Facial flushing, shortness of breath/dyspnea*) Amiodarone HCl (Cordarone) (*Corneal microdeposits are noted in almost all patients treated for >6 months [can lead to blurry vision], hypotension, nausea, fever, bradycardia, constipation, headache, decreased appetite, nausea, vomiting, numbness of fingers/toes, photosensitivity, muscular incoordination;* Bretylium tosylate (Bretylol) (*Transitory hypertension followed by postural and supine hypotension in 50% of patients observed as dizziness, lightheadedness, faintness, vertigo*)
Class IV Calcium channel lockers	Blocks calcium influx; slows conduction velocity, decreases myocardial contractility (negative inotropic), and increases refraction in the AV node	Verapamil HCl (Calan) (*Constipation, dizziness, lightheadedness, headache, asthenia [loss of strength, energy]*) Diltiazem (Cardizem) (*Peripheral edema, dizziness, lighheadedness, headache, bradycardia, asthenia [loss of strength, weakness], nausea, constipation, flushing, altered EKG*)

Cardiac dysrhythmias frequently follow a myocardial infarction (heart attack) or result from hypoxia (lack of oxygen to body tissues), hypercapnia (increased carbon dioxide in the blood), excess catecholamines, or electrolyte imbalance. Antidysrhythmics are grouped into four classes.

1. Fast (sodium) channel blockers. Fast (sodium) channel blockers are 1A (I) (quinidine and procainamide), 1B (II) (lidocaine), and IC (III) (encainide, flecainide).
2. Beta blockers. Beta blockers were discussed previously in this chapter and discussed in Chapter 15. This includes propanolol (Inderal).
3. Prolong repolarization. Prolonged repolarization is the time when the electrical impulse returns to normal and is ready to fire again. These include bretylium (Bretylol) and amiodarone (Cordarone).
4. Slow (calcium) channel blockers. Slow (calcium) channel blockers were discussed previously in this chapter and include verapamil (Calan, Isoptin) and diltiazem (Cardizem).

Antihypertensive drugs

Antihypertensive drugs are used to treat hypertension. Hypertension is classified as follows.

There are two types of hypertension.

1. Essential hypertension. Essential hypertension affects 90% of patients who are hypertensive and is caused by conditions other than those related to renal and endocrine disorders.
2. Secondary hypertension. Secondary hypertension affects 10% of patients who are hypertensive and is caused by secondary disorders of the renal and endocrine systems.

The exact cause of essential hypertension is unknown. However, there are nine factors that contribute to hypertension. These are:

- Family history of hypertension.
- Hyperlipidemia.
- African-American descent.
- Diabetes.
- Obesity.
- Aging.

- Stress.
- Diet.
- Excessive smoking and alcohol ingestion.

There are three stages of hypertension. Along with normal blood pressure (systalic and distalic) these are

1. Normal <120 and <80
2. Pre-hypertension: 120–129/80–89 mm Hg.
3. Stage 1 hypertension: 140–159/90–99 mm Hg.
4. Stage 2 hypertension: at or greater than 160–179/100–109 mm Hg.

KIDNEYS AND BLOOD PRESSURE

The kidneys use the renin-angiotensin system to maintain blood pressure. The renin-angiotensin system increases blood pressure by retaining sodium and water. Once baroreceptors in the aorta and carotid sinus detect adequate blood pressure, the baroreceptors signal the vasomotor center in the medulla to signal the renin-angiotensin system to excrete sodium and water, thereby lowering the blood pressure.

Hypertension is treated using a stepped-care approach. Each step uses a different group of antihypertensive drugs to control hypertension. There are four steps.

Step 1: Diuretic, beta blocker, calcium blocker, angiotensin-converting enzyme (ACE)
Step 2: Diuretic with beta blocker, sympatholytics
Step 3: Direct-acting vasodilator; sympatholytic with diuretic
Step 4: Adrenergic neuron blocker; combinations from Steps 1, 2, and 3.

COMBINING ANTIHYPERTENSIVE DRUGS

An antihypertensive drug can be used alone or in combination with one or more drugs that fall into one of five categories.

Diuretics

Diuretics promote sodium depletion, which decreases extracellular fluid volume. It is the first-line drug for treating mild hypertension. Hydrochlorothiazide

(HydroDIURIL), a thiazide, is the most frequently prescribed diuretic to control mild hypertension.

Thiazides are not used in patients who have renal insufficiency. Loop diuretics, such as furosemide (Lasix), are usually recommended for these patients because they do not depress renal flow.

Diuretics are not used if hypertension is the result of renal-angiotensin-aldosterone involvement because these drugs tend to elevate the serum renin level. Hydrochlorothiazides are combined with beta blockers, and angiotensin-converting enzyme (ACE) inhibitors. ACE inhibitors tend to increase serum potassium (K) levels. When they are combined with the thiazide diuretic, serum potassium loss is minimized.

Sympathetic depressants (sympatholytics)

Sympatholytics (see Chapter 15) are divided into five groups. These are

- Beta-adrenergic blockers: (acebutolol HCL (Sectral), atenolol (Tenormin), metoprolol (Lopressor), Nadolol (Corgard), propranolol (Inderal).
- Centrally acting sympatholytics (adrenergic blockers): clonidine HCl (Catapres) methyldopa (Aldomet).
- Alpha-adrenergic blockers: phentolamine (Regitine); doxazosin mesylate (Cardura), terazosin HCl (Hytrin).
- Adrenergic neuron blockers (peripherally acting sympatholytics): guanethidine monosulfate (Ismelin), resperine (Serpasil).
- Alpha- and beta-adrenergic blockers: carteolol HCl (Cartrol, Ocupress).

Direct-acting arteriolar vasodilators

Direct-acting arteriolar vasodilators are Step 3 drugs that act by relaxing the smooth muscles of the blood vessels—mainly the arteries—causing vasodilation. Direct-acting arteriolar vasodilators promote an increase in blood flow to the brain and kidneys. Diuretics can be given with direct-acting vasodilators to decrease edema. Reflex tachycardia is caused by vasodilation and the decrease in blood pressure. Beta blockers are frequently prescribed with arteriolar vasodilators to decrease the heart rate, counteracting the effect of reflex tachycardia. Nitroprusside and diazoxide are prescribed for acute hypertensive emergencies.

A list of drugs utilized in the treatment of hypertension is provided in the Appendix. Detailed tables show doses, recommendations, expectations, side effects, contraindications, and more; available on the book's Web site (see URL in Appendix).

Angiotensin antagonists

Drugs in this group inhibit angiotensin-converting enzyme (ACE) which, in turn, inhibits the formation of angiotensin II (vasoconstrictor) and blocks the release of aldosterone. When aldosterone is blocked, peripheral resistance is lowered.

Calcium channel blockers

These drugs dilate coronary arteries and arterioles and decrease total peripheral vascular resistance by vasodilation.

STEPPED-CARE TREATMENT

The prescribed method of treating hypertension begins with a nonpharmacological approach such as lifestyle changes: losing weight, reducing sodium intake, limiting alcohol intake, smoking cessation, and increasing physical activity.

If blood pressure remains elevated, then treatment moves to the next step. The patient is administered diuretics or beta-blockers.

If blood pressure still remains high, then the dose of diuretics or beta-blockers is increased or a calcium channel blocker, ACE inhibitor, angrotension II blocker, or combination drug replaces or is added to the treatment plan.

If blood pressure does not decrease, the patient is given a diuretic with a beta-blocker or a second drug is added such as a calcium channel blocker, ACE inhibitor, alpha blocker, or centrally acting sympatholytic.

If blood pressure still does not decrease, two or three additional drugs are administered to the patient. These include alpha blockers, direct-acting vasodilators, or adrenergic neuron blockers.

A list of drugs utilized in the treatment of high blood pressure is provided in the Appendix. Detailed tables show doses, recommendations, expectations, side effects, contraindications, and more; available on the book's Web site (see URL in Appendix).

ANGIOTENSIN ANTAGONISTS, ACE INHIBITORS, ANGIOTENSIN II BLOCKERS

Angiotensin antagonists (angiotensin-converting enzyme inhibitors) and ACE inhibitors inhibit the formation of angiotensin II (vasoconstrictor) and block the release of aldosterone. Aldosterone promotes sodium retention and potassium excretion. When aldosterone is blocked, sodium is excreted along with water and potassium is retained. These drugs cause little change in cardiac output or heart rate and lower peripheral resistance. They can be used in patients with elevated serum renin levels.

They are used primarily to treat hypertension; some of the agents are also effective in treating heart failure. Examples of these drugs include benazepril (Lotensin), captopril (Capoten), enalapril maleate (Vasotec), enalaprilat (Vasotec IV), lisinopril (Prinivil, Zestril), and ramipril (Altace).

Losartan (Cozaar), valsartan (Diovan), and irbesartan (Avapro) are Angiotensin II blockers that block angiotension II at the receptor site. ACE inhibitors and angiotensin II receptor antagonists are less effective for treating hypertension in African-American persons. They both may cause angioedema. Angioedema is very similar to urticaria, with which it often coexists and overlaps. The swellings occurs especially in the lips and other parts of the mouth and throat, the eyelids, the genitals, and the hands and feet. Angioedema is life-threatening if swelling in the mouth or throat makes it difficult to breathe. Less often the sheer amount of swelling means that so much fluid has moved out of the blood circulation that blood pressure drops dangerously.

CLALCIUM CHANNEL BLOCKERS

As discussed previously in this chapter, calcium channel blockers decrease calcium levels and promote vasodilation. Calcium channel blockers include verapamil (Calan), diltiazem (Cardiazem), nifedipine (Procardia), amlodipine (Norvasc), felodipine (Plendil), nicardipine HCl (Cardene), and nisoldipine (Sular, Nisocor).

Calcium channel blockers can be combined with ACE inhibitors. Such combinations include benazepril with amlodipine (Lotrel), enalapril with diltiazem (Teczem), enalapril with felodipine (Lexxel), and trandolapril with verapamil (Tarka).

A list of ACE inhibitor drugs in the Appendix. Detailed tables show doses, recommendations, expectations, side effects, contraindications, and more; available on the book's Web site (see URL in Appendix).

DIURETICS

Diuretics lower blood pressure and decrease peripheral and pulmonary edema in congestive heart failure and renal or liver disorders by inhibiting sodium and water reabsorption from the kidney tubules resulting in increased urine flow (diuresis).

Most sodium and water reabsorption occurs throughout the renal tubular segments. Diuretics affect one or more of these segments. Every one and one-half hours the kidneys (glomeruli) clean the body's extracellular fluid (ECF).

Small particles—such as electrolytes, drugs, glucose, and waste products from protein metabolism—are filtered in the glomeruli during this process. Sodium and water are the largest filtrate substances. Larger products—such as protein and blood—are not filtered with normal renal function. Instead, they remain in the circulation.

Nearly all filtered sodium is reabsorbed. Half occurs in the proximal tubules, approximately 40% in the loop of Henle, about 7% in the distal tubules, and the remaining in the collecting tubules.

Diuretics, such as Mannitol, that act on the tubules closest to the glomeruli have the greatest effect in causing sodium loss in the urine (natriuresis).

Diuretics have an antihypertensive effect by promoting sodium and water loss. They block sodium and chloride reabsorption causing a decrease in fluid volume, a lowering of blood pressure, and a decrease of edema. If sodium is retained, water is also retained in the body and blood pressure increases.

Many diuretics cause loss of other electrolytes, including potassium, magnesium, chloride, and bicarbonate. The diuretics that promote potassium excretion are classified as potassium-wasting diuretics. Potassium-sparing diuretics promote the reabsorption of potassium. Combination diuretics have been marketed that have both actions.

There are five categories of duretics that remove water and sodium.

Thiazide and thiazide-like diuretics

Thiazide diuretics include: chlorothiazide (Diuril), hydrochlorothiazide (HydroDIURIL, HCTZ), bendroflumethiazide (Naturetin), benzthiazide Aquatag, (Hydrex), hydroflumethiazide (Saluron, Diucardin); methychlothiazide (Aquatensen, Enduron), Polythiazide (Renese-R), trichlormethiazide (Metahydrin, Naqua); Thyzaide-like diuretics: chlorthalidone (Hygroton), indapamide (Lozol), metolazone (Zaroxolyn), and quinethazone (Hydromox).

Loop or high-ceiling diuretics

Loop or high-ceiling diuretics include bumetanide (Bumex), ethacrynic acid (Edecrin), furosemide (Lasix), and toresemide (Demadox).

Osmotic diuretics

Osmotic diuretics include Mannitol and urea (Ureaphil).

Carbonic anhydrase inhibitors

Carbonic anhydrase inhibitors include acetazolamide (Diamox), dichlorphenamide (Darnide, Oratrol), and methazolamide (Neptazane).

Potassium-sparing diuretics

Potassium-sparing diuretics include amiloride HCl (Midamor); spironolactone (Aldactone), and triamterene (Dyrenium). Combination diuretics include: amiloride HCl and hydrochlorothiazide (Moduretic); spironolactone and hydrochlorothiazide (Aldactazide), and triamterene and hydrochlorothiazide (Dyazide, Maxzide).

THIAZIDE DIURETICS

Thiazides influence the distal convoluted renal tubule beyond the loop of Henle to promote sodium, chloride, and water excretion. Thiazides are used in the treatment of hypertension and peripheral edema, but are not effective for immediate diuresis and should be used mainly with patients with normal kidney function.

Thiazides cause a loss of sodium, potassium, and magnesium and promote calcium reabsorption. They affect glucose tolerance and should be used with caution in clients with diabetes mellitus. Monitor laboratory tests for electrolytes and glucose.

Side effects and adverse reactions of thiazides are electrolyte imbalances, hyperglycemia, hyperuricemia (elevated serum uric acid level), and hyperlipidemia (elevated blood lipid levels). They affect the metabolism of carbohydrates.

Other side effects include dizziness, headaches, nausea, vomiting, constipation, and rarely urtacaria (hives) and blood dyscrasias.

A list of thiazides diuretic drugs is provided in the Appendix. Detailed tables show doses, recommendations, expectations, side effects, contraindications, and more; available on the book's Web site (see URL in Appendix).

LOOP OR HIGH-CEILING DIURETICS

Loop or high-ceiling diuretics act on the ascending loop of Henle by inhibiting chloride transport of sodium into the circulation. Sodium, potassium, calcium, and magnesium are lost. Loop or high-ceiling diuretics have little effect on blood sugar, but increase the uric acid level.

Loop or high-ceiling diuretics are potent and cause marked depletion of water and electrolytes. They are more potent than thiazides and two to three times more effective when inhibiting reabsorption of sodium. However, loop or high-ceiling diuretics are less effective as antihypertensive agents.

Loop or high-ceiling diuretics can increase renal blood flow up to 40%. This drug is commonly the choice for patients who have decreased kidney function or end-stage renal disease.

Loop or high-ceiling diuretics cause excretion of calcium and have a great saluretic (sodium-losing) affect that causes rapid diuresis, decreases vascular fluid volume, and decreased cardiac output and blood pressure.

Loop or high-ceiling diuretics causes a vasodilatory effect and increase renal blood flow before diuresis. The most common side effects are fluid and electrolyte imbalances such as hypokalemia, hyponatremia, hypocalcemia, hypomagnesemia, and hypochloremia. Hypochloremic metabolic alkalosis may result. Orthostatic hypotension can also occur. Thrombocytopenia, skin disturbances, and transient deafness are seen rarely. Prolonged use can cause thiamine deficiency.

A list of loop diuretic drugs is provided in the Appendix. Detailed tables show doses, recommendations, expectations, side effects, contraindications, and more; available on the book's Web site (see URL in Appendix).

OSMOTIC DIURETICS

Osmotic diuretics increase the concentration (osmolality) of the plasma and fluid in the renal tubules. Sodium, chloride, potassium (to a lesser degree), and water are excreted. Osmotic diuretics are used to prevent kidney failure, decrease intracranial pressure (ICP) (cerebral edema), and decrease intraocular pressure (IOP) as is the case with glaucoma.

Mannitol is a potent potassium-wasting osmotic diuretic used in emergencies to treat intraocular pressure. Mannitol is also used with cisplatin and carboplatin in cancer chemotherapy to induce a frank diuresis for decreased side effects of treatment.

Mannitol is the most frequently prescribed osmotic diuretic. The side effects and adverse reactions include fluid and electrolyte imbalance, pulmonary edema from rapid shift of fluids, nausea, vomiting, tachycardia from rapid fluid loss, and acidosis.

CARBONIC ANHYDRASE INHIBITORS

The carbonic anhydrase inhibitors block the action of the enzyme carbonic anhydrase which is needed to maintain the acid-base balance (hydrogen and bicarbonate ion balance). Inhibition of this enzyme causes increased sodium, potassium, and bicarbonate excretion. Prolonged use can result in metabolic acidosis.

Carbonic anhydrase inhibitors include acetazolamide dichlorphenamide (Diamox), and methazolamide (Daranide).

Carbonic anhydrase inhibitors are used to decrease intraocular pressure in patients with open-angle (chronic) glaucoma and are not used in narrow-angle or acute glaucoma. Other uses include inducing diuresis, management of epilepsy, and treatment of high-altitude or acute mountain sickness.

Carbonic anhydrase inhibitors can cause fluid and electrolyte imbalance, metabolic acidosis, nausea, vomiting, anorexia, confusion, orthostatic hypotension, and crystalluria. Hemolytic anemia and renal calculi can also occur. Carbonic anhydrase inhibitors are contraindicated in the first trimester of pregnancy.

A list of drugs for carbonic anhydrase inhibitors is provided in the Appendix. Detailed tables show doses, recommendations, expectations, side effects, contraindications, and more; available on the book's Web site (see URL in Appendix).

POTASSIUM-SPARING DIURETICS

Potassium-sparing diuretics act primarily in the collecting distal duct renal tubules to promote sodium and water excretion and potassium retention. The drugs interfere with the sodium-potassium pump that is controlled by mineralocorticoid hormone aldosterone (sodium retained and potassium excreted). Potassium is reabsorbed and sodium is excreted.

Potassium-sparing diuretics are weaker than thiazides and loops and are used as mild diuretics or in combination with antihypertensive drugs. Continuous use of potassium-wasting diuretics requires a daily oral potassium supplement because potassium, sodium, and body water are excreted through the kidneys. However, potassium supplements are not used when the patient takes potassium-sparing diuretics.

When potassium-sparing diuretics are used alone they are less effective in reducing body fluid and sodium than when used in combination. They are usually combined with a potassium-wasting diuretic, such as a thiazide or loop. The combination intensifies the diuretic effect and prevents potassium loss. The main side effect of these drugs is hyperkalemia.

Caution should be used with patients who have poor kidney function. Urine output should be at least 600 mL per day. Patients should not use potassium supplements while taking this group of diuretics. If given with an ACE inhibitor, hyperkalemia could become severe or life-threatening because both drugs retain potassium. Gastrointestinal disturbances (anorexia, nausea, vomiting, diarrhea) can occur.

A list of potassium-sparing diuretic drugs is provided in the Appendix. Detailed tables show doses, recommendations, expectations, side effects, contraindications, and more; available on the book's Web site (see URL in Appendix).

Circulatory Disorders

Circulatory disorders impair the flow of blood throughout the body. Circulatory drugs are used to restore and maintain circulation. There are four groups of circulatory drugs.

1. Anticoagulants and antiplatelets (antithrombotics). Anticoagulants and antiplatelets prevent platelets from clumping together and lower the risk that a patient will develop blood clots.
2. Thrombolytics. Thrombolytics are sometimes called clot busters because they attack and dissolve blood clots that have already formed.
3. Antilipemics. Antilipemics decrease blood lipid concentrations.
4. Peripheral vasodilators. Peripheral vasodilators dilate vessels narrowed by vasospasm.

ANTICOAGULANTS AND ANTIPLATELET

A clot is a thrombus that has formed in an arterial or venous vessel and is caused by decreased circulation (blood stasis). Anticoagulants such as warfarin and heparin inhibit clot formation but do not dissolve clots that have already formed.

Anticoagulants are given to patients who are at risk for deep venous thrombosis and pulmonary embolism. These patients may have had a myocardial infarction (MI, heart attack), a cerebrovascular accident (CVA or stroke), or have an artificial heart valve.

Antiplatelet drugs such as aspirin, dipyridamole (Persantine), and sulfinpyrazone (Anturane) are prescribed for the prevention and formation of blood clots (platelet aggregation).

Patients who have chronic or acute atrial fibrillation are also given anticoagulants to prevent the formation of mural thrombi (blood clots in the heart).

Anticoagulants can be administered orally (coumadin) or parenterally (heparin) to combine with antithrombin III, thus inactivating thrombin and other clotting factors. This prevents the formation of a fibrin clot.

Anticoagulants are poorly absorbed through the GI mucosa and destroyed by liver enzymes so it is given subcutaneously or intravenously. Anticoagulants can be given as an IV bolus or infusion. Clotting time is prolonged and partial thromboplastin time (PTT) and activated partial thromboplastin time (aPTT) are monitored during therapy.

Anticoagulants decrease platelet count causing thrombocytopenia. The antidote for heparin is protamine sulfate, which is given intravenously.

When IV therapy is to be discontinued, oral warfarin (Coumadin) or dicumarol is administered simultaneously. However, you must monitor lab values as heparin is gradually stopped and coumadin is added. The dose of Coumadin is adjusted based on PT values.

The International Normalized Ratio (INR) is the laboratory test used to monitor patients on anticoagulant therapy. Normal INR is 1.3 to 2.0 and patients on warfarin therapy are maintained at an INR of 2.0 to 3.0. Monitoring the lab values at regular intervals is required for the duration of drug therapy.

Patients should also be observed for petechiae and ecchymosis, tarry stools, and hematemesis which all could be indicative of occult (hidden) bleeding. The antidote for the oral anticoagulants is Vitamin K (phytonadione) (AquaMEPHYTON).

Low Molecular Weight Heparins (LMWHs) are derivatives of standard heparin and include enoxaparin sodium (Lovenox) and dalteparin sodium (Fragmin). They are used for prevention of deep venous thrombosis (DVT).

Low Molecular Weight Heparins can be administered at home because PTT monitoring is not necessary. They are given subcutaneously in the abdomen twice a day. The average treatment is for 7 to 14 days. The half life of LMWH is two to four times longer than that of heparin. Patients should not take antiplatelet drugs such as aspirin while taking LMWHs. Bleeding is less likely to occur and overdose is rare. However, protamine sulfate is the antidote if necessary and the dose is 1 mg of protamine for every 1 mg of LMWH given.

A list of anticoagulant low molecular weight drugs is provided in the Appendix. Detailed tables show doses, recommendations, expectations, side effects, contraindications, and more; available on the book's Web site (see URL in Appendix).

Thrombolytics

When a blood clot is mobilized, it is called a thrombus or embolus. It moves through blood vessels eventually causing a blockage—called a thromboembolism—resulting in decreased blood flow (ischemia) that causes death (necrosis) of tissues in the effected area. Thromboembolisms disintegrate naturally in about two weeks through the fibrinolytic mechanism, which breaks down fibrin.

Thrombolytics are drugs that promote the fibronolytic mechanism if administered within 4 hours following an acute myocardial infarction (AMI). An acute myocardial infarction (heart attack) can be caused by a thromboembolism blocking a coronary artery. This results in decreased circulation to that part of the heart. The ischemic (without oxygen) tissue becomes necrotic (dies) if left without an oxygen supply. Thrombolytics prevent or minimize necrosis that results from the blocked artery and therefore decreases hospitalization time. After thrombolytic treatment, the patient is evaluated for cardiac bypass or coronary angioplasty procedures.

Thrombolytics are also used for pulmonary embolism, deep vein thrombosis, and noncoronary arterial occlusion from an acute thromboembolism.

Commonly used thrombolytics are streptokinase, urokinase, tissue plasminogen activator (t-PA, Alteplase), anisoylated plasminogen streptokinase activator complex (APSAC, Anistreplase), and reteplase (Retavase).

All of these drugs induce fibrin breakdown (fibrinolysis).

Allergic reactions can complicate thrombolytic therapy. Anaphylaxis (vascular collapse) occurs more frequently with streptokinase than with the other thrombolytics.

Reperfusion dysrhythmia or hemorrhagic infarction can result if thrombolytics break up the clot after an MI. The major complication using thrombolytics is hemorrhage. The hemorrhage is stopped by using aminocaproic acid (Amicar) to inhibit plasminogen activation. The use of heparin with thrombolytic medications is commonly done and can prevent formation of new clots but requires intensive care and close monitoring of the patient.

A list of thrombolytic drugs is provided in the Appendix. Detailed tables show doses, recommendations, expectations, side effects, contraindications, and more; available on the book's Web site (see URL in Appendix).

Antilipemics

Antilipemics are drugs that lower abnormal blood lipid levels (see Table 19-4). Lipids, composed of cholesterol, triglycerides, and phospholipids, are bound to

Table 19-4. Serum lipid values.

Lipids	Normal Value (mg/dL)	Low Risk (mg/dL)	Level of Risk for CAD Moderate Risk	Level of Risk for CAD High Risk (mg/dL)
Cholesterol	150–240	<200	200-240	>240
Triglycerides	40–190	Values vary with age		>190
Lipoproteins LDL	60–160	<130	130–159	>160
Lipoproteins HDL	29–77	>60	35–50	<35

lipoproteins (see Table 19-5) and are transported in the body. These lipoproteins are classified as:

- Chylomicrons
- Very low-density lipoproteins (LDL)
- High-density lipoproteins (HDL).

The HDL (friendly or "good" lipoproteins) has a higher percentage of protein and fewer lipids. HDL removes cholesterol from the bloodstream and delivers cholesterol to the liver. The other three lipoproteins are composed of cholesterol

Table 19-5. Hyperlipidemia: Lipoprotein Phenotype Types II and IV are commonly associated with coronary artery disease.

Type	Major Lipids
I	Increased chylomicrons and increased triglycerides. Uncommon.
IIA	Increased low-density lipoprotein (LDL) and increased cholesterol.
IIB	Increased very low-density lipoprotein (VLDL), increased LDL, increased cholesterol and triglycerides. Very common.
III	Moderately increased cholesterol and triglycerides. Uncommon.
IV	Increased VLDL and markedly increased triglycerides. Very common.
V	Increased chylomicrons, VLDL, and triglycerides. Uncommon.

and triglycerides and contribute to atherosclerotic plaque in the blood vessels ("bad" lipoproteins).

When cholesterol, triglycerides, and LDL are elevated, the patient is at increased risk for coronary artery disease.

Before antilipemics are administered, patients are treated with nonpharmacological methods to reduce cholesterol and saturated fats in their diet. Total fat intake should be 30%. The patient is also encouraged to exercise. Hereditary factors have a great influence on cholesterol levels and are considered non-modifiable risk factors.

Antilipemics include cholestyramine (Questran), colestipol (Colestid), clofibrate (Atromid-S), gemfibrozil (Lopid), nicotinic acid or niacin (Vitamin B2).

Clofibrate is not used for long-term treatment because of its many side effects such as cardiac dysrhythmias, angina, thromboembolism, and gallstones.

Nicotinic acid is effective in lowering cholesterol levels, but it too has numerous side effects including GI disturbances, flushing of the skin, abnormal liver function (elevated serum liver enzymes), hyperglycemia, and hyperuricemia. Required large doses make it intolerable for most patients.

Probucol is poorly absorbed and is not as effective as the other antilipemic drugs. Probucol also causes diarrhea and is contraindicated in patients with cardiac dysrhythmias.

Cholestyramine lowers cholesterol levels, but causes constipation and peptic ulxcer.

Statin drugs inhibit the enzyme HMG CoA reductase in cholesterol biosynthesis. They inhibit cholesterol synthesis in the liver, decrease the concentration of cholesterol, decrease the LDL, and slightly increase the HDL cholesterol.

Reduction of LDL is seen in as early as two weeks.

Statins include atorvastatin calcium (Lipitor), cerivastatin (Baycol), fluvastatin (Lescol), lovastatin (Mevacor), pravastatin sodium (Pravachol), and simvastatin (Zocor).

A list of antihyperlipemic HMG-COa reductase inhibitor drugs is provided in the Appendix. Detailed tables show doses, recommendations, expectations, side effects, contraindications, and more; available on the book's Web site (see URL in Appendix).

PERIPHERAL VASCULAR DISEASE

A common problem in the elderly is peripheral vascular disease. It is characterized by numbness and coolness of the extremities, intermittent claudication (pain and weakness of limbs when walking and symptoms are absent at rest), and possible leg ulcers. The primary cause is hyperlipemia resulting in athero- sclerosis and arteriosclerosis. The arteries become occluded.

Peripheral vasodilators increase blood flow to the extremities and are used for venous and arterial disorders. They are more effective for disorders resulting from vasospasm (Raynaud's disease) than from vessel occlusion or arteriosclerosis (arteriosclerosis obliterans, thromboangiitis obliterans [Buerger's disease]). Some of the drugs that promote vasodilation include tolazoline (Priscoline), an alpha- adrenergic blocker (Chapter 15); isoxsuprine (Vasodilan) and nylidrin (Arlidin), beta-adrenergic agonists (Chapter 15); and cyclandelate (Cyclan), nicotinyl alcohol, and papaverine (Cerespan, Genabid), direct-acting peripheral vasodila- tors. The alpha blocker prazosin (Minipress) and the calcium channel blocker nifedipine (Procardia) have also been used.

A list of vasodilator drugs is provided in the Appendix. Detailed tables show doses, recommendations, expectations, side effects, contraindications, and more; available on the book's Web site (see URL in Appendix).

Summary

The cardiovascular system consists of the heart, blood vessels, and blood that are used to distribute oxygen, nutrients, and hormones and transports waste products so they can be removed from the body.

Cardiac drugs regulate heart contraction, heart rate, and heart rhythm and reg- ulate blood flow to the heart muscle. There are three groups of cardiac drugs: glycosides, antianginals, and antidysthythmics.

Glycosides are known as digitalis glycosides. They inhibit the sodium- potassium pump and increase intracellular calcium. As a result, there is an increase in cardiac muscle contraction, decrease in the heart rate, and a decrease in conduction of electrical stimulus to the heart.

Antianginal drugs are used to treat angina pectoris by increasing blood flow either by increasing oxygen supply or by decreasing oxygen demand of the heart. Antidysrhythmics are drugs that restore normal cardiac rhythm and are used to treat cardiac dysrhythmias.

Antihypertensive drugs are used to treat hypertension by using a stepped-care approach where groups of antihypertensive drugs are used in succession if blood pressure isn't at first decreased. Angiotensin antagonists are used primarily to treat hypertension and some are also effective in treating heart failure.

Diuretics lower blood pressure and decrease peripheral and pulmonary edema in congestive heart failure. In renal or liver disorders diuretics inhibit sodium and water reabsorption from the kidney tubules resulting in an increase in urine flow.

Circulatory disorders impair the flow of blood throughout the body. Circulatory drugs are used to restore and maintain circulation. There are four groups of circulatory drugs: anticoagulants and antiplatelets prevent blood clots from forming, thrombolytics dissolve blood clots, antilipemics decrease blood lipids, and peripheral vasodilators dilate vessels narrowed by vasospasm.

Quiz

1. Vasodilators work by
   (a) reducing cardiac afterload.
   (b) dilating the arterioles of the kidneys.
   (c) improving circulation to the skeletal muscles.
   (d) all of the above.

2. What type of angina occurs over the course of a day?
   (a) Stable
   (b) Preinfarction
   (c) Class angina
   (d) Distal angina

3. Beta-blockers
   (a) decrease the workload of the heart and decrease the heart's oxygen demands.
   (b) increase the workload of the heart and decrease the heart's oxygen demands.
   (c) decrease the workload of the heart and increase the heart's oxygen demands.
   (d) None of the above

4. Repolarization is the time when the electrical impulses return to normal.
   (a) True
   (b) False

5. Thiazides are not used with patients who have renal insufficiency.
   (a) True
   (b) False

6. Many diuretics cause a loss of
   (a) potassium.
   (b) magnesium.
   (c) bicarbonate.
   (d) all of the above.

7. Loop diuretics increase renal blood flow before diuresis.
   (a) True
   (b) False

8. Carbonic anhydrase inhibitors
   (a) decrease intraocular pressure in patients with open-angle glaucoma.
   (b) decrease intraocular pressure in patients with narrow-angle glaucoma.
   (c) decrease intraocular pressure in patients with acute glaucoma.
   (d) increase intraocular pressure in patients with open-angle glaucoma.

9. Potassium-sparing diuretics act primarily in the collecting distal duct renal tubules to promote sodium and water excretion and potassium retention.
   (a) True
   (b) False

10. Osmotic diuretics increase the concentration of the plasma and fluid in the renal tubules.
    (a) True
    (b) False

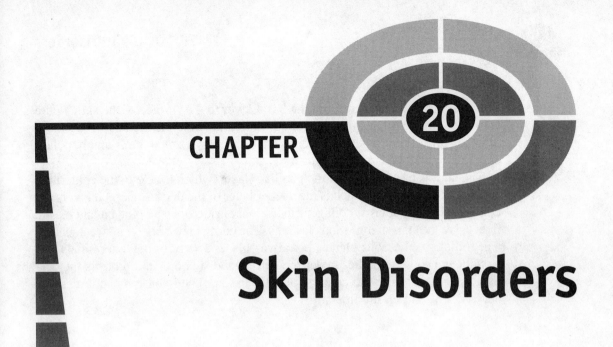

Skin Disorders

The least appreciated organ in your body is your skin. Yet your skin is your first line of defense against infection. Injury to your skin can have far more resounding repercussions than leave an unflattering blemish. It can be life threatening.

There are many disorders that can affect your skin including acne, dry skin, a rash, injuries such as cuts, scrapes, puncture wounds, and burns. Some disorders are annoying while others endanger your existence.

You'll learn about common disorders in this chapter and about the medications used to help treat those disorders.

A Brief Look at the Skin

Skin is the largest organ of the body. It is composed of two major layers: the epidermis, which is the outer layer; and the dermis, which is beneath the epidermis. The skin protects the body from the environment, aids in controlling the body's temperature, and prevents the body's fluid loss.

The epidermis has four layers: the basal layer (stratum germinativum), which is the deepest layer covering the dermis, the spinous layer (stratus spinosum); the outer layer; and the cornified layer (stratum corneum).

Epidermal cells migrate from the basal layer to the surface of the skin where cells die. Their cytoplasm is converted to keratin, which is the hard, rough texture that forms keratinocytes. Eventually keratinocytes slough off and new layers of epidermal cells migrate upward.

The dermis has two layers: the papillary layer, which is next to the epidermis; and the reticular layer, which is the deeper layer of the dermis. Dermal layers are comprised of fibroblasts, collagen fibers, and elastic fibers. Collagen and elastic fibers give the skin strength and elasticity. The dermal layer contains sweat glands, hair follicles, sebaceous glands, blood vessels, and sensory nerve terminals.

Subcutaneous tissue lies under the dermis and supports and protects the dermis. Subcutaneous tissue consists of fatty tissue, blood and lymphatic vessels, nerve fibers, and elastic fibers.

Skin Disorders

The skin is the site of several common disorders that include *acne vulgaris,* psoriasis, eczema dermatitis, contact dermatitis, drug-induced dermatitis, and burns. Some disorders result from viral infections such as herpes simplex and herpes zoster. Some result from fungal infections such as tinea pedis (athlete's foot) and tinea capitis (ringworm).

Lesions may also appear on the skin as macules (flat with varying colors), papules (raised, palpable, and less than 1 cm in diameter), vesicles (raised, filled with fluid, and less than 1 cm in diameter), or plaques (hard, rough raised, and flat on top).

Nearly all the disorders can be treated using mild or aggressive drug therapy in the form of topical creams, ointments, pastes, lotions, and solutions—some of which are available over the counter.

ACNE VULGARIS

Acne vulgaris, commonly called acne, is inflammation of the pilosebaceous glands. These are the glands which produce oil for the hair. Acne is more likely to occur in adolescent males and is associated with testosterone level and the ingestion of "greasy" foods—food containing trans-fatty acids (TFA). TFA are synthetic alterations of naturally fatty acids and are present in processed foods, candies, and potato chips.

Table 20-1. Medication for systemic therapy.

Non-Hormonal Treatment	Hormonal Treatment
Antibiotics, oral	Corticosteroids
Tetracycline	Anti-inflammatory actions: high dose
Erythromycin	Androgen suppressant action: low dose
Minocycline	Sex hormones (for women only)
Trimethoprim-sulfamethoxazole	Estrogen (oral contraceptive medication)
Isotretinoin, oral	Antiandrogens

Inflammation of the pilosebaceous glands form papules, nodules, and cysts on the face, neck, shoulders, and back as a result of keratin plugs at the base of the pilosebaceous oil glands near the hair follicles.

The increase in androgen production that occurs during adolescence increases the production of sebum, an oily skin lubricant. Sebum combines with keratin to form a keratin plug. An individual has little control over acne except to eat a nutritionally healthy diet and practice good hygiene. Acne is significantly influenced by age, heredity, stress, hormonal changes, and onset of puberty. All of these are beyond the patient's control.

Acne is treated by gently applying a cleansing agent several times a day to the skin. Vigorous scrubbing should be avoided. In addition, the patient can administer topical anti-acne medication such as keratolytics. These include benzoyl peroxide, resorcinol, and salicylic acid that dissolves keratin, the outer layer of the epidermis.

The patient should undergo systemic treatment if he or she has a severe case of *acne vulgaris* that results in scarring, has persistent hyperpigmentation, or when topical treatment fails (see Table 20-1).

A list of drugs utilized in the treatment of skin disorders is provided in the Appendix. Detailed tables show doses, recommendations, expectations, side effects, contraindications, and more; available on the book's Web site (see URL in Appendix).

PSORIASIS

Psoriasis is a chronic skin disorder characterized by erythematous papules and plaques covered with silvery scales appearing on the scalp, elbows, palms of the hands, knees, and soles of the feet. This is caused by an accelerated growth of epidermal cells—more than five times its normal rate. Less than 3% of the population of the United States is affected by psoriasis. More caucasians are affected than African-Americans and onset occurs between 10 and 30 years old.

Patients who have psoriasis are treated with antipsoriatic medications that loosen erythematous papules and plaques. However, patients usually experience periods of exacerbation and remission.

Psoriasis scales are loosened with keratolytics (salicylic acid, sulfur). Topical glucocorticoids are used for mild psoriasis. Other topical preparations that are effective for psoriasis include anthralin (Anthra-Derm, Lasan) and coal tar (Estar, PsoriGel).

Applications of 1% anthralin may cause erythema to occur and can stain clothing, skin, and hair. Coal tar products are available in shampoos, lotions, and creams. However, they have an unpleasant odor and can cause burning and stinging. Systemic toxicity does not occur with anthralin and coal tar.

Calcipotriene (Dovonex), a synthetic vitamin D_3 derivative, is used to suppress cell proliferation, but it may cause local irritation, hypercalciuria, and hypercalcemia (increased calcium levels in urine).

Methotrexate, an anti-cancer drug, slows cellular growth and is prescribed to decrease the acceleration of epidermal cell growth in severe psoriasis. Etretinate (Tegison) is used for severe pustular psoriasis when other medications have failed. Etretinate has an anti-inflammatory effect and inhibits keratinization and proliferation of the epithelial cells.

Ultraviolet A (UVA) may also be used to suppress mitotic (cell division) activity. Photochemotherapy, a combination of ultraviolet radiation with a psoralen derivative, methoxsalen (photosensitive drug), is used to decrease proliferation of epidermal cells. This is called psoralen and ultraviolet A (PUVA) and permits lower doses of drug and ultraviolet A to be used.

See Antipsoriatic in the Appendix. Detailed tables show doses, recommendations, expectations, side effects, contraindications, and more; available on the book's Web site (see URL in Appendix).

WARTS

A wart is a benign lesion characterized as a hard, horny nodule that may appear anywhere on the body, but particularly on the hands and feet. Warts are removed by freezing, electrodesiccation, or surgical excision.

Salicyclic acid, podophyllum resin, and cantharidin are three medications commonly used to remove warts. Salicylic acid promotes desquamation. However, salicylic acid is also absorbed through the skin and can result in salicylism (toxicity).

Podophyllum resin is used to remove venereal warts, but is not as effective against the common wart. Podophyllum also can be absorbed through the skin resulting in toxic symptoms such as peripheral neuropathy, blood dyscrasias, and kidney impairment. Podophyllum can cause teratogenic effects and should not be used during pregnancy.

Cantharidin (Cantharone, Verr-Canth) is used to remove the common wart, but can be harmful to the normal skin. Cantharidin is applied topically, allowed to dry, and covered with a nonporous tape for 24 hours. This treatment is repeated in a week or two.

DERMATITIS

Dermatitis is a skin eruption that is caused by medications (drug-induced dermatitis) or by a chemical agent coming in touch with the skin (contact dermatitis).

Drug-induced dermatitis is characterized by skin lesions that can be a rash, urticaria, papules, vesicles or life-threatening skin eruptions such as erythema multiforme (red blisters over a large portion of the body) or Stevens-Johnson syndrome (large blisters in the oral and anogenital mucosa, pharynx, eyes, and viscera). As a result of having a hypersensitive reaction to a drug, the patient may form sensitizing lymphocytes.

If the patient received multiple drug therapy, the last drug administered to the patient may have caused hypersensitivity and skin eruptions. Drug-induced dermatitis may take a few minutes, several hours, or a day for urticaria (hives) to appear. Certain drugs such as penicillin are known to cause hypersensitivity.

Other drug-induced dermatitis includes discoid lupus erythematosus (DLE) and exfoliative dermatitis. Hydralazine hydrochloride (Apresoline), isoniazid (INH), phenothiazines, anticonvulsants, and antidysrhythmics such as procainamide (Pronestyl) may cause lupus-like symptoms. If lupus-like symptoms occur, the drug should be discontinued.

Certain antibacterials and anticonvulsants may cause exfoliative dermatitis, resulting in erythema of the skin, itching, scaling, and loss of body hair.

Contact dermatitis, also called exogenous dermatitis, is caused by chemical or plant irritation and is characterized by a skin rash with itching, swelling, blistering, oozing, or scaling at the affected skin sites. The chemical contact may include cosmetics, cleansing products (soaps and detergents), perfume, clothing, dyes, and topical drugs. Plant contacts include poison ivy, poison oak, and poison sumac.

Nonpharmacological treatment of contact dermatitis includes avoiding direct contact with the causative irritant. The patient should use protective gloves and clothing if the chemical agent is associated with his or her employment.

At the first sign of contact dermatitis, clean the skin area immediately. Patch testing may be needed to determine the causative factor. Apply wet dressings containing Burow's solution (aluminum acetate), lotions such as calamine that contain zinc oxide, calcium hydroxide solution, and glycerin. Calamine lotion may contain the antihistamine diphenhydramine and is used primarily for plant irritations. If itching persists, antipruritics (topical or systemic diphenhydramine [Benadryl]) may be used. Topical antipruritics should not be applied to open wounds or near the eyes or genital area.

Other medications used as antipruritics are:

- Systemic drugs such as cyproheptadine hydrochloride (Periactin) and trimeprazine tartrate (Temaril).
- Antipruritic baths of oatmeal such as Alpha-Keri.
- Solutions of potassium permanganate, aluminum subacetate, or normal saline.
- Glucocorticoid ointments, creams, or gels.

Topical glucocorticoids can aid in alleviating dermatitis (see Table 20-2). These include dexamethasone (Decadron) cream, hydrocortisone ointment or cream, methylprednisolone acetate (Medrol) ointment, triamcinolone acetonide (Aristocort), and flurandrenolide (Cordran).

Topical glucocorticoids are systemically absorbed into the circulation depending on whether it is a cream or lotion, drug concentration, drug composition, and skin area to which the glucocorticoid is applied.

Absorption is greater at the face, scalp, eyelids, neck, axilla, and genitalia with prolonged use of the topical drug and if the drug is continuously covered with a dressing. Prolonged use of topical glucocorticoids can cause thinning of the skin with atrophy of the epidermis and dermis, and purpura from small-vessel eruptions.

ALOPECIA (MALE PATTERN BALDNESS)

Alopecia occurs when the hair shaft is lost and the hair follicle cannot regenerate. This results in permanent hair loss. Alopecia is associated with a familial history and the aging process. Some patients experience alopecia earlier than others.

Some medications can cause temporary alopecia. These include anticancer (antineoplastic) agents, gold salts, sulfonamides, anticonvulsants, aminoglycosides, and nonsteroideal antiflammatory drugs (NSAIDs) such as indomethacin.

Table 20-2.   Topical glucocorticoids.

Potency	Drug Name	Drug Form
High	Amcinonide 0.1% (Cyclocort)	Cream, ointment
	Betamethasone dipropionate 0.05% (Dirposone)	Cream, ointment, lotion
	Desoximetasone 0.25% (Topicort)	Cream, ointment
	Desocimetasone 0.05%	Gel
	Diflorasone diacetate 0.05% (Florone)	Cream, ointment
	Halcinonide 0.1% (Halog)	Cream, ointment
	Triamcinolone acetonide 0.5% (Aristcort A, Kenalog)	Cream, ointment
Moderate	Betamethasone benzoate 0.025% (Benisone)	Cream, ointment
	Betamethasone valerate 0.1% (Valisone)	Cream, ointment, lotion
	Desoximetasone 0.05% (Topicort LP)	Cream, gel
	Flucinolone acetonide 0.025% (Fluonid)	Cream, ointment
	Flurandrenolide 0.025% (Cordran, Cordran SP)	Cream, ointment, lotion
	Halcinonide 0.025% (Halog)	Cream, ointment
	Hydrocortisone valerate 0.2% (Westcort)	Cream, ointment
	Mometasone furoate 0.1% (Elocon)	Cream, ointment, lotion
	Triamcinolone acetonide (0.025%–0.1% (Aristocort A, Kenalog)	Cream, ointment, lotion
Low	Dexamethasone 0.1% (Decadron)	Cream
	Desonide 0.05% (Tridesilon)	Cream
	Fluocinolone acetonide 0.02% (Fluonid)	Solution
	Hydrocortisone 0.25%, 0.5%, 1.0%, 2.5% (Cortef, Hytone)	Cream, ointment
	Methylprednisolone acetate 0.25%, 1.0% (Medrol)	Ointment

Severe febrile illnesses, pregnancy, myxedema (condition resulting from hypothyroidism), and cancer therapies are conditions contributing to temporary hair loss.

A 2% minoxidil (Rogaine) solution has been approved by the FDA for treating alopecia. Minoxidil causes vasodilation. This increases cutaneous blood flow and stimulates hair-follicle growth. However, alopecia returns within 3 to 4 months after the patient stops using minoxidil. Systemic absorption of minoxidil is minimal and adverse reactions seldom occur.

BURNS

A burn causes lesions that break down skin exposing the body to infection. There are three causes of burns: heat (thermal), electricity (electrical), and chemicals. All cause the same kind of skin lesion.

Burns are classified by degree, which is based on the tissue depth of the burn. There are three burn classifications: first-degree, second-degree, and third degree. Burns are assessed by the percentage of body area that has been burned. This is commonly referred to as the Rule of Nines (see Table 20-3). For example, if a patient's left leg is burned, then 18% of the patient's body is burned.

First-degree (superficial) burns

First-degree burns affect only the epidermis (outer layer) of skin. The burn site is red, painful, dry, and with no blisters such as seen in a mild sunburn. Rarely

Table 20-3.   Rule of nines.

Body Area	Percentage Assessed
Head	9%
Front Torso	18%
Back Torso	18%
Right Arm	9%
Left Arm	9%
Right Leg	18%
Left Leg	18%
Groin	1%

is there any long-term tissue damage and it usually results in an increase or decrease in the skin color.

Treatment involves placing a cold, wet compress on the burned area in order to constrict blood vessels and reduce swelling and pain. Less tissue damage occurs if the burned area is cooled quickly. Remove clothing immediately and flush the burned area with water if a chemical agent caused the burn.

Don't apply greasy ointments, butter, or a dressing to the burned area. This inhibits heat loss and increases tissue damage. Bacitracin with polymyxin B (Polysporin) and similar over-the-counter antibiotics should be used.

Second-degree (partial thickness) burns

Second-degree burns expose the epidermis and part of the dermis layer of skin. The burn site appears red, blistered, and may be swollen and painful.

These burns can be quite painful and can become infected easily. They should be cleaned with a non-abrasive solution, treated with antibiotic ointment such as silver sulfadiazine (Silvadine), protected with a non-stick dressing, and the patient should be given an analgesic based on the amount of area burned and the pain experienced.

Third-degree (full thickness) burns

Third-degree burns destroy the epidermis and dermis and may also damage underlying nerve, bones, muscles, and tendons. The burn site appears white or charred and the patient has no sensation in the area since the nerve endings are destroyed.

Third-degree burns can be very painful because they are generally mixed (that is, second- and third-degree). Analgesics are used to manage the pain (see Chapter 16). Burn patients are susceptible to infection. With the skin gone, the patient is exposed to infection.

Third-degree burns are treated by first removing the charred skin (eschar) which is called debridement. This is a painful procedure. The patient is then given multiple antibiotics to prevent infections. The patient is also at risk for fluid and electrolyte imbalances (see Chapter 10) and at high risk for stress ulcers (see Chapter 18). Burn patients must be assessed for possible smoke inhalation. If it exists, the patient is treated with respiratory medications (see Chapter 14).

Burned areas must be cleansed with sterile saline solutions and an antiseptic such as povidone-iodine (Betadine). Broad-spectrum topical antibiotics are then applied to burn areas. These include antibacterials such as mafenide acetate

(Sulfamylon), silver sulfadiazine (Silvadene), silver nitrate 0.5% solution, and nitrofurazone (Furacin).

Third-degree burns are best managed in a designated burn center by a burn specialist or surgeon.

A list of drugs utilized in the treatment of burns is provided in the Appendix. Detailed tables show doses, recommendations, expectations, side effects, contraindications, and more; available on the book's Web site (see URL in Appendix).

ABRASIONS AND LACERATIONS

The most common skin injuries are abrasions and lacerations that are the result of accidents such as "road rash." This is caused by the body scraping along the roadway such as in a motorcycle accident. Patients who receive an abrasion or laceration are exposed to the same risk as a burn patient.

The site of the abrasion and laceration must be cleansed very carefully and treated with topical and sometimes systemic antibiotics and analgesics. Incomplete cleansing can result in tattoo-type scars.

Lacerations, commonly referred to as cuts, are interruptions in the integrity of the skin and should be monitored for signs of infection after they are cleaned and treated with antibiotics. Infection will cause the wound to appear red, swollen, and have purulent drainage (pus) and persistent pain.

Most minor cuts and abrasions are treated by cleaning the area with hydrogen peroxide or betadine and the applying a topical antibiotic such as Neosporin.

Some lacerations need to be sutured to close the open areas of the skin or topical skin adhesives are used to bring the edges together. Before suturing, the area must be flushed with copious amounts of normal saline. Sutures remain in place for about 7–10 days before they dissolve or are removed.

Puncture wounds do not cause a large area of visible injury to the skin but can carry a risk of damage to underlying tissues and infection. Puncture wounds should be cleansed carefully and monitored for signs of infection. The need for a tetanus toxoid booster immunization should be assessed.

Summary

Skin is the largest organ of the body composed of two major layers—the epidermis and dermis. Skin controls body temperature, provides protection against infection, the environment, and prevents the loss of bodily fluids.

There are many skin disorders. The more common are *acne vulgaris,* psoriasis, warts, dermatitis, alopecia, burns, abrasions, and lacerations.

Acne vulgarisis is an inflammation of the pilosebaceous glands and is treated by using a cleansing agent and applying topical anti-acne medication.

Psoriasis is a chronic skin disorder characterized by erythematous papules and plaques covered with silvery scales appearing on the scalp, elbows, palms of the hands, knees, and soles of the feet. Psoriasis is treated by using antisopriatic medication to loosen the psoriasis scales.

A wart is a benign lesion characterized as a hard, horny nodule on the hands and feet. Warts are removed by freezing, electrodesiccation, or surgical excision using topical treatments salicyclic acid, podophyllum resin, and cantharidin.

Dermatitis is a skin eruption that is caused by medications (drug-induced dermatitis) or by a chemical agent coming in touch with the skin (contact dermatitis). Dermatitis can be treated by using topical glucocorticoids.

Alopecia is male pattern baldness and occurs when the hair shaft is lost and the hair follicle cannot regenerate. Minoxidil (Rogaine) returns hair growth, but alopecia returns within 3 to 4 months after the patient stops using the drug.

A burn causes lesions that break-down skin and expose the body to infection. Burns are classified by degree, which is based on the tissue depth of the burn. There are three burn classifications: first-degree (superficial), second-degree (partial-thickness), and third degree (full-thickness) burns. Burns are treated by cleaning the burn site, removing charred skin, and then administering anti-infectives to prevent infection.

An abrasion is a scrape and a laceration is a cut. Both are cleaned and treated with topical antibiotics.

Quiz

1. *Acne vulgaris* is associated with
   (a) foods containing trans-fatty acids (TFA).
   (b) testosterone level.
   (c) genetics.
   (d) all of the above.

2. Keratolytics
   (a) loosen psoriasis scales.
   (b) are used to treat burn patients.
   (c) remove warts.
   (d) protect lesions from becoming infected.

3. Contact dermatitis is caused by
   (a) pollen.
   (b) sunlight.
   (c) plants.
   (d) none of the above.

4. First-degree burns affect only the epidermis of skin.
   (a) True
   (b) False

5. Podophyllum resin is used to remove venereal warts.
   (a) True
   (b) False

6. Absorption of topical glucocorticoids is greater at the
   (a) axilla.
   (b) feet.
   (c) eyelids.
   (d) all of the above.

7. A patient who has burns over 36% of his body may have a burned right leg and right arm
   (a) True
   (b) False

8. A wound that appears red, swollen, and has purulent drainage (pus) and persistent pain is said to be
   (a) infected.
   (b) healed.
   (c) starting to heal.
   (d) nearly healed.

9. The patient has little control over acne vulgaris.
   (a) True
   (b) False

10. Second-degree burns destroy the epidermis and dermis and may also damage underlying nerve, bones, muscles, and tendons.
    (a) True
    (b) False

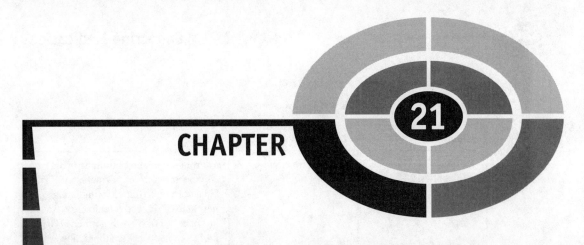

Endocrine Medications

When the hormones kick in and the adrenals begin pumping, practically nothing can stand in your way. However, you can quickly feel out of sorts and behave strangely if your body doesn't produce enough hormones or produces too many.

Hormones are messengers that influence how tissues, organs, and other parts of your body function. An overproduction of hormones causes an overreaction such as growing too tall. An underproduction of hormones causes an underreaction such as producing insufficient insulin to metabolize glucose.

In this chapter, you'll learn about disorders caused by hormone imbalance and you"ll learn about the drugs used to correct the imbalance.

A Brief Look at the Endocrine System

Glands of the endocrine system produce hormones that are distributed throughout the body in circulating blood. Hormones, synthesized from amino acids and cholesterol, affect cellular activity of tissues and organs.

There are two types of hormones: proteins (which are also known as small peptides) and steroids. Steroids are secreted from the adrenal glands and the gonads.

Endocrine glands are ductless glands that include the pituitary (hypophysis), thyroid, parathyroid, adrenals, gonads, and pancreas. Table 21-1 lists endocrine glands, their location, and the hormone(s) secreted by the gland.

Table 21-1.   Endocrine glands and their secretions.

Gland	Location	Secretes
Pituitary (hypophysis) Anterior (adenophypophysis)	Base of the brain	Thyroid-stimulating hormone (TSH) Adrenocorticotropic hormone (ACTH) Gonadotropins (follicle-stimulating hormone (FSH) and luteinizing hormone (LH). Growth hormone (GH), prolactin, melanocyte-stimulating hormone (MSH)
Posterior (neurohypophysis)		Antidiuretic hormone (ADH), vasopressin, oxytocin
Thyroid gland	Anterior to the trachea (Two lobes)	Thyroxine (T4) and triodothyroinine (T3)
Parathyroid gland	Lie on the dorsal surface of the thyroid gland (4 glands—2 pairs)	Parathormone (PTH)
Adrenal glands	Top of each kidney (2 sections—medulla is inner and 2 cortex surrounds medulla)	Cortex secretes corticosteroids (glucosteroids and mineralcorticoids); Small amounts of androgen, estrogen, and progestin.
Pancreas	Left of and behind the stomach (exocrine and endocrine gland)	Exocrine secretes digestive enzymes into the duodenum; Endocrine has cell clusters called islets of Langerhans; alpha islet cells produce glucagons; beta cells secrete insulin

Drugs and Hormones

Think of hormones as messengers that can increase or decrease tissue, organ, and cellular activities by the amount of hormones that are carried by the blood. Sometimes, through aging or disease, an inappropriate amount of hormones are produced causing the patient to experience adverse reactions.

Hormonal drug therapy is used to return the patient to hormonal balance by either replacing the missing hormone or by inhibiting the secretion of the hormone. Hormonal drug therapy is used for hormones produced by the pituitary, thyroid, parathyroid, and adrenal glands.

DRUGS AND THE PITUITARY GLAND

Growth hormone (GH) is secreted by the pituitary gland to influence growth. Gigantism (during childhood) and acromegaly (after puberty) can occur with GH hypersecretion. They are frequently caused by a pituitary tumor. If the tumor cannot be destroyed by radiation, or bromocriptine, a prolactin-release inhibitor can inhibit the release of GH from the pituitary. Octreotide (Sandostatin) is a potent synthetic somatostatin used to suppress growth hormone release. It is very expensive and gastrointestinal side effects are common.

If the pituitary gland produces too little GH, the patient will not reach a normal height. This is referred to as GH deficiency. Patients with this deficiency undergo GH replacement using Somatrem (protropin) and somatropin (Humatrope) to replenish the missing GH and enable normal growth to occur.

The posterior pituitary gland secretes antidiuretic hormone (ADH) and oxytocin. ADH is a vasopressin. Oxytocin is released to start labor contractions. ADH promotes water reabsorption from the renal tubules to maintain water balance in the body's fluids. A deficiency of ADH, called diabetes insipidus (DI), causes the kidneys to excrete large amounts of water. This leads to severe fluid volume deficit and electrolyte imbalances.

Diabetes insipidus can also be caused by head injury and brain tumors resulting in trauma to the hypothalamus and pituitary gland. You must monitor fluid and electrolyte balance in patients who have diabetes insipidus. ADH replacement may be needed.

Some of the drugs used for pituitary disorders include desmopressin acetate (DDAV), desmopressin (Stimate), lypressin (Diapid), vasopressin (aqueous) (Pitressin), vasopressin tannate/oil (Pitressin Tannate).

A list of anterior pituitary hormone and posterior pituitary hormone drugs are provided in the Appendix. Detailed tables show doses, recommendations, expectations, side effects, contraindications, and more; available on the book's Web site (see URL in Appendix).

DRUGS AND THE ADRENAL GLAND

There are two adrenal glands—located near the top of each kidney. The adrenal gland is comprised of two parts: the adrenal medulla and the adrenal cortex.

The adrenal cortex produces glucocorticoids (cortisol) and mineralocorticoids (aldosterone). Corticosteroids promote sodium retention and potassium excretion. Corticotropin (Acthar) is an ACTH drug that is used to diagnosis adrenal gland disorders.

Corticotropin (Acthar) is also used to treat adrenal gland insufficiency and as an anti-inflammatory drug in the treatment of allergic reactions such as anaphylaxis shock.

ACTH given intravenously increases the serum cortisol levels in 30 to 60 minutes if the adrenal gland is properly functioning. ACTH will eventually stimulate cortisol production if pituitary insufficiency causes steroid deficiency.

Table 21-2 shows the effects of an adrenal gland that produces too much (hypersecretion) or too little hormone (hyposecretion). Adrenal hyposecretion is called Addison's disease and hypersecretion is called Cushing's syndrome.

ACTH is a hormone released by the anterior pituitary gland that influences the glucocorticoids that are secreted by the adrenal gland. Glucocorticoids affect carbohydrate, protein, and fat metabolism in addition to muscle and blood cell activity.

Table 21-2.   Effects of adrenal hyposecretion and hypersecretion.

Body System	Hyposecretion	Hypersecretion
Metabolism Glucose Protein Fat	Hypoglycemia Muscle weakness	Hyperglycemia Muscle wasting; thinning of the skin; fat accumulation in face, neck, and trunk (protruding abdomen, buffalo hump); hyperlipidemia; high cholesterol
Central Nervous System	Apathy, depression, fatigue	Increased neural activity; mood elevation; irritability; seizures
Gastrointestinal	Nausea, vomiting, abdominal pain	Peptic ulcers
Cardiovascular	Tachycardia, hypotension, cardiovascular collapse	Hypertension; edema; heart failure
Eyes	None	Cataract formation
Fluids and Electrolytes	Hypovolumia; hyponatremia; hyperkalemia	Hypervolemia; hypernatremia; hypokalemia
Blood cells	Anemia	Increased red blood cell count and neutrophils; impaired clotting

Glucocorticoids can cause sodium absorption from the kidney that result in water retention, potassium loss, and increased blood pressure. Cortisol, the primary glucocorticoid, has anti-inflammatory, anti-allergic, and antistress effects.

Glucocorticoid therapy is used in trauma, surgery, infections, emotional upsets, and anxiety. Most glucocorticoid drugs are synthetically produced and are administered orally, IM, IV, topically (see Chapter 20), intranasally (see Chapter 14), and as aerosol inhalers (see Chapter 14).

Glucocorticoid drugs include beclomethasone dipropionate (Vanceril), betamethasone (Celestone), cortisone acetate (Cortone Acetate), dexamethasone (Decadron), fludrocortisone acetate (Florinef Acetate), hydrocortisone (Hydrocortone), methylprednisoline (Medrol, Solu-Medrol, Depo-Medrol), prednisolone, and prednisone. The adrenal medulla synthesizes, stores, and releases epinephrine and norepinephrine. Hypersecretion causes prolonged or continual sympathetic nervous system responses. A lack of secretion from the adrenal medulla has no significant effects.

DRUGS AND THE THYROID GLAND

The thyroid gland secretes two hormones that regulate protein synthesis, enzyme activity, and stimulate mitochondrial oxidation. These are thyroxine (T4) and tri-iodothyronine (T3). The thyroid gland secretes 20% of the circulating T3. The remaining 80% comes from degradation of T4 hormone. Approximately 40% of T4 is degraded and becomes T3.

T3 and T4 are carried in the blood by thyroxine-binding globulin (TBG) and albumin, which protects the hormones from being degraded. T3 is more potent than T4. Only unbound free T3 and T4 are active and produce a hormonal response.

A decreased amount of T3 and T4 is produced in a condition called hypothyroidism. This is caused by a disorder of the thyroid gland or a secondary lack of TSH secretion. Hyperthyroidism is an increase in circulatory T4 and T3 caused by an overactive thyroid gland or an excessive output of thyroid hormones.

Hypothyroidism

Primary hypothyroidism is characterized by a decrease in T4 and an increase in TSH levels. Primary hypothyroidism is caused by acute or chronic inflammation of the thyroid gland, radioiodine therapy, excess intake of antithyroid drugs, and surgery.

Myexedema is severe hypothyroidism characteristic by lethargy, apathy, memory impairment, emotional changes, slow speech, deep coarse voice, edema of the eyelids and face, thick dry skin, cold intolerance, slow pulse, constipation, weight gain, and abnormal menses.

In children, hypothyroidism can have a congenital (cretinism) or prepubertal (juvenile hypothyroidism) onset.

Hypothyroidism is treated by administering levothyroxine sodium (Levothroid, Synthroid), which increases levels of T3 and T4. Levothyroxine sodium (Levothroid, Synthroid) is also used to treat simple goiter and chronic lymphocytic (Hashimoto's) thyroiditis.

Lyothyronine (Cytomel) is a synthetic T3 that is used for short-term treatment of hypothyroidism. It isn't used for maintenance therapy because lyothyronine has a short half-life and duration.

Liotric (Euthroid, Thyrolar) is a mixture of levothyroxine sodium and liothyronine sodium with no significant advantage over levothyroxine sodium. Thyroid and thyroglubin (Proloid) are seldom used.

A list of drugs utilized in the treatment of hypothyroidism is provided in the Appendix. Detailed tables show doses, recommendations, expectations, side effects, contraindications, and more; available on the book's Web site (see URL in Appendix).

Hyperthyroidism

Hyperthyroidism is an increase in circulating T4 and T3 levels resulting from an overactive thyroid gland or excessive output of thyroid hormones. Hyperthyroidism may be mild with few symptoms or severe leading to vascular collapse and death.

Graves' disease or thyrotoxicosis is the most common type of hyperthyroidism and is caused by a hyperfunctioning thyroid gland. Graves' disease is characterized by a rapid pulse (tachycardia), palpitations, excessive perspiration, heat intolerance, nervousness, irritability, exopthalmos (bulging eyes), and weight loss. Treatment involves surgical removal of a portion of the thyroid gland (subtotal thyroidectomy), radioactive iodine therapy, or antithyroid drugs that inhibit either the synthesis or the release of thyroid hormones.

Antithyroid drugs reduce the excessive secretion of T4 and T3 by inhibiting thyroid secretion. Thiourea derivatives (thioamides) are the drugs of choice used to decrease thyroid production.

Propylthiouracid (PTU) and methylthiouracil (Tapazole) are effective thioamide antithyroid drugs used for treating thyrotoxic crisis and in preparation for subtotal thyroidectomy. Methimazole does not inhibit peripheral conversion of T4 to T3 as does PTU, but it is 10 times more potent and has a longer half-life than PTU. Prolonged use of thioamides may cause a goiter because of the increased TSH secretion that inhibits T4 and T3 synthesis. Minimal doses should be given when indicated to avoid goiter formation.

Strong iodide preparations such as Lugol's solution are used to suppress thyroid function in patients having a subtotal thyroidectomy for Graves's disease. Sodium iodide administered intravenously is useful for the management of thyrotoxic crisis.

A list of drugs utilized in the treatment of hyperthyroidism is provided in the Appendix. Detailed tables show doses, recommendations, expectations, side effects, contraindications, and more; available on the book's Web site (see URL in Appendix).

DRUGS AND THE PARATHYROID GLANDS

The parathyroid glands secrete parathyroid hormone (PTH) that regulate calcium levels in the blood. A decrease in serum calcium stimulates the release of PTH. A decrease of PTH is called hypoparathyroidism and an increase in PTH is hyperparathyroidism.

Hypoparathyroidism is treated with PTH drugs and hyperparathyroidism is treated with calcitonin. Calcitonin decreases serum calcium levels by promoting renal excretion of calcium.

PTH deficiency can cause hypocalcemia, which is a deficit of serum calcium. Hypocalcemia can also be caused by vitamin D deficiency, renal impairment, or diuretic therapy.

Hypocalcemia is treated with PTH replacement that corrects the calcium deficit by promoting calcium absorption from the GI tract, promotes calcium reabsorption from the renal tubules, and activates Vitamin D. Calcitriol is a vitamin D analogue that promotes calcium absorption from the GI tract and secretion of calcium of bone to the bloodstream.

Hyperparathyroidism is caused by malignancies of the parathyroid glands or ectopic PTH hormone secretion from lung cancer, hyperthyroidism, or prolonged immobility during which calcium is lost from bone.

DRUGS AND THE PANCREAS

The pancreas secretes insulin that is used to metabolize glucose. The patient contracts diabetes mellitus if insufficient insulin is produced. Diabetes mellitus is a chronic disease resulting from deficient glucose metabolism caused by insufficient insulin secretion from the beta cells of the pancreas. Table 21-3 illustrates hypo-glycemic and hyperglycemic reactions caused by a deficient glucose metabolism.

There are two types of diabetes mellitus: Type I and Type II.

Type 1 diabetes mellitus

Type 1 diabetes mellitus is referred to as insulin-dependent diabetes mellitus (IDDM) or juvenile-onset diabetes because Type 1 diabetes mellitus usually begins in childhood or adolescence. In Type 1 diabetes mellitus, the pancreas produces little or no insulin.

Type 1 diabetes mellitus is characterized by a sudden onset that occurs more frequently in populations descended from Northern European countries (Finland, Scotland, Scandinavia) than in those from Southern European countries, the Middle East, or Asia.

Approximately 3 in 1000 people in the United States develop Type 1 diabetes and are dependent on regular insulin injections.

Type 2 diabetes mellitus

Type 2 diabetes mellitus, sometimes called age-onset or adult-onset diabetes, is the common form of diabetes mellitus that effects approximately 5% of Americans under the age of 50 and 15% of those 50 and older. More than 90% of the diabetics in the United States have Type 2 diabetes mellitus.

Patients with Type 2 diabetes mellitus are often overweight and don't exercise. They can produce insulin but are unable to use it effectively. Type 2

Table 21-3. Hypoglycemic reactions and diabetic ketoacidosis.

Reaction	Signs and Symptoms
Hypoglycemic reaction (insulin shock)	Headache, lightheadedness, nervousness, apprehension, tremor, excess perspiration; cold, clammy skin, tachycardia, slurred speech, memory lapse, confusion, seizures Blood sugar <60 mg/dL
Diabetic ketoacidosis (hyperglycemic reaction)	Extreme thirst, polyuria, fruity breath odor, Kussmaul breathing (deep, rapid, labored, distressing, dyspnea), rapid, thready pulse, dry mucous membranes, poor skin turgor Blood sugar level >250 mg/dL

diabetes mellitus is more common in people of Aboriginal, Hispanic, and African-American descent. People who have emigrated to the West from India, Japan, and Australian, more likely to develop Type 2 diabetes mellitus than those who remain in their original countries.

Type 2 diabetes mellitus is considered a milder form of diabetes mellitus because of its slow onset (sometimes developing over the course of several years) and because it can usually be controlled with diet and oral medication. Type 2 diabetes mellitus is also called noninsulin-dependent diabetes (NIDDM), a term that is somewhat misleading. Many people with Type II diabetes mellitus can control the condition with diet and oral medications. However, insulin injections are sometimes necessary if treatment with diet and oral medication is not adequate.

Uncontrolled and untreated Type 2 diabetes mellitus is as serious as Type 1 diabetes mellitus.

Gestational diabetes mellitus

Gestational diabetes mellitus develops during pregnancy and resolves after delivery. Gestational diabetes mellitus develops during the second or third trimester of pregnancy in about 2% of pregnancies and is treated by diet. However, insulin injections may be required. Women who have gestational diabetes mellitus are at higher risk for developing Type 2 diabetes mellitus within 5–10 years.

SIGNS AND SYMPTOMS OF DIABETES MELLITUS

The signs and symptoms of diabetes are polyuria (increased urine output), polydipsia (increased thirst), and polyphagia (increased hunger). Certain drugs increase blood sugar and can cause hyperglycemia in prediabetic persons. These include glucocorticoids (cortisone, prednisone), thiazide diuretics (hydrochlorothiazide [HydroDIURIL]), and epinephrine. Usually the blood sugar returns to normal after the drug is discontinued.

INSULIN

Insulin is a protein that cannot be administered orally because GI secretions destroy the insulin structure. Insulin is therefore administered subcutaneously in a special insulin syringe (see Chapter 6). The site and depth of the injection affects the absorption and is greater when given in the deltoid and abdominal areas than when given in the thighs and buttocks. Heat and massage can increase subcutaneous absorption. Cooling the area can decrease absorption.

Insulin can also be delivered via insulin pump. An insulin pump is surgically implanted in the abdomen and delivers an insulin infusion and bolus doses with meals either intraperitoneally or intravenously.

Insulin can also be administered intranasally to provide a rapid-onset effect for a short duration although this method is expensive and rarely used.

Insulin injectors deliver insulin under high pressure through the skin into fatty tissue without a needle. Insulin injectors can cause bruising, pain, and burning and are not indicated for children or the elderly. Insulin injectors are expensive.

Insulin types

There are three standard types of insulin:

- Rapid-acting (regular or Lispro [Humalog] insulin), onset $1/2$ to 1 hour, peak 2 to 4 hours, and a duration of 6 to 8 hours
- Intermediate-acting (NPH, Humulin N, Lente, and Humulin L insulin), onset 1–2 hours, peak 6–12 hours, duration 18–24 hours
- Long-acting (Ultralente insulin), onset 5–8 hours, peak 14–20 hours, duration 30–36 hours

There are also combinations that include Humulin 70/30 (NPH 70%, regular 30%) and Humulin 50/50 (NPH 50%, regular 50%).

Unopened insulin vials are refrigerated until needed. Once an insulin vial has been opened it may be kept at room temperature for 1 month or in the refrigerator for 3 months. An open insulin vial should not be put in the freezer, placed in direct sunlight, or in a high-temperature area.

A list of drugs utilized in the treatment of diabetes is provided in the Appendix. Detailed tables show doses, recommendations, expectations, side effects, contraindications, and more; available on the book's Web site (see URL in Appendix).

ORAL ANTIDIABETICS

Oral antidiabetic drugs such as sulfonylureas are administered to patients who have Type 2 diabetes mellitus to stimulate beta cells to secrete insulin. This results in an increase in insulin cell receptors, enabling cells to bind to insulin during glucose metabolism. Sulfonylureas are chemically related to sulfon-amides but lack antibacterial activity.

Sulfonylureas are classified as first- and second-generation drugs and each generation is divided into short-acting, intermediate-acting, and long-acting antidiabetics.

First-generation sulfonylureas are:

- Tolbutamide (Orinase)
- Acetohexamide (Dymelor)
- Tolazamide (Tolinase)
- Chlorpropamide (Diabinese)

Second-generation sulfonylureas include

- Glipizide (Glucotrol)
- Glyburide nonmicronized (DiaBeta, Micronase)
- Glimepiride (Amryl)

Second-generation sulfonylureas increase tissue response to insulin and decrease glucose production by the liver. This results in greater hypoglycemic potency at smaller doses. Second-generation sulfonylureas have a longer dura-tion of action and cause few side effects, but should not be used if the patient has liver or kidney dysfunction.

Nonsulfonylureas are new drugs that affect the hepatic and GI production of glucose. For example, metformin (Glucophage) is a nonsulfonylurea biguanide compound that acts by decreasing hepatic production of glucose from stored glycogen. The result is a reduced increase in serum glucose following a meal and limits the degree of post-prandial (after a meal) hyperglycemia.

Metformin (Glucophage) also decreases the absorption of glucose from the small intestine and may increase insulin receptor sensitivity as well as peripheral glucose uptake at the cellular level. Metformin does not produce hypoglycemia or hyperglycemia and can cause GI disturbances. Metformin can be used alone. When combined with a sulfonylurea, however, it is useful in cases resistant to oral antidiabetics.

Alpha-glucosidase inhibitors (acarbose [Precose]) inhibit alpha glucosidase, the digestive enzyme in the small intestine that is responsible for the release of glucose from the complex carbohydrates in the diet. By inhibiting alpha glu-cosidase, carbohydrates cannot be absorbed and instead, pass into the large intestine. Acarbose has no systemic effects, is not absorbed into the body in sig-nificant amounts, and does not cause a hypoglycemic reaction.

Thiazolidinediones such as Pioglitazone (Actos), decrease insulin resistance and help muscle cells to respond to insulin and use glucose more effectively. Thiazolidinediones may be used in addition to sulfonylurea, metformin, or insulin for insulin-resistant patients. Pioglitazone (Actos) has no significant side effects or adverse effects.

Rapaglinide (Prandin) is used alone or in combination with metformin as a short-acting similar to sulfonylureas, however Rapaglinide does not cause a hypoglycemic reaction.

GLUCAGON

Glucagon is a hyperglycemic hormone secreted by the alpha cells of the islets of Langerhans in the pancreas and increases blood sugar by stimulating glycogenolysis (glycogen breakdown) in the liver.

Glucagon protects the body cells, especially those in the brain and retina, by providing the nutrients and energy needed to maintain body function. Glucagon, available for parenteral use, treats insulin-induced hypoglycemia when other methods of providing glucose are not available. Glucagon can increase blood glucose level in patients who are semiconscious or unconscious and unable to ingest carbohydrates.

Oral diazoxide (Proglycem) increases blood sugar by inhibiting insulin release from the beta cells and stimulating release of epinephrine (Adrenalin) from the adrenal medulla. Oral diazoxide (Proglycem) is used to treat chronic hypoglycemia caused by hyperinsulinism due to islet cell cancer or hyperplasia, but not for hypoglycemic reactions. Patients don't experience hypotension when taking oral diazoxide (Proglycem).

A list of antidiabetic second generation drugs is provided in the Appendix. Detailed tables show doses, recommendations, expectations, side effects, contraindications, and more; available on the book's Web site (see URL in Appendix).

Summary

Glands of the endocrine system produce hormones that are distributed throughout the body by blood vessels. Hormones are messengers that influence how tissues, organs, and other parts of your body function. Glands can overproduce or underproduce hormones causing parts of the body to behave inappropriately.

Hormonal drug therapy is used to return the patient to hormonal balance by either replacing the missing hormone or by inhibiting the secretion of the hormone. Hormonal drug therapy is used for hormones produced by the pituitary, thyroid, parathyroid, and adrenal glands.

The pituitary gland secretes the growth hormone. Octreotide (Sandostatin) is used to suppress growth hormone release. Somatrem (protropin) and somatropin (Humatrope) are used to replenish missing growth hormone.

The adrenal glands produce a number of hormones. Cortiocotropin (Acthar) is used to treat adrenal gland insufficiency.

The thyroid gland secretes two hormones that regulate protein synthesis and enzyme activity and to stimulate mitochondrial oxidation. These are Thyroxine (T4) and triiodothyronine (T3). Levothyroxine sodium (Levothroid, Synthroid) is used to increase the production T3 and T4. Thiourea derivatives (thioamides) inhibit T3 and T4.

The parathyroid glands secrete parathyroid hormone (PTH) that regulate calcium levels in the blood. Calcitonin increases the level of PTH.

The pancreas secretes insulin that is used to metabolize glucose. Insulin is used to treat a decreased output of insulin by the pancreas.

Quiz

1. An overproduction of GH results in
   (a) acromegaly.
   (b) gigantism.
   (c) abnormal growth.
   (d) all of the above.

2. ADH replacement is needed in trauma to the
   (a) hypothalamus and pituitary gland.
   (b) pancreas.
   (c) liver.
   (d) adrenal gland.

3. Addison's disease is caused by
   (a) underproduction of the adrenal gland.
   (b) overproduction of the adrenal gland.
   (c) overproduction of the pancreas.
   (d) underproduction of the pancreas.

4. Glucocorticoids therapy is used in trauma, surgery, infections, emotional upsets and anxiety.
   (a) True
   (b) False

5. Lyothyronine (Cytomel) is a synthetic T3 that is used for short-term treatment of hypothyroidism.
   (a) True
   (b) False

6. Graves' disease is caused by
   (a) overproduction of the thyroid gland.
   (b) underproduction of the thyroid gland.
   (c) overproduction of the parathyroid gland.
   (d) underproduction of the parathyroid gland.

7. In Type 1 diabetes mellitus, the pancreas produces little or no insulin.
   (a) True
   (b) False

8. Type 2 is considered a milder form of diabetes mellitus because
   (a) the pancreas secretes a normal amount of insulin after the patient gives birth.
   (b) it affects only children.
   (c) it has a slow onset and is usually controlled with diet and oral medication.
   (d) none of the above.

9. Diabetes insipidus (DI) is a deficiency of ADH.
   (a) True
   (b) False

10. Hormonal drug therapy inhibits the secretion of a hormone.
    (a) True
    (b) False

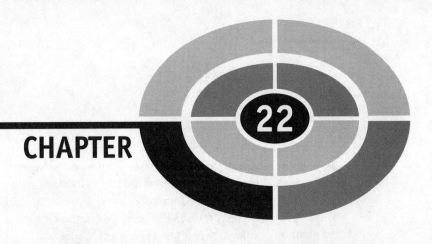

CHAPTER 22

Disorders of the Eye and Ear

Most of us become anxious whenever anything happens to our vision or hearing and tend to avoid reporting the condition to our healthcare professional fearing devastating news—we're going blind or deaf.

The truth is that common eye and ear disorders rarely result in loss of sight and hearing once the disorder is diagnosed and treated with the proper medication. Some conditions heal themselves and others are cured with a few weeks of treatment.

This chapter takes a look at common disorders that affect the eyes and the ears and discusses drugs that are used to treat those disorders.

Eye Disorders

The eye has three layers. The first layer contains the cornea and sclera. The second layer contains the choroid, iris, and ancillary body. The third layer contains the retina that connects to the brain through the optic nerve.

There are three common disorders of the eye: glaucoma, conjunctivitis, and corneal abrasion.

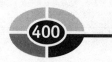

GLAUCOMA

The eye is under constant intraocular pressure (IOP) that increases in patients who have glaucoma. This increased pressure damages the optic nerve resulting in decreased peripheral vision and eventually blindness.

About three million Americans have glaucoma, 120,000 of them have lost their eyesight. Glaucoma is the leading cause of blindness. There are two types of glaucoma: chronic (primary) open-angle glaucoma (POAG) and acute closed-angle glaucoma.

Chronic open-angle glaucoma

Chronic open-angle glaucoma is the most common form of glaucoma. The "open" drainage angle of the eye can become blocked leading to a gradual increase in eye pressure. If this increased pressure results in optic nerve damage, it is known as chronic open-angle glaucoma. The optic nerve damage and vision loss usually occurs so gradually and painlessly that you are not aware of trouble until the optic nerve is already badly damaged.

Angle-closure glaucoma

Angle-closure glaucoma results when the drainage angle of the eye narrows and becomes completely blocked. In the eye, the iris may close off the drainage angle and cause a dangerously high eye pressure. When the drainage angle of the eye suddenly becomes completely blocked, pressure builds up rapidly, and this is called acute angle-closure glaucoma. The symptoms include severe eye pain, blurred vision, headache, rainbow haloes around lights, nausea, and vomiting. Unless an ophthalmologist treats acute angle-closure glaucoma quickly, blindness can result. When the drainage angle of the eye gradually becomes completely blocked, pressure builds up gradually, and this is called chronic angle-closure glaucoma. This form of glaucoma occurs more frequently in people of African and Asian ancestry, and in certain eye conditions.

Acute angle-closure glaucoma is a medical emergency. If IOP is not reduced within hours of onset, the patient's vision can be permanently damaged.

CONJUNCTIVITIS

Conjunctivitis, commonly known as pink eye, is an inflammation of the thin, clear membrane that covers the white part of the eye and the eyelids (the conjunctiva). This inflammation causes the white of the eye and the inside of eyelids to become pink or red. The patient's eyes may be itchy or painful.

There are four types of conjunctivitis. These are:

1. Viral conjunctivitis. Viral conjunctivitis affects only one eye causing excessive eye watering and a light discharge from the eye.
2. Bacterial conjunctivitis. Bacterial conjunctivitis affects both eyes causing a heavy greenish discharge.
3. Allergic conjunctivitis. Allergic conjunctivitis also affects both eyes causing itching and redness and excessive tearing. The patient may also experience an itchy and red nose.
4. Giant papillary conjunctivitis. Giant papillary conjunctivitis (GPC) affects both eyes causing contact lens intolerance, itching, heavy discharge, and tearing and red bumps on the underside of the eyelids.

CORNEAL ABRASION

A corneal abrasion is a cut or scratch on the cornea, which is the clear, protective membrane covering the colored part of the eye (iris). Corneal abrasion can be caused by sand, dust, dirt, and shavings from materials such as metal. Fingernails, tree branches, rubbing your eyes, and even contact lenses can also scratch the cornea. Some patients have a weak outer layer of the cornea that can sustain an abrasion for no apparent reason.

Most corneal abrasions heal properly with the proper treatment. However, if the treatment isn't successful, the abrasion can reappear months following the originally injury.

Corneal abrasions are painful because of the sensitivity of the cornea. Patients may feel as if there is sand in their eye. Their eyes become teary and red. Their vision is blurry and light hurts their eyes (photophobia). Corneal abrasions have been known to cause headaches.

Fluorescein sodium and fluress (fluorescein sodium and benoxinate HCl) are used to diagnose corneal abrasions and to locate lesions or foreign objects in the eye.

Fluorescein is a dye used to demonstrate defects in corneal epithelium and is excreted in nasal secretions if the lacrimal (tear) duct is patent.

When fluorescence strips are used to examine the eye:

- Corneal scratches turn bright red.
- Foreign bodies are surrounded by a green ring.
- Loss of conjunctiva appears orange yellow.

Fluress is a dye and a local anesthetic and is used for short corneal and conjunctival procedures such as removing foreign bodies from the eye.

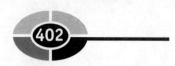

Eye Medication

Eye disorders are treated by using one of a variety of medications (Table 22-1).

Topical Anesthetics

Topical anesthetics are used to anesthetize the eye for comprehensive eye examinations and for removal of foreign bodies from the eye. Onset occurs in about 1 minute and lasts for 15 minutes. During this time, the blink reflex is temporarily lost and the corneal epithelium is temporarily dried. The patient is required to wear a protective eye patch until the effects of the drug wear off.

Anti-infectives and Antimicrobials

Anti-infectives and antimicrobials are administered for eye infections such as conjunctivitis. These drugs can cause local skin and eye irritation. You learned about anti-infective and antimicrobial medication in Chapter 12 and Chapter 13.

Lubricants

Lubricants are used to alleviate the discomfort that is associated with dry eyes and to moisten contact lenses and artificial eyes. Lubricants are also used to maintain the integrity of the epithelial surface and to moisten the eye during anesthesia and unconsciousness.

Miotics

Miotics lower intraocular pressure in open-angle glaucoma allowing increased bloodflow to the retina. This results in less retinal damage and prevents the loss of vision. There are two types of miotics: direct-acting cholinergics and cholinesterase inhibitors. Direct-acting cholinergics pupillary constrict and cholinesterase inhibitors pupillary constrict. Patients who take miotics might experience headache, eye pain, decreased vision, brow pain, and less frequently hyperemia of the conjunctivia (red eye). Miotics can be systemically absorbed resulting in the patient experiencing nausea, vomiting, diarrhea, frequent urination, precipitation of asthma attacks, increased salivation, diaphoresis, muscle weakness, and respiratory difficulty.

Carbonic Anhydrase Inhibitors

Carbonic anhydrase inhibitors are used as a long-term treatment for open-angle glaucoma by decreasing intraocular pressure by interfering with the production of aqueous humor. Patients who take carbonic anhydrase inhibitors can experience lethargy, anorexia, drowsiness, paresthesia, depression, polyuria, nausea, vomiting, hypokalemia, and renal calculi. It is because of these adverse side effects that patients frequently discontinue taking carbonic anhydrase inhibitors. Carbonic anhydrase inhibitors are contraindicated in the first trimester of pregnancy and for patients who are allergic to sulfonamides.

Osmotics

Osmotics are preoperative and postoperative medications used to reduce intraocular pressure by decreasing vitreous humor volume. They are also used in the emergency treatment of closed-angle glaucoma. Patients who are administered osmotics can experience headache, nausea, vomiting, and diarrhea. Elderly patients can become disoriented.

Anticholinergic mydriatics and cycloplegics

Anticholinergic mydriatics and cycloplegics are used in diagnostic procedures and ophthalmic surgery. Anticholinergic mydriatics dilate the pupils. Cycloplegics paralyze eye muscles. Patients who are treated with these medications experience tachycardia, photophobia, dryness of the mouth, edema, conjunctivitis, and derematitis. You learned about anticholinergics in Chapter 15.

A list of eye disorder drugs is provided in the Appendix. Detailed tables show doses, recommendations, expectations, side effects, contraindications, and more; available on the book's Web site (see URL in Appendix).

Patient Education for Eye Medication

It is important that patients understand the effects of their eye disorder and the effects of the medication treating the condition. Patients are anxious about eye disorders fearing that they could lose their vision.

Demonstrate the proper technique to administer eye drops and ointment. Be sure that the patient knows how to maintain a sterile technique so the eyedropper does not become contaminated.

Tell the patient about expected side effects such as blurry vision and that administering the medication at bedtime can avoid problems that could arise from temporary loss of vision.

The patient should record each time they administer the medication. This is especially important for patients who are confused or forgetful and could accidentally receive an overdose of the medication. The patient should not stop taking the medication without consulting his or her healthcare provider.

Table 22-1. Ophthalmic medications.

Antibacterials	Antifungals	Antivirals	Anti-inflammatories
Chloramphenicol (Chlormycetin Ophthalmic)	Natamycin (Natacyn Ophthalmic)	Idoxuridine (IDU)	Dexamethasone
Ciprofloxacin (Cipro)		Trifluridine (Viroptic)	Diclofenac Na (Voltaren)
Erythromycin		Vidarabine monohydrate (Vira-A)	Suprofen (Profenal)
Gentamicin sulfate (Garamycin Ophthalmic)			Ketorolac tromethamine (Acular)
Norfloxacin (Chibroxin)			Olopatadine HCl Ophthalmic solution
Tobramycin (Nebcin, Tobrex)			Medrysone (HMS Liquifilm)
Silver nitrate 1% (used in neonates to prevent ophthalmia neoatorum)			Prednisolone acetate
			Prednisolone Na phosphate
Tetracycline HCL (Achromycin Ophthalmic)			Combination: TobraDex (tobramycin 0.3% and dexamethasone 0.1%)
Miotics: Cholinergics and beta-adrenergic blockers	**Indirect-acting cholinesterase inhibitors: Short acting**	**Beta-adrenergic blockers**	**Carbonic anhydrase inhibitors**
Acetylcholine Cl (Miochol)	Physostigmine salicylate (Osopto Eserine)	Betaxolol HCl (Betoptic)	Acetazolamide (Diamox)
Carbachol intraocular (Miostat)		Levobunolol HCl	Brinzolamideophthalmic sus. 1%
Pilocarpine HCl (Isopto Carpine)		Timolol maleate (Timoptic)	Dichlorphenamide (Daranide)
Pilocarpine nitrate (Ocusert Pilo-20)			Dorzolamide (Trusopt)
Echothiophate iodide (Phospholine Iodide)			Methazolamide (Neptazane)

Table 22-1. Ophthalmic medications. *(continued)*

Antibacterials	Antifungal	Antiviral	Antiinflammatories
Osmotics	**Mydriatics and Cycloplegics**		
Glycerin	Atropine sulfate		
Isosorbide (Ismotic)	Cyclopentolate HCl		
Mannitol (Osmitrol)	Dipivefrin HCl		
Urea (Ureaphil)	Epinephrine HCl		
	Epinephrine borate		
	Homatropine hydrobromide (Isopto Homatropine)		
	Scopolamine hydrobromide		
	Tropicamide (Mydriacyl Ophthalmic)		

Ask the patient to wear a medical alert bracelet if they are taking glaucoma medications or if they are allergic to any medication.

Ear Disorders

The ear consists of three parts: the external, middle, and inner ear. The external ear consists of the pinna and the external auditory canal that transmits sound to the middle ear. The middle ear has an air-filled cavity that contains auditory ossicles, which are the malleus, incus, and stapes. The auditory ossicles forward the sound to the inner ear where the eardrum is located. Pressure on both sides of the eardrum is equalized by the eustachian tube that connects to the nasopharynx. The eardrum could rupture if pressure becomes unequal. The inner ear also contains a series of canals called the labyrinths that are made up of the vestibule, cochlea, and semicircular canals. The vestibule maintains equilibrium and balance and the cochlea is the principal hearing organ.

Common ear disorders are cerumen (ear wax) impaction, otitis external, otitis media (infections of the external and middle ear), and vestibular disorders of the inner ear.

CERUMEN IMPACTION

Cerumen (ear wax) is produced by glands in the outer portion of the ear canal. Cerumen moves down the canal to the external os (opening) where the cerumen is washed away. When this process fails, cerumen becomes impacted and must be loosened by using ceruminolytics such as a hydrogen peroxide solution (3% diluted to $1/2$ strength with water). The ear canal is irrigated with ceruminolytics, which flushes cerumen deposits out of the ear canal. Patients who have chronic cerumen impaction are treated with drops of olive oil or mineral oil or by Cerumenex and Debrox. Cerumenex is available by prescription and Debrox is an over-the-counter medication.

OTITIS EXTERNA AND OTITIS MEDIA

Otitis externa and otitis media are infections of the external and middle ear, respectively. These disorders are treated with analgesics and antibiotics. Antibiotics are discussed in Chapter 13. Analgesics are discussed in Chapter 16. Table 22-2 contains commonly used antibiotics for ear infections. Most ear infections are caused by a virus and should not be treated with an antibiotic.

VESTIBULAR DISORDERS

The most frequently reported symptoms of vestibular disorders are dizziness, unsteadiness or imbalance when walking, vertigo, and nausea. These symptoms may be quite mild, lasting minutes, or quite severe, resulting in total disability.

Because the vestibular system interacts with many other parts of the nervous system, symptoms may also be experienced as problems with vision, muscles, thinking, and memory. In addition, people with vestibular disorders may suffer headache and muscular aches in the neck and back, increased tendency to suffer from motion sickness, and increased sensitivity to noise and

Table 22-2.   Common medications used to treat ear infections.

External Ear	Internal Ear
Acetic acid and aluminum acetate (Otic Deomboro)	Amoxicillin (amoxil, Augmentin)
	Ampicillin trihydrate (Polycillin)
Boric acid (Ear-Dry), Carbamide peroxide (Debrox)	Cefaclor (Ceclor)
Chloramphenical (Chloromycetin Otic)	Erythromycin (E-Mycin)
	Penicillin (Pentids, Pen-V)
Polymyxin B	Sulfonamides (Azulfidine, Bactrim)
Tetracycline (Achromycin)	Clarithromycin (biaxin)
Trolamine polypeptide oleate-condensate (Cerumenex)	Amoxicillin and potassium clavulanate (Augmentin)
	Loracarbef (Lorabid)

bright lights. Patients with vestibular disorders often report fatigue and loss of stamina and an inability to concentrate. Difficulty with reading and speech may occur during times of fatigue. When these symptoms are constant and disabling, they may be accompanied by irritability, loss of self-esteem, and/or depression. Meniere's disease, labyrinthitis, and inner ear infections should cause vestibular disorders.

EAR PAIN

Ear pain usually resolves itself between 48 and 72 hours from the onset of the pain. However, analgesics such as acetaminophen or ibuprofen should be administered to relieve the pain in the interim.

EAR CONGESTION

Ear congestion can be caused by the improper drainage of the eustachian tube. This can be relieved by administering antihistamine-decongestant medications such as Actifed, Allerest, Dimetapp, Drixoral, Novafed, Ornade, and Triaminic, all of which are available over the counter.

Patient Education for Ear Medication

Patients should understand that they should not place any foreign objects into their ear canal including Q-Tips. Ceruminolytics should be used to remove cerumen. Patients who are prone to swimmer's ear (otitis externa) should keep the ear canal dry by placing two drops of alcohol in the ear canal.

Many medications used to treat ear disorders are sensitive to light. Therefore, they should be kept in a light-resistant container.

All antibiotics must be taken for the prescribed length of time (10–14 days). The patient should not stop taking antibiotics once the pain has subsided.

The patient should report any change in hearing. Some patients may not report the loss to their healthcare professional because they consider the loss of hearing as part of aging or due to exposure to environmental noises.

Summary

There are three common eyes disorders: glaucoma, conjunctivitis, and corneal abrasion. Glaucoma is characterized by an increase in intraocular pressure that, if left untreated, can damage the optic nerve and lead to blindness.

Conjunctivitis is inflammation of the thin, clear membrane that covers the white part of the eye and the eyelids. There are four types of conjunctivitis: viral conjunctivitis, bacterial conjunctivitis, allergic conjunctivitis, and giant papillary conjunctivitis. A corneal abrasion is a cut or scratch on the cornea caused by debris, fingernails, contact lenses, or rubbing the eye. Most corneal abrasions heal with the proper treatment.

Eye disorders are treated using a topical anesthetic, antiinfectives, antimicrobials, lubricants, miotics, carbonic anhydrase inhibitors, osmotics, anticholinergic mydriatics, and cycloplegics.

There are four common ear disorders: cerumen impaction, otitis external, otitis media, and vestibular disorders. Cerumen impaction is the overproduction of earwax. Otitis externa and otitis media are infections of the external and middle ear, respectfully. Vestibular disorders include Meniere's disease, labyrinthitis, and inner ear infections.

Cerumen impaction is treated by administering ceruminolytics to flush the cerumen from the canal. Otitis externa and otitis media are treated with analgesics. If a bacterial infection is suspected, antibiotics may be ordered.

Quiz

1. What type of conjunctivitis causes a heavy greenish discharge?
   - (a) Viral conjunctivitis
   - (b) Bacterial conjunctivitis
   - (c) Allergic conjunctivitis
   - (d) None of the above.

2. What type of conjunctivitis causes itching and redness and excessive tearing?
   - (a) Viral conjunctivitis
   - (b) Bacterial conjunctivitis
   - (c) Allergic conjunctivitis
   - (d) None of the above.

3. What medication lowers intraocular pressure?
   - (a) Choloinesterase inhibitors
   - (b) Direct-acting cholinergics
   - (c) Miotics
   - (d) All of the above.

4. Blurry vision is an expected side effect of some eye medications.
   - (a) True
   - (b) False

5. Topical anesthetics are used to anesthetize the eye for a comprehensive eye examination.
   - (a) True
   - (b) False

6. Which medication is used to treat cerumen impaction?
   - (a) Hydrogen peroxide solution
   - (b) Olive oil
   - (c) Debrox
   - (d) All of the above.

7. Two drops of alcohol in the ear canal helps to prevent swimmer's ear.
   - (a) True
   - (b) False

8. Which medication relieves ear congestion?
   (a) Allerest
   (b) Phenergan
   (c) Novafed
   (d) All of the above.

9. Ear pain usually resolves itself between 48 hours and 72 hours from the onset of the pain.
   (a) True
   (b) False

10. A virus causes nearly all ear infections.
    (a) True
    (b) False

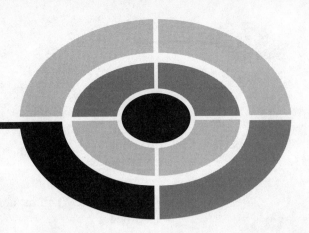

Final Exam

1. A patient who requires a higher dose to achieve the same therapeutic effect is said to
   (a) be cured.
   (b) be addicted to the drug.
   (c) have developed a tolerance to the drug.
   (d) None of the above

2. A patient who is allergic to shellfish is not likely to be allergic to some medications.
   (a) True
   (b) False

3. What type of injection is used to prevent medication from leaking back onto the tissue?
   (a) IM
   (b) Z-Track
   (c) SC
   (d) None of the above

4. Order: 1000 mL of IV fluid q12h. Available: 1000 mL of IV fluid and microdrip tubing. How many gtts per minute will the nurse regulate the IV?
   (a) 83 gtt/min
   (b) 83.3 gtt/min
   (c) 8.33 gtt/min
   (d) .833 gtt/min

5. Peppermint may relieve migraine headaches when rubbed on the forehead.
   (a) True
   (b) False

6. Water-soluble vitamins are excreted in urine shortly after they are absorbed.
   (a) True
   (b) False

7. Blenderized enteral feedings are
   (a) lactose-free liquid.
   (b) powered mixed with milk.
   (c) liquids that are individually prepared based on the nutritional needs of the patient.
   (d) powered mixed with water.

8. When administering enteral feedings, the patient may become dizzy if:
   (a) large amounts of solution is administered rapidly.
   (b) the solution is too concentrated.
   (c) the patient is supine (lying flat on back).
   (d) none of the above.

9. Which of the following medications prevents the formation of blood clots?
   (a) Analgesic
   (b) Antipyretic
   (c) Anticoagulant
   (d) All of the above

10. A infant does not receive a full dose of the drug given to its mother when the infant breastfeeds.
    (a) True
    (b) False

11. The desired action of a medication is called its
    (a) medication reaction.
    (b) safety action.
    (c) addictive action.
    (d) therapeutic effect.

12. What may be given to a patient prior to administering bad tasting medication?
     (a) Nothing
     (b) Water
     (c) Ice chips
     (d) None of the above

13. When installing drops in a 7-year-old child,
     (a) pull earlobe downward and back.
     (b) pull earlobe upward and back.
     (c) pull earlobe upward and forward.
     (d) pull earlobe downward and forward.

14. A patient reports taking herbal medications and complains of having palpitations. The nurse suspects the patient may be taking which herb?
     (a) ma huang
     (b) comfrey
     (c) chamomile
     (d) ginkgo

15. Vitamin K is the antidote for coumadin.
     (a) True
     (b) False

16. Which of the following isn't a sign of inflammation?
     (a) redness
     (b) warmth
     (c) headache
     (d) swelling

17. All antibiotics kill all bacteria
     (a) True
     (b) False

18. A runny nose is not caused by nasal congestion
     (a) True
     (b) False

19. A correct dose of medication for a pediatric patient is determined by
     (a) the patient's weight.
     (b) the patient's height.
     (c) the patient's age.
     (d) the patient's sex.

20. An undesired outcome of a medication is called
    (a) an emergency.
    (b) risk factor.
    (c) an adverse reaction to a medication.
    (d) a side effect to a medication.

21. Order: 1000 mL D5Wq 8 hrs. Using tubing that delivers 15 gtts/mL the nurse will regulate the IV to _____ gtts/min?
    (a) 31 gtts/min
    (b) 31.25 gtts/min
    (c) 310 gtts/min
    (d) 10 gtts/min

22. What vitamin is acquired through sunlight?
    (a) Vitamin A
    (b) Vitamin E
    (c) Vitamin D
    (d) Vitamin C

23. A serum potassium level higher than normal is called
    (a) hyperkalemia.
    (b) hypokalemia.
    (c) hypernatremia.
    (d) none of the above.

24. Potassium is not necessary for conduction of nerve impulses:
    (a) True
    (b) False

25. Blood in the pleural cavity is called
    (a) pneumothorax.
    (b) hemothorax.
    (c) hydrothorax.
    (d) all of the above.

26. A healthy, well-nourished person has a nutritional level to last 4 days before they begin to show signs of malnutrition.
    (a) True
    (b) False

27. Antibiotics may fight bacteria by
    (a) inhibiting the ability to make protein called protein synthesis.
    (b) inhibiting the growth of a cell wall.
    (c) disrupting or altering the permeability of the membrane.
    (d) all the above.

28. What triggers respiration in a patient who has emphysema?
    (a) A decrease in CO_2
    (b) A decrease in O_2
    (c) An increase in O_2
    (d) An increase in CO_2

29. Naloxone (Narcan) is the antidote to an overdose of opioid narcotics
    (a) True
    (b) False

30. When administering a vaccination, which of the following would you have on hand?
    (a) Immune globulin
    (b) Whole blood
    (c) Plasma
    (d) Epinephrine

31. A malfunctioning of the esophageal sphincter causes
    (a) dizziness.
    (b) GERD.
    (c) rickets.
    (d) none of the above.

32. How many doses of nitroglycerin should a patient take for an angina attack?
    (a) 3
    (b) 5
    (c) 1
    (d) None

33. Thiazides should not be used with patients who have renal insufficiency.
    (a) True
    (b) False

34. The nurse should not massage the site after giving a heparin injection.
    (a) True
    (b) False

35. Order: Duricef 0.4g On hand: Duricef 200 mg capsules. How many capsules should the nurse give?
    (a) 1 capsule
    (b) 2 capsules
    (c) 5 capsules
    (d) 20 capsules

36. Comfrey causes swelling associated with abrasions and sprains.
    (a) True
    (b) False

37. Electrolytes are found in
    (a) intracellular fluid.
    (b) interstitial fluid.
    (c) intravascular fluid.
    (d) all of the above.

38. A pain diary may be helpful for
    (a) HIV patients.
    (b) patients whose pain has been relieved.
    (c) patients who expect to be in pain.
    (d) patients who are in chronic pain.

39. A newborn whose mother is HIV positive should be treated for HIV unless the newborn shows signs and symptoms of HIV.
    (a) True
    (b) False

40. A patient's condition after medication is administered is compared to
    (a) baseline patient data.
    (b) drug manufacturer's statistics.
    (c) the condition of other patients who have received the same medication.
    (d) statistics provided by the hospital.

41. The nurse should pinch the skin when giving an insulin injection.
    (a) True
    (b) False

42. Herbal therapies
    (a) do not require FDA approval.
    (b) are safe to self-medicate as long as the patient is undergoing conventional therapy.

    (c) require a prescription from a specially certified physician.

    (d) None of the above

43. The ingredient in a drug that gives it shape is called

    (a) filler.

    (b) excipient.

    (c) D-active.

    (d) particle.

44. All drugs are not absorbed immediately when they are administered.

    (a) True

    (b) False

45. A patient shows he or she knows how to self-medicate by

    (a) explaining the film on self-medication.

    (b) explaining to the patient's family how to medicate.

    (c) knowing the name of the medication.

    (d) demonstrating to the nurse how to self-medicate.

46. Using a prescribed pain management routine

    (a) helps prevent a patient from becoming dependent on a drug.

    (b) helps the patient afford the medication.

    (c) increases the risk of becoming drug dependent.

    (d) is most likely to give the patient pain relief.

47. What can inadvertently cause a patient to receive an insufficient dose of a medication?

    (a) Genetic substitution of a brand medication

    (b) Allergies

    (c) Obesity

    (d) Under weight

48. Ordered: 1 liter of NS q 7h. Available: 1 liter of NS and IV tubing with a drip factor of 10. You would regulate the IV at 24 gtts/min.

    (a) True

    (b) False

49. Potassium levels are higher intracellularly than extracellularly.

    (a) True

    (b) False

50. NNRTs arrests the progression of rheumatoid arthritis.
    (a) True
    (b) False

51. Superinfection is
    (a) an infection that spreads to more than one organ.
    (b) infection caused by a bacterium that has become resistant to antibiotics.
    (c) a hospital acquired infection.
    (d) none of the above.

52. Rhinitis is
    (a) nose surgery.
    (b) insertion of an NG tube.
    (c) a sinus infection.
    (d) a common cold.

53. Patients with emphysema lack the
    (a) Trypsin protein
    (b) $beta_1$-antitrypsin protein
    (c) $alpha_1$-antitrypsin protein
    (d) Trypsin-7 protein

54. Smooth muscles are stimulated by
    (a) muscarinic receptors.
    (b) antimuscarinic receptors.
    (c) barrel receptors.
    (d) all of the above.

55. Nonpharmacological pain relief treatments are based on the
    (a) Pain Oppression theory.
    (b) Pain Suppression theory.
    (c) Brain Suppression theory.
    (d) Gate Control theory.

56. Cell-mediated immunity uses T-leukocytes referred to as natural killer cells.
    (a) True
    (b) False

57. Parietal cells produce
    (a) hydrochloric acid in the gall bladder.
    (b) hydrochloric acid in the liver.
    (c) hydrochloric acid in the stomach.
    (d) none of the above.

58. Many diuretics cause loss of
    (a) potassium.
    (b) magnesium.
    (c) bicarbonate.
    (d) all of the above.

59. IM glucocorticoids resin is used to remove veneral warts.
    (a) True
    (b) False

60. Graves' disease is caused by
    (a) overactive thyroid gland.
    (b) underactive thyroid gland.
    (c) overactive parathyroid gland.
    (d) underactive parathyroid gland.

61. HIV is transmitted via
    (a) injection of infected blood or blood products.
    (b) sexual contact.
    (c) maternal–fetal transmission.
    (d) all of the above.

62. Music cannot help relieve pain.
    (a) True
    (b) False

63. Pain occurring from skeletal muscles, fascia, ligaments, vessels, and joint is called
    (a) neuropathic pain.
    (b) visceral pain.
    (c) chronic pain.
    (d) none of the above.

64. Antibiotics fight off viruses.
    (a) True
    (b) False

65. Calcium is not necessary for conduction of nerve impulses.
    (a) True
    (b) False

66. Ordered is Ceclor 2 mg/kg for a child who weighs 20 lbs. Available is Ceclor 20 mg/2 ml. You would administer 1.8 ml.
    (a) True
    (b) False

67. A piggyback infusion is connected to
    (a) the IV tubing.
    (b) the patient's arm.
    (c) the patient's leg.
    (d) none of the above.

68. A nurse may administer medication to a patient that is prepared by another licensed practitioner.
    (a) True
    (b) False

69. St. John's Wort has action similar to
    (a) sage.
    (b) Prozac.
    (c) psyllium.
    (d) kava kava.

70. What vitamin is given to help alleviate symptoms of neuritis caused by isoniazid therapy for TB?
    (a) Vitamin A
    (b) Vitamin E
    (c) Vitamin D
    (d) None of the above.

71. Vitamin A may be used to treat acne
    (a) True
    (b) False

72. Insulin and glucose administered parenterally
    (a) force potassium out of the cell.
    (b) force potassium into the cell.
    (c) correct the acidosis balance.
    (d) None of the above.

73. It is dangerous to suddenly interrupt parenteral nutrition therapy
    (a) True
    (b) False

74. Which of the following symptoms are possible side effects of an antibiotic?
    (a) Rash
    (b) Fever
    (c) Hives and itching
    (d) All of the above

75. The saddle block is never used during childbirth.
    (a) True
    (b) False

76. The HI virus enters the cell through the CD4 molecule on the cell surface.
    (a) True
    (b) False

77. Prolonged exposure to a drug decreases the excretion of the drug from the body.
    (a) True
    (b) False

78. If a medication order is unclear, the nurse should
    (a) ask a colleague to explain it.
    (b) review it with the patient.
    (c) ask the prescriber to clarify the order.
    (d) try to figure it out.

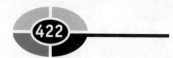

79. A pregnant patient tells the nurse she is taking Gingko to keep her mind sharp. The nurses best response would be,
    (a) "That's fine. It should help."
    (b) "Take it in small doses."
    (c) "You should not take any herbal therapies while you are pregnant."
    (d) "Check the label carefully before you take it."

80. Monomeric is a very expensive enteral solution.
    (a) True
    (b) False

81. During what phase of the inflammation response do the red blood cells infiltrate the injured tissue?
    (a) Anti-inflammatory phase
    (b) Vascular phase
    (c) Delayed phase
    (d) None of the above

82. Ringing in the ear can be a side effect of salicylates.
    (a) True
    (b) False

83. What chemical mediators bring about the inflammatory response by causing vasodilatation, smooth muscle relaxation, capillary permeability, and sensitized nerve cells within the affected area to pain?
    (a) PCN
    (b) sulfonamides
    (c) prostaglandins inhibitors
    (d) prostaglandins

84. Compliance is
    (a) the ability of the lungs to be contracted.
    (b) the ability of the lungs to be distended.
    (c) the ability of the lungs to exchange gases.
    (d) all of the above.

85. Beta-adrenergic blockers
    (a) decrease blood pressure.
    (b) decrease heart rate.
    (c) cause bronchoconstriction.
    (d) All of the above

86. Chamomile can be taken by a patient who is allergic to ragweed.
    (a) True
    (b) False

87. Valerian has a therapeutic effect similar to
    (a) ginseng.
    (b) zingiber.
    (c) Benadryl.
    (d) none of the above.

88. The concentration of a hyptonic intravenous solution does not have the same concentration as intracellular fluid.
    (a) True
    (b) False

89. The nurse should instruct the patient to monitor for adverse side effects of herbal therapies.
    (a) True
    (b) False

90. If the patient cannot absorb oral medication ordered by the provider, the nurse should
    (a) use a rectal suppository.
    (b) postpone administering medication.
    (c) insert a GI tube.
    (d) call the physician.

91. What can be used to relieve swelling associated with abrasions and sprains?
    (a) Ginseng
    (b) Comfrey
    (c) Zingiber
    (d) Valerian

92. A good source of dietary potassium is
    (a) bread
    (b) milk
    (c) eggs
    (d) bananas

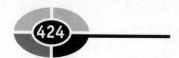
93. Spinach is a source of iron.
    (a) True
    (b) False

94. A drug that causes a nonspecific physiological response is called
    (a) an agonist.
    (b) a metabolite.
    (c) a protein.
    (d) a molecule.

95. A medical diagnosis
    (a) is the same as a nursing diagnosis.
    (b) identifies the patient's disease or medical condition.
    (c) is a problem statement that identifies the potential or actual health problem.
    (d) None of the above

96. A patient undergoing withdrawal from hashish can be treated by
    (a) administering a lower dose of hashish.
    (b) administering a sedative.
    (c) doing nothing.
    (d) prescribing exercise.

97. Healthcare providers never use drugs for recreational purposes.
    (a) True
    (b) False

98. If the dose of a transdermal patch is more than the prescriber's medication order,
    (a) cut the patch to an appropriate length.
    (b) contact the prescriber.
    (c) do nothing.
    (d) apply the patch anyway.

99. The nursing process is a circular process.
    (a) True
    (b) False

100. Commonly used medications for relieving headaches are aspirin, acetaminophen, and ibuprofen.
    (a) True
    (b) False

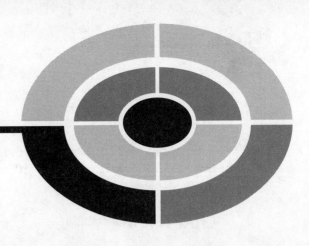

Answers to Quiz and Final Exam Questions

CHAPTER 1

1. b	2. b	3. d	4. b	5. b
6. d	7. b	8. c	9. b	10. a

CHAPTER 2

1. b	2. c	3. c	4. b	5. a
6. d	7. b	8. a	9. b	10. a

CHAPTER 3

| 1. b | 2. b | 3. d | 4. b | 5. b |
| 6. a | 7. a | 8. d | 9. a | 10. b |

CHAPTER 4

| 1. c | 2. d | 3. c | 4. b | 5. a |
| 6. a | 7. a | 8. a | 9. a | 10. a |

CHAPTER 5

| 1. c | 2. c | 3. a | 4. b | 5. a |
| 6. c | 7. b | 8. b | 9. a | 10. b |

CHAPTER 6

| 1. c | 2. b | 3. a | 4. a | 5. a |
| 6. a | 7. b | 8. a | 9. b | 10. a |

CHAPTER 7

| 1. b | 2. d | 3. a | 4. a | 5. a |
| 6. c | 7. a | 8. b | 9. b | 10. a |

CHAPTER 8

| 1. d | 2. b | 3. d | 4. a | 5. b |
| 6. c | 7. b | 8. c | 9. a | 10. a |

CHAPTER 9

| 1. b | 2. c | 3. b | 4. a | 5. a |
| 6. a | 7. b | 8. d | 9. b | 10. a |

CHAPTER 10

| 1. b | 2. b | 3. d | 4. a | 5. b |
| 6. c | 7. a | 8. b | 9. a | 10. a |

CHAPTER 11

| 1. b | 2. b | 3. a | 4. b | 5. a |
| 6. d | 7. a | 8. d | 9. a | 10. a |

CHAPTER 12

| 1. c | 2. c | 3. a | 4. a | 5. a |
| 6. b | 7. a | 8. d | 9. b | 10. a |

CHAPTER 13

| 1. b | 2. a | 3. d | 4. b | 5. a |
| 6. d | 7. b | 8. d | 9. a | 10. a |

CHAPTER 14

| 1. b | 2. b | 3. c | 4. a | 5. a |
| 6. c | 7. a | 8. c | 9. a | 10. a |

CHAPTER 15

| 1. b | 2. a | 3. a | 4. a | 5. a |
| 6. d | 7. a | 8. b | 9. a | 10. a |

CHAPTER 16

| 1. a | 2. d | 3. d | 4. a | 5. a |
| 6. d | 7. a | 8. b | 9. a | 10. a |

CHAPTER 17

1. c	2. a	3. d	4. a	5. a
6. c	7. b	8. d	9. b	10. a

CHAPTER 18

1. b	2. d	3. c	4. a	5. a
6. c	7. a	8. b	9. b	10. a

CHAPTER 19

1. d	2. b	3. a	4. a	5. a
6. d	7. a	8. a	9. a	10. a

CHAPTER 20

1. d	2. a	3. c	4. a	5. a
6. c	7. b	8. a	9. a	10. b

CHAPTER 21

1. d	2. a	3. a	4. a	5. a
6. a	7. a	8. c	9. a	10. b

CHAPTER 22

1. b	2. c	3. d	4. a	5. a
6. d	7. a	8. d	9. a	10. a

FINAL EXAM

1. c	2. b	3. b	4. a	5. b
6. a	7. c	8. a	9. c	10. a
11. d	12. c	13. b	14. a	15. a
16. c	17. b	18. b	19. a	20. c
21. a	22. c	23. a	24. b	25. b
26. b	27. d	28. a	29. a	30. d
31. b	32. a	33. a	34. a	35. b
36. b	37. d	38. d	39. a	40. a
41. a	42. a	43. a	44. a	45. d
46. d	47. c	48. a	49. a	50. a
51. b	52. d	53. c	54. a	55. d
56. a	57. c	58. d	59. b	60. a
61. d	62. b	63. d	64. b	65. b
66. a	67. a	68. b	69. b	70. d
71. a	72. b	73. a	74. d	75. b
76. a	77. b	78. c	79. c	80. a
81. d	82. a	83. d	84. b	85. d
86. b	87. c	88. a	89. a	90. d
91. b	92. b	93. a	94. a	95. b
96. d	97. b	98. b	99. a	100. a

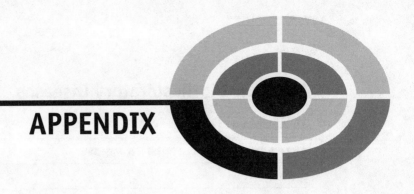

APPENDIX

Drug-Specific Tables

Note: All of these tables are available on the book's Web site:
www.books.mcgraw-hill.com/authors/kamienski

CHAPTER 14: Respiratory Diseases

Antihistamine (H_1 blocker)

Alpha Adrenergic Agonist Nasal Decongestant

Systemic Decongestant

Intranasal Glucocorticoids

Antitussives

Expectorants

Beta-Adrenergic

Adrenergic Agonist

Anticholinergics

Methylxanthine

Leukotrine Modifiers and LT Synthesis Inhibitors

Mast Cell Stabilizer

CHAPTER 15: Nervous System Drugs

Amphetamine-Like Drugs

Ergot Alkaloids and Related Compounds

Serotonin Agonists: Triptans

Sedative-Hypnotic—Benzodiazepine—Schedule IV

Sedative-Hypnotic: Barbiturates and Others

Inhalation and Intravenous Anesthetics

Local Anesthetics

Adrenergics

Beta Blockers

Direct-Acting Cholinergic

CHAPTER 15 *(continued)*

Anticholinergic/Parasympatholytic

Anticholinergic: GI

Anticholinergic-Antiparkinsonism Drugs

Anticholinergic-Antiparkinsonism

Cholinesterase Inhibitor/Indirect Cholinergic

Other: COMT Inhibitor

Anxiolytics, Skeletal Muscle Relaxant, Anticonvulsant

Centrally Acting Muscle Relaxants

Depolarizing Muscle Relaxants (Adjunct to Anesthesia)

Peripherally Acting Muscle Relaxant

Dopaminergics

Dopamine Agonists

MAO-B Inhibitor

Barbiturates

Benzodiazepines (Anxiolytics)

Phenothiazine (Alipathic)

Nonphenothiazine

Tricyclic Antidepressant

CHAPTER 16: Narcotic Agonists

Non-Narcotic Analgesic

Narcotic Agonist-Opiate Analgesic

Opioid Agonist

Narcotic Agonist-Antagonists

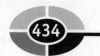

CHAPTER 17: Immunologic Agents

Nonnucleoside Reverse Transcriptase Inhibitor (NNRTI) Antiretroviral

Nucleoside Reverse Transcriptase Inhibitor (NRTI) Antiretroviral

Protease Inhibitors Antiretroviral

Fusion Inhibitors

CHAPTER 18: Gastrointestinal System

Anticholinergic

Serotonin Antagonist

Antihistamine

Antidiarrheals

GI Stimulant-Laxative

GI Osmotic: Laxative/Antacid, Anticonvulsant, Electrolyte

Proton Pump Inhibitor (PPIs)

Antiulcers: Histamine$_2$ Blocker

CHAPTER 19: Cardiac Circulatory Medications

Cardiac Glycoside

Nitrates

Calcium Channel Blocker

Fast (Sodium) Channel Blocker I

Direct-Acting Arteriolar Vasodilators

ACE Inhibitors

Thiazide Diuretic

Loop Diuretic

CHAPTER 19 *(continued)*

Carbonic Anhydrase Inhibitors

Potassium-Sparing Diuretic

Anticoagulant Low Molecular Weight

Thrombolytic

Antihyperlipemic HMG-CoA Reductase Inhibitor

Vasodilator

CHAPTER 20: Skin Disorders

Acne Vulgaris (Systemic Preparation)

Antipsoriatic

Antiinfective

CHAPTER 21: Endocrine Medications

Anterior Pituitary Hormone

Posterior Pituitary Hormone

Hypothyroidism

Hyperthyroidism

Antidiabetic Drugs

Antidiabetic: Second Generation Sulfonylurea

CHAPTER 22: Disorders of the Eye and Ear

Direct-Acting Miotic (Cholinergics)

Osmotic (Osmotic Diuretic, Antiglaucoma, Antihemolytic)

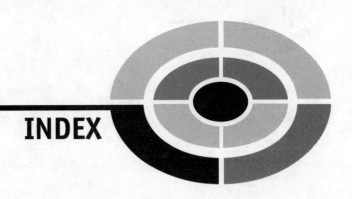

INDEX

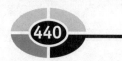

Index

Index

Index

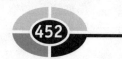

Index

Index

ABOUT THE AUTHORS

Mary Kamienski, PhD, RN, FAEN, FNP, CEN, is the Director of the Center for Lifelong Learning at the University of Medicine and Dentistry of New Jersey School of Nursing, and teaches advanced practice and undergraduate registered nursing students.

Jim Keogh is on the faculty of St. Peter's College and Columbia University. He is the author of more than 60 books, including McGraw-Hill's *Microbiology Demystified* and *Java Demystified*.